Peripheral Neuropathies

Peripheral Neuropathies

A Practical Approach

Mark Bromberg

Department of Neurology, University of Utah, Salt Lake City, UT, USA

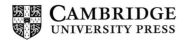

CAMBRIDGE
UNIVERSITY PRESS

CAMBRIDGE
UNIVERSITY PRESS

University Printing House, Cambridge CB2 8BS, United Kingdom

Cambridge University Press is part of the University of Cambridge.

It furthers the University's mission by disseminating knowledge in the pursuit of
education, learning and research at the highest international levels of excellence.

www.cambridge.org
Information on this title: www.cambridge.org/9781107092181

© Mark B. Bromberg 2018

First published 2018

Printed in the United Kingdom by TJ International Ltd. Padstow Cornwall

A catalogue record for this publication is available from the British Library

Library of Congress Cataloging-in-Publication Data
Names: Bromberg, Mark, author.
Title: Peripheral neuropathies : a practical approach / Mark Bromberg.
Description: Cambridge, United Kingdom; New York: Cambridge University Press, 2018. |
Includes bibliographical references and index.
Identifiers: LCCN 2017051826 | ISBN 9781107092181 (hardback)
Subjects: | MESH: Peripheral Nervous System Diseases
Classification: LCC RC409 | NLM WL 520 | DDC 616.85/6–dc23
LC record available at https://lccn.loc.gov/2017051826

ISBN 978-1-107-09218-1 Hardback

Every effort has been made in preparing this book to provide accurate and up-to-date information which
is in accord with accepted standards and practice at the time of publication. Although case histories are
drawn from actual cases, every effort has been made to disguise the identities of the individuals
involved. Nevertheless, the authors, editors and publishers can make no warranties that the
information contained herein is totally free from error, not least because clinical standards are
constantly changing through research and regulation. The authors, editors and publishers
therefore disclaim all liability for direct or consequential damages resulting from the use of
material contained in this book. Readers are strongly advised to pay careful attention to
information provided by the manufacturer of any drugs or equipment that they plan to use.

Contents

Contents

Preface and Abbreviations

Peripheral neuropathy is a general term, which refers to disorders of the peripheral nervous system. The peripheral nervous system consists of all nerves distal to the spinal cord, and includes nerve fibers that either originate in the spinal cord (motor neurons) or terminate in the spinal cord (sensory nerves). It also includes autonomic nerve fibers. The pattern of nerve involvement in peripheral neuropathies includes:

- Radiculopathies
- Plexopathies
- Mononeuropathies
- Polyneuropathies

Polyneuropathies represent the largest group, and the term "poly" refers to generalized and homogenous involvement of many nerves, and usually following a distal to proximal pattern. There are a large number of underlying causes (many of which remain unidentified despite efforts), and, unfortunately, few polyneuropathies can be stopped or reversed with treatment.

Disorders of peripheral nerves are relatively common, but it is difficult to determine true prevalence numbers for different types of neuropathies as study designs and reporting metrics are not uniform. Prevalence estimates include: polyneuropathy in people >55 years of age ~8,000/100,000; diabetic neuropathy 300/100,000; hereditary neuropathy 8–41/100,000; and carpal tunnel syndrome 5,800/100,000 for women and 600/100,00 for men (Martyn and Hughes, 1997).

The evaluation process of a patient with a neuropathy has many possible approaches. This book is based on personal experience using a structured approach. This approach is not wholly unique, but is applied here in a rigorous fashion for each type of neuropathy (Barohn, 1998). This book is written to be concise and readily usable, and covers relatively common types of neuropathies, and hence descriptions and discussions are focused. Chapters are organized in sections. The first section is basic background information on peripheral nerve anatomy and pathology, followed by structured approaches to the clinical and electrodiagnostic evaluation, and

concludes with informative laboratory tests. While no classification scheme of neuropathies is entirely satisfactory, clinical sections are organized by the patterns of nerve involvement listed above. Chapter content for each type of neuropathy is based on underlying pathology, clinical features, diagnostic evaluation (including electrodiagnostic and informative laboratory tests), and ends with management and treatment options.

References have been chosen to be maximally informative for a topic, and not to support every feature listed. There is an extensive literature on all aspects of peripheral neuropathies, and many articles represent observations, case reviews, or small patient series, and thus many statements and conclusions in the literature may not be based on sound evidence. Selected references concentrate on evidence-based data, or those with a focus on data from high-level studies.

The book is written to be helpful to a spectrum of clinicians, those in training (neurology and rehabilitation residents, fellows in clinical neurophysiology and neuromuscular medicine), and practitioners, whether they perform electrodiagnostic studies or evaluate and manage the clinical aspects of peripheral neuropathies.

Abbreviations have been kept to a minimum, and the following, which are familiar to the intended audience, are defined here at the outset:

CMAP	compound muscle action potential
EMG	needle electromyography
IVIG	intravenous immune globulin
MRC	Medical Research Counsel
MRI	magnetic resonance imaging
SNAP	sensory nerve action potential

References

Barohn RJ. Approach to peripheral neuropathy and neuronopathy. *Semin Neurol.* 1998;18:7–18.

Martyn CN, Hughes RA. Epidemiology of peripheral neuropathy. *J Neurol Neurosurg Psychiatry.* 1997;62:310–8.

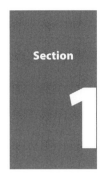

Section

1

Approach to the Evaluation of Peripheral Neuropathies

The process of evaluating a peripheral neuropathy can be divided into five elements: the first is having in mind an understanding of the anatomical arrangement of the peripheral nervous system; the second is having in mind the spectrum of pathologic processes that can affect nerves; the third is using an organized approach in history-taking to understand what the patient experiences, which leads to an initial formulation of the pattern of nerve involvement that is confirmed or changed based on neurologic examination abnormalities; the fourth is estimating underlying nerve pathology by electrodiagnostic or other testing; and the fifth is selecting informative laboratory tests to help determine underlying causes.

This section covers these elements, with most emphasis on the history and electrodiagnostic studies, as they define what nerve elements are involved and unlikely underlying pathology. A structured approach is efficient because it leads to a rational selection of laboratory tests. In comparison, a shotgun approach to testing is costly, with uninformative tests or false positive results. Despite a considered evaluation, an underlying cause cannot be reached in 20–30% of neuropathies (England and Asbury, 2004; Farhad et al., 2016)

References

England JD, Asbury AK. Peripheral neuropathy. *Lancet.* 2004;363:2151–61.

Farhad K, Traub R, Ruzhansky KM, Brannagan TH, III. Causes of neuropathy in patients referred as "idiopathic neuropathy." *Muscle Nerve.* 2016;53: 856–61.

Approach to the Evaluation of
Peripheral Neuropathies

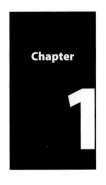

Peripheral Nerve Anatomy

Introduction

Peripheral nerve anatomy includes two levels: gross arrangement of nerve roots, plexuses and individual (named) nerves; and microscopic structures of nerve fibers and whole nerve structures. An understanding at both levels is a key element in localization of the site of involvement, and also in planning and interpreting electrodiagnostic studies.

Gross Anatomic Arrangement

The peripheral nervous system is composed of somatic and autonomic nerves. Somatic nerves consist of large- to medium-diameter myelinated fibers, while autonomic nerves consist of unmyelinated fibers. Somatic nerve fibers are much fewer in number compared to autonomic nerves, but most clinical symptoms and signs of peripheral neuropathies are attributable to pathology of somatic nerves (Figure 1.1). While autonomic nerves are frequently affected, symptoms are vague and signs are difficult to elicit without special autonomic laboratory testing equipment. This section focuses on somatic nerves.

Somatic Sensory Nerves

Sensory (afferent) nerve fibers are pseudo-unipolar with the cell body in the dorsal root ganglia and a peripheral process that begins with receptors in skin, joint capsule, or muscle, and a central process that terminates in the spinal cord or medulla of the brainstem (Figure 1.2). The root segment, from the cell body to entry into the cord, is important because the pathology associated with inflammatory or immune-mediated neuropathies frequently involves this segment and may cause a breakdown of the blood–nerve (root) barrier, marked by increased cerebrospinal fluid protein. Further, damage restricted to a root (such as a radiculopathy) will affect sensory perception of stimuli in a nerve's dermatome (see below), but will not affect sensory nerve conduction studies, as

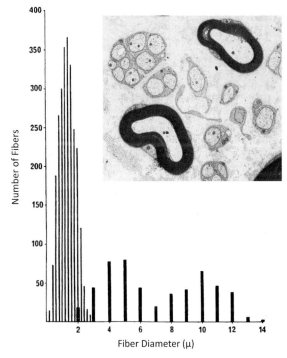

Figure 1.1 Histogram of nerve fiber diameters (µ) showing lesser numbers of large-diameter myelinated fibers (2–14 µ) compared to small-diameter myelinated and unmyelinated fibers (<1–3 µ). Inset is electron micrograph of a nerve in cross-section showing large myelinated and unmyelinated fibers.
From *Handbook of Peripheral Neuropathy*, Taylor & Francis, with permission.

the peripheral segment remains connected to the cell body. Conversely, damage to nerve segments distal to the dorsal root ganglia will affect sensory perception and result in abnormal sensory nerve conduction studies. This gives rise to the terms "preganglionic" and "postganglionic" lesions.

Somatic Motor Nerves

Motor (efferent) nerve fibers are unipolar with the cell body in the anterior horn of the spinal cord and

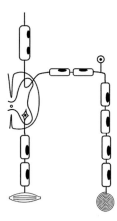

Figure 1.2 Diagram of large-diameter myelinated somatic nerve fibers. Sensory nerve fibers (right side) have cell bodies in dorsal root ganglia and begin from receptors in the skin, joint capsule, or muscle and terminate in the spinal cord. Motor nerves (left side) have cell bodies in the spinal cord and end in muscle at the neuromuscular junction.

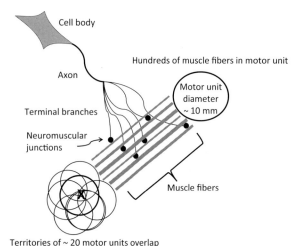

Figure 1.3 Diagram of the motor unit. The cell body is located in the spinal cord; the axon ends in terminal branches in muscle; each branch innervates a single muscle fiber at a neuromuscular junction. Each motor unit consists of hundreds of muscle fibers with a cross-sectional diameter of 5–10 mm. About 20 motor units partially overlap at any site (x) in a muscle.

a peripheral axon that terminates in muscle at neuromuscular junctions (Figure 1.2). Each motor axon branches hundreds of times within a muscle, and each terminal branch innervates a muscle fiber (Figure 1.3). Nerve action potentials are converted to muscle fiber action potentials at the neuromuscular junction, and while the process is complex, transmission is normally 100 percent secure. This functional entity is the "motor unit," consisting of the alpha motor neuron, axon, and all innervated muscle fibers.

Nerve Roots and Plexuses

At intervals along the spinal cord, sensory (dorsal) rootlets and motor (ventral) rootlets periodically join as dorsal and ventral roots, and both roots come together within the dural space to form spinal nerves, which pass through the dura (dorsal root ganglia lie outside of the dura). The spinal nerves then come together to form the plexuses. In the cervical region, nerve roots from segments C5–T1 contribute to the brachial plexus; in the thoracic region, nerve roots from segments T2–L1 remain as roots; while in the lumbosacral region roots, L2–S4 join to form the lumbosacral plexus. Each sensory nerve root innervates an area of skin called a dermatome, and each motor nerve root innervates a portion of a muscle called a myotome. Distal to the plexuses, individual named nerves form and innervate large areas of skin and whole muscles, while in the thoracic region nerve roots remain separate to innervate truncal skin and muscle.

In the brachial plexus (Figure 1.4), the arrangement of nerve branching is: dorsal and ventral roots fuse to form spinal nerves; spinal nerves divide into posterior and anterior rami; anterior rami from C5 and C6 spinal nerves join to form the upper trunk; the spinal nerve from C7 forms the posterior trunk, and spinal nerves from C8 and T1 form the lower trunk; each trunk forms anterior and posterior divisions; three cords emerge – the lateral cord from the anterior division of the upper and middle trunks, the posterior cord from the union of the posterior divisions, and the medial cord from the anterior division of the lower trunk; and finally the terminal or named nerves, which include proximally the musculocutaneous and axillary nerves, and distally the median, ulnar, and radial nerves. There may be rostral or caudal shifts of root contributions (prefixed or postfixed, respectively), but these do not affect the arrangement of nerves in the plexus (Ferrante, 2004).

The lumbosacral plexus combines the lumbar and sacral plexuses (Figure 1.5). In the lumbar plexus, the arrangement of nerve branching is: dorsal and ventral roots form spinal nerves; spinal nerves divide into posterior and anterior rami; anterior rami from L1–L4 plus a nerve from T12 form the iliohypogastric, ilioinguinal, genitofemoral, and obturator nerves, and

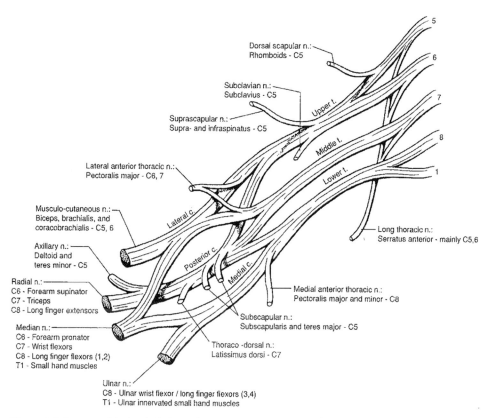

Dorsal scapular n.:
Rhomboids - C5

Subclavian n.:
Subclavius - C5

Suprascapular n.:
Supra- and infraspinatus - C5

Upper t.

5

6

7

8

1

Middle t.

Lower t.

Lateral anterior thoracic n.:
Pectoralis major - C6, 7

Lateral c.

Musculo-cutaneous n.:
Biceps, brachialis, and
coracobrachialis - C5, 6

Axillary n.:
Deltoid and
teres minor - C5

Posterior c.

Medial c.

Radial n.:
C6 - Forearm supinator
C7 - Triceps
C8 - Long finger extensors

Median n.:
C6 - Forearm pronator
C7 - Wrist flexors
C8 - Long finger flexors (1,2)
T1 - Small hand muscles

Long thoracic n.:
Serratus anterior - mainly C5,6

Medial anterior thoracic n.:
Pectoralis major and minor - C8

Subscapular n.:
Subscapularis and teres major - C5

Thoraco -dorsal n.:
Latissimus dorsi - C7

Ulnar n.:
C8 - Ulnar wrist flexor / long finger flexors (3,4)
T1 - Ulnar innervated small hand muscles

Figure 1.4 Diagram of the brachial plexus showing termination in named nerves.
From S Oh, MD, with permission.

branches from L4–L5 contribute to the sacral plexus; and posterior rami gives rise to the lateral femoral cutaneous nerve and the femoral nerve. In the sacral plexus, the arrangement of nerve branching is: the anterior rami contribute to the pudendal, levator ani nerves, the obturator nerve, and the sciatic nerve; and the posterior rami contribute to the gluteal nerves and the sciatic nerve (which includes fibular/peroneal and tibial nerves).

Peripheral Nerves

Individual named nerves emerge from the plexuses (Figures 1.4 and 1.5), and most are mixed nerves with both sensory and motor nerve fibers, and also include autonomic fibers. Cutaneous sensory nerves are branches joining mixed nerves, usually from distal areas of skin, but some join at proximal sites (cutaneous sensory branches in the forearm and leg). Motor nerves branch to muscles, and contain both motor and muscle afferent nerve fibers (from muscle spindles and tendon organs), in an approximate

50 percent:50 percent ratio. Thus, the term "motor branch" is technically inaccurate, but clinical deficits that result from motor nerve injuries primarily relate to loss of motor nerve fibers, and it is not possible to accurately gauge changes in function due to loss of muscle-afferent nerve fibers.

Nerve Variability

Dermatomes and myotomes are reasonably consistent among individuals and serve as the basis of localization of lesions. For individual dermatomes, boundaries overlap with adjacent dermatomes and published dermatomal maps may vary, and thus the effects of sensory nerve lesions may not conform to maps. Most myotomes include innervation of several muscles, and conversely, most muscles receive innervation from several roots. Further, there may be rare variability among individuals for cervical roots being shifted one root segment rostral or cauday (prefixed and postfixed plexus, respectively). Nerve fibers may follow variant (anomalous) pathways as they leave the plexus and

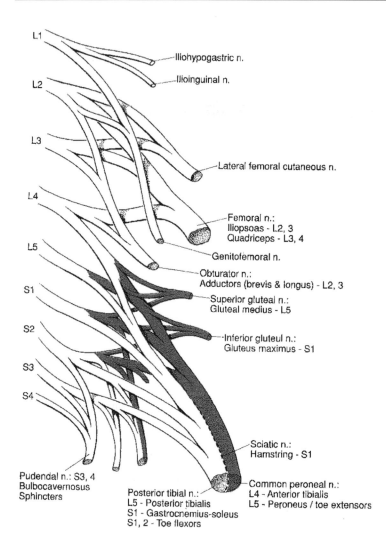

Figure 1.5 Diagram of the lumbosacral plexus showing termination in named nerves. From S Oh, MD, with permission.

L1

Iliohypogastric n.

Ilioinguinal n.

L2

L3

Lateral femoral cutaneous n.

L4

Femoral n.:
Iliopsoas - L2, 3
Quadriceps - L3, 4

L5

Genitofemoral n.

Obturator n.:
Adductors (brevis & longus) - L2, 3

Superior gluteal n.:
Gluteal medius - L5

S1

S2

Inferior gluteal n.:
Gluteus maximus - S1

S3

S4

Sciatic n.:
Hamstring - S1

Pudendal n.: S3, 4
Bulbocavernosus
Sphincters

Posterior tibial n.:
L5 - Posterior tibialis
S1 - Gastrocnemius-soleus
S1, 2 - Toe flexors

Common peroneal n.:
L4 - Anterior tibialis
L5 - Peroneus / toe extensors

move distally to muscles (most anomalies involve motor fibers). Several variants are common and can influence interpretation of electrodiagnostic studies (Gutmann, 1993; Oh, 2003). There are also rare variant muscle innervation patterns where a different nerve innervates a muscle.

Martin-Gruber Anastomosis

The Martin-Gruber anastomosis is the most common variant (15–31 percent of individuals), and involves variable numbers of ulnar motor axons initially descending with the median nerve and crossing to join the ulnar nerve in the forearm (crossings of sensory nerve fibers is rare). Several patterns are described:

- Type I involves ulnar axons crossing over from the median nerve in the forearm with normal termination in muscles in the hand, demonstrated by a lower hypothenar CMAP to stimulation of the ulnar nerve at the elbow than at the wrist. The loss of proximal CMAP amplitude could be mistakenly interpreted as conduction block in the forearm.

- Type II involves ulnar fibers to the first dorsal interosseous muscle crossing over from the median nerve in the forearm, demonstrated by a larger amplitude first dorsal interosseous CMAP to ulnar nerve stimulation at the wrist than at the elbow. This is the most common type, but does not cause confusion during routing nerve conduction studies, which are recorded from hypothenar muscles.

- Type III involves crossings of ulnar fibers to the thenar muscles in the forearm. It is apparent when the thenar CMAP to stimulation at the elbow is greater than to stimulation at the wrist. This variant is the least common, but in the setting of carpal tunnel syndrome can lead to a very fast median forearm conduction velocity despite a prolonged distal latency (see Chapter 8).

Accessory Fibular/Peroneal Nerve

Innervation of the extensor digitorum brevis muscle is usually by the deep fibular/peroneal nerve, but a common variant (20 percent of individuals) is for a portion of the muscle to be innervated by an accessory fibular/peroneal nerve, a branch of the superficial fibular/peroneal nerve that leaves the common fibular/peroneal nerve near the fibular head and travels posterior to the deep fibular/peroneal nerve. This pattern affects nerve conduction studies and could be mistakenly interpreted as conduction block in the middle of the leg (see Chapter 11).

Variant Innervation Patterns

Rare variants include median fibers crossing from the ulnar nerve in the forearm and variations in innervation of intrinsic hand muscles (called Riche-Cannieu anastomoses). These include all thenar muscles innervated by the median nerve or all hypothenar muscles innervated by the median nerve.

Microscopic Anatomic Arrangement

Axons

Axons are the electrical conducting elements. While they are viewed as cylinders of axoplasma, they are not uniform in diameter and are narrower at specialized regions, nodes of Ranvier, and also taper over their length (Figure 1.6). The axon membrane has ion channels distributed in varying proportions along its length, in high concentrations at the nodes. Metabolic maintenance of the axon is dependent upon processes in the cell body, and it is to be appreciated that axonal processes can be very long – up to a meter in length. Disease processes that "tax" these processes likely account for the length-dependent pattern of many neuropathies. Axons do not function independent of myelin, and axon and myelin must be considered as a

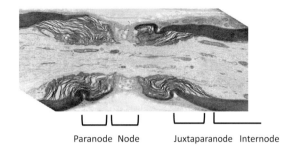

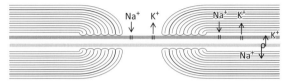

Paranode Node   Juxtaparanode Internode

Figure 1.6 Composite picture showing structural elements at the node of Ranvier and adjacent regions. Top: micrograph of node and paranodal region. Middle: distribution of node, paranodal, juxtaparanodal, and internodal regions. Lower: distribution of sodium and potassium channels (Na$^+$ represents sodium transient persistent current channels; K$^+$ represents potassium slow fast current channels) and sodium (Na$^+$)/potassium (K$^+$) pump.

functional unit. Thus, neuropathies that affect myelin may secondarily affect the axon, and vice versa.

Myelin

Somatic nerve axons are individually myelinated, while unmyelinated axons are myelinated in groups, called Remak bundles (Figure 1.1). Myelin represents the extended membrane of Schwann cells, and many Schwann cells are distributed along the axon. For myelinated axons, compact myelin is tightly wrapped around the axon in Schwann cell segments, with the length of myelin covering proportional to axon diameter (segments 0.5–1.4 mm long for axons 0.5–1.4 microns in diameter). Nerve fiber action potentials are regenerated at nodes of Ranvier, and longer myelinated segments of larger-diameter nerves account for their faster conduction velocities.

Node of Ranvier

The nodal region includes the juxtaparanodal and paranodal segments (Figure 1.6). Compact myelin changes at the node of Ranvier as it clinches tightly around the axon, and the axon becomes reduced in diameter at the paranode and the node. The types and distributions of ion channels vary, with more voltage-gaited sodium channels at the nodal region and more

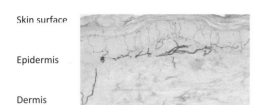

Figure 1.7 Normal pattern of unmyelinated fibers in the intraepidermal region of skin.
From University of Utah Cutaneous Pathology Laboratory, with permission.

voltage-gaited potassium channels in the paranodal region, and there are differences between fast and slow ion channels. There are also many proteins at the node that are essential for axon-myelin structure and function. The proteins can serve as epitopes for antibody-mediated immune attacks at the node (see Chapter 2).

Fascicules

Nerve fibers are organized in bundles (fascicles) within nerves. Nerve fibers can cross from one fascicule to another or stay relatively localized within a fascicle, and both patterns occur. What is important is that there is a somatotopic organization of sensory and motor nerves, especially over distal portions of nerves (Stewart, 2003). A clinical implication for an intrinsic fascicular organization is that a lesion at a proximal site affecting a fascicule can result in sensory and motor deficits in a restricted distribution of skin or muscle that can appear to result from a more distal lesion site. Specific examples are discussed in appropriate chapters.

Endoneurium, Perineurium, Epineurium

The endoneurium is a sheath around myelinated fibers and contains fibrous connective tissue and collagen. Bundles of endoneurium are in turn covered in by perineurium, which forms the fascicles. Groups of fascicles are surrounded by epineurium. Blood vessels penetrate the epineurium and then the perineurium, and capillaries lie within the endoneurium. Increased amounts of endoneurial fluid represent the basis for bright signals on magnetic resonance neurography.

Motor Unit

A motor unit consists of all muscle fibers innervated by a motor axon. An accurate number of muscle fibers included in a motor unit cannot be assessed in human muscle, but from animal experiments the number is found to be in the hundreds, and likely varies among muscles. The territory of a motor unit in a muscle is 5–10 mm across, and thus the territories of 10–15 motor units may overlap at any cross-sectional site in a muscle, with muscle fibers of one motor unit intermingled with fibers from other motor units (Figure 1.3).

Intraepidermal Nerve Terminals

Neuropathies can include damage or loss of small myelinated and unmyelinated nerve fibers. Loss of these fibers cannot be detected in the SNAP, but can be assessed on nerve biopsies, and the density of terminal branches of unmyelinated fibers in the skin can be determined in skin biopsies. Skin biopsies can be obtained from either 3-mm punch samples or skin blister preparations. Intraepidermal nerve terminal branches can be observed by staining with pan-axonal marker protein gene product 9.5 (PGP 9.5). Biopsies are customarily taken from ankle and thigh levels, where normative values are available for comparisons. The normal arrangement in skin is an orderly array of uniform diameter fibers with simple branching (Figure 1.7), whereas pathologic changes are reduced density and focal areas of swelling (Figure 2.6; Figure 1.7). Criteria for the preparation and interpretation of skin biopsies are available (EFNS, 2010).

References

European Federation of Neurological Societies/Peripheral Nerve Society Guideline on the use of skin biopsy in the diagnosis of small fiber neuropathy. Report of a joint task force of the European Federation of Neurological Societies and the Peripheral Nerve Society. *J Peripher Nerv Syst.* 2010;15:79–92.

Ferrante MA. Brachial plexopathies: classification, causes, and consequences. *Muscle Nerve.* 2004;30:547–68.

Gutmann L. AAEM minimonograph #2: important anomalous innervations of the extremities. *Muscle Nerve.* 1993;16:339–47.

Oh SJ. *Clinical Electromyography: Nerve Conduction Studies.* 3rd ed. Philadelphia: Lippincott Williams & Wilkins; 2003.

Stewart JD. Peripheral nerve fascicles: anatomy and clinical relevance. *Muscle Nerve.* 2003;28:525–41.

Chapter 2

Peripheral Nerve Pathology

Introduction

Peripheral nerve pathology can present clinically as nerve dysfunction (negative symptoms and signs) with loss of sensory perception and weakness due to disconnection from receptors or muscle fibers, or as hyperfunction (positive symptoms) with pain and other disagreeable sensations from sensory fibers, or fasciculations and cramps due to spontaneous or exaggerated motor nerve discharges. Nerve pathology can occur at the nerve cell body or anywhere along a nerve fiber. Within the body, the distribution can be in individual named nerves, multiple individual nerves, mixed sensory and motor nerves, or sensory only and motor only nerves. Underlying pathologic processes are determined from limited numbers of cases (nerve biopsy, postmortem examination with death usually from other causes) or from experimental animal models. It is important to appreciate that the role of electrophysiologic studies is to "estimate" underlying pathology, but in the absence of tissue pathology can only be inferred. However, the distribution of pathology along a nerve means that biopsy of a distal nerve segment may not include clinically relevant sites.

Nerve Damage

Causes of nerve pathology include direct and indirect trauma, biochemical insults (toxic or metabolic), or immune-mediated damage. Nerve trauma can be classified by degrees: (1) neurapraxia indicates inability to propagate a signal but the nerve is structurally intact; (2) axonotmesis indicates damage to the axon but surrounding connective tissue is intact; (3) neurotmesis indicates separation of axon and connective tissue with complete structural disruption (Campbell, 2008; Robinson, 2015). Nerve damage from trauma depends upon the nature of physical forces, and can occur focally or anywhere along a nerve. Toxic or metabolic insults can affect the cell body, causing death of the whole axon, or tax cellular metabolic processes affecting longer nerves initially and progressively shorter nerves over time. Immune-mediated damage can affect the cell body, multiple sites along a nerve or among fibers, or at the node of Ranvier.

Axonal Damage

After axonotmesis and neurotmesis, degeneration of distal axons begins within 24–36 hours after injury, but within this time period distal portions of nerve remain electrically excitable (Chaudhry and Cornblath, 1992). Regeneration at nerve ends occurs spontaneously after biochemical or traumatic injury, and involves many protein elements (Chen et al., 2007). Nerve growth cones emerge from the proximal segment and grow distally. This appears in nerve biopsies as clusters of thinly myelinated regenerating axons (Figure 2.1). With intact endoneurium, advancing axons have a chance to reach target tissue. With greater nerve disruption (neurotmesis), the degree of successful reinnervation depends on tissue obstacles (scar tissue) and the extent of the gap (if present) that the nerve fiber has to traverse, and aberrant sprouts may enter functionally unrelated endoneurial tubes or lead to neuromas (tangles of nerve endings). Under the best of circumstances, nerve regeneration advances 1–2 mm/day, and is more rapid in proximal segments and in younger individuals. In general, after severe axonal loss, any functional reinnervation will occur within 18–24 months (Robinson, 2015).

Myelin Damage

Myelin is formed from the Schwann cell membrane, and, with nerve injury, Schwann cells lose contact with degenerating axons, and dedifferentiate and proliferate (Chen et al., 2007; Gaudet et al., 2011). The Schwann cell myelin membrane breaks up into small

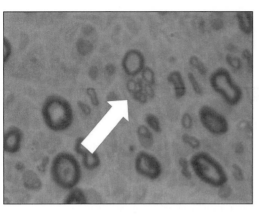
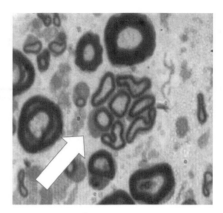

Figure 2.1 Nerve biopsy cross-sections showing clusters of regenerating nerves (white arrows). Photomicrographs from Y. Harati, MD, with permission.

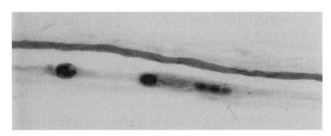
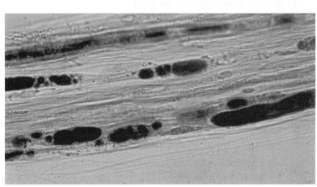

Figure 2.2 Nerve biopsies showing myelin ovoids. Upper panel is teased fiber preparation showing normal fiber above and fiber with myelin ovoids below. Lower panel is longitudinal section showing several fibers with myelin ovoids.
Photomicrographs from Y. Harati, MD, with permission.

ovoids, which participate in autophagocytosis, and Schwann cells serve as phagocytic cells (Figure 2.2). Macrophages also participate in phagocytosis. Schwann cells secrete factors that promote nerve growth, but the effect diminishes after two months. When contact is reestablished with the axon, Schwann cells redifferentiate and remyelinate the axon, but the myelin is thinner and the intermodal length reduced, resulting in slower saltatory conduction, and, as a consequence, conduction velocities are permanently slowed.

Nodal Damage

Pathology specific to the node of Ranvier is also referred to as nodopathies (Uncini and Kuwabara, 2015). Proteins at the nodes can be immunologic target sites in immune-mediated neuropathies causing nodal conduction block with relatively little structural damage (Figure 2.3). Alternatively, focal axonal damage can occur at the node.

Painful neuropathies are felt to result from alterations in ion channels, and are called channelopathies.

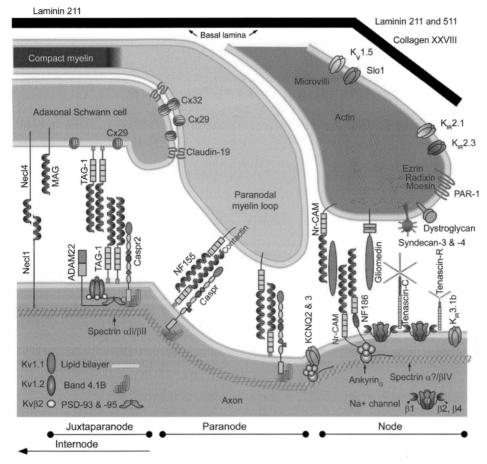

Figure 2.3 Diagram of molecular components at the node of Ranvier that may be immunogenic and contribute to altered nerve conduction in inflammatory neuropathies (precise molecular organization largely unknown). (Willison, Scherer, Neurology, 2014, with permission.) Nr-CA Composite of node of Ranvier showing node flanked by paranodal regions with several proteins neurofascin (NF) 186 and 155 and Contact-associated protein, TAG1 (CNTN1) – Casper complex. Inset is immunefluorescence photomicrograph showing antibody attachment to CNTN1-Casper complex 26218529.

Mutations in the Nav1.7 sodium channel gene causing a gain of function have been found in both small myelinated and unmyelinated sensory fibers and at multiple sites along the nerve, including nociceptive receptors, nodes of Ranvier, dorsal root ganglion cells, and at central processes (Bennett and Woods, 2014). Mutations lead to nerve and dorsal root hyperexcitability with enhanced firing frequency and spontaneous activity, presumably resulting in noxious sensory perceptions. Skin biopsies show reduced intraepidermal nerve fiber densities. Inactivating mutations in Nav1.7 sodium channels can result in congenital insensitivity to pain and loss of function mutations (erythromelalgia).

Focal Conduction Block

Focal conduction block refers to the blockage of nerve action potentials across restricted regions of an axon, with normal conduction proximal and distal to the region. The number of fibers that need to be blocked to show as a block with nerve conduction tests is not known. Conduction block may occur as a result of demyelination over a number of consecutive segments or from functional changes at the node of Ranvier. Focal conduction block is encountered in hereditary neuropathy with predisposition to pressure palsies (HNPP), in immune-mediated neuropathies such as multifocal neuropathies with conduction block, and

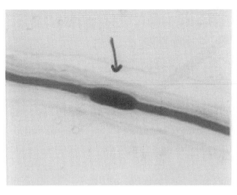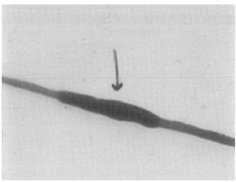

Figure 2.4 Teased fiber showing focal enlargement of myelin (tomacula). Photomicrographs from Y. Harati, MD, with permission.

also in normal nerves at sites of pressure (entrapment sites) such as the median nerve at the wrist (carpal tunnel syndrome), ulnar nerve at the elbow (ulnar palsy) and fibular/peroneal nerve at the knee (foot drop).

Hereditary Neuropathy with Predisposition to Pressure Palsies

HNPP is an autosomal dominant disorder where focal conduction block occurs after mild trauma to nerves that is reversible over hours to days, although there can be an accumulation of nerve damage. It is associated with a duplication of the peripheral myelin protein 22 (PMP 22) or point mutations. Pathologically, there are nerve segments with thickened myelin, called tomacula, which are associated with axonal constrictions (Farrar et al., 2014) (Figure 2.4). There is evidence for chronic hyperpolarization of the axon, and it is hypothesized that mild mechanical stress (pressure) further hyperpolarizes axons, leading to focal conduction block.

Compression-Entrapment Neuropathies

Pathology of focal neuropathies at common sites of entrapment is difficult to study because clinical features of chronicity, limb postures, and work exposure cannot be accurately duplicated in experimental models. Early factors include reduced epineural blood flow due to regional compression pressure, followed by epi- and endoneural edema, and altered myelin and axonal transport (Slater, 1999). There may be changes in the degree of axonal polarization contributing to slow conduction and conduction block. Eventually,

there is thickening of all neural elements leading to increases in nerve cross-sectional area and alterations in blood flow in the nerve segment visible on nerve imaging. There can be rearrangement of myelin and axonal loss.

Multifocal Neuropathies with Conduction Block

Multifocal neuropathies with conduction block are immune-mediated neuropathies with unique features of focal conduction block distributed along segments of nerve involving either only motor or both motor and sensory fibers. Over time, there can be progressive axonal loss. Factors causing conduction block are immune interactions at nodes of Ranvier with changes in axonal polarization, alterations in sodium channels, and altered sodium/potassium pump function and varying degrees of demyelination and remyelination (Franssen, 2014).

Length-Dependent Axonal Loss

Both autonomic and somatic peripheral nerves have long axons, up to one meter in length, which imposes a high metabolic demand on the cell bodies. Alterations in cell body metabolism may account in part for the clinical feature of length-dependent pathology in many polyneuropathies. The long length of lower-extremity axons makes them particularly vulnerable to metabolic alterations leading to a dying-back pattern, and a similar pattern occurs in upper-extremity nerves when shorter lengths are affected (stocking-glove distribution). Causative factors include metabolic derangements (diabetes and the metabolic syndrome,

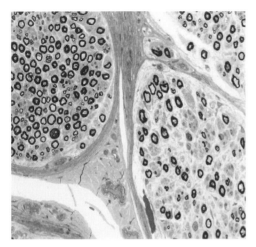

Figure 2.5 Nerve biopsy cross-section showing spectrum of axonal loss. Fascicle upper left with near-normal fiber density; fascicles right side with marked loss of fibers.
Photomicrographs from Y. Harati, MD, with permission.

uremia), neurotoxic drugs (chemotherapeutic drugs), and toxins (drugs, metals, alcohol). Axonal loss is felt to be the primary pathologic process, but demyelination at multiple foci may also occur as a secondary process. Loss of fast-conducting large fibers explains mildly slowed conduction velocities in primary axonal neuropathies, but there may also be myelin loss and repair. Many polyneuropathies affect sensory perception before and to greater degrees than motor function. The reasons are not fully clear, but, in addition to loss of large sensory and motor fibers, there is loss of small sensory fibers before loss of large fibers (Dyck et al., 2013).

Nerve biopsy shows axonal loss of small and large fibers, axonal degeneration and regeneration (and some fascicles may be affected to greater degrees than others) (Figure 2.5), and demyelination and remyelination. Biophysiological abnormalities in diabetes include changes in sodium conductance, reduced sodium/potassium pump function, and an alteration in axon transport (both ortho- and retrograde) (Arnold et al., 2013). Skin biopsy findings are the loss of intraepidermal nerve terminals (Mellgren et al., 2013).

Small Fiber Neuropathies

Small fiber neuropathies are defined as involving no large fibers, and nerve conduction studies will be normal (Chan and Wilder-Smith, 2016). Whole nerve biopsies may be less informative as small fiber loss will be less apparent. Skin biopsies are less invasive and more likely to show abnormalities in the form of reduced intraepidermal fiber density and axonal swellings (Figure 2.6).

Vasculitic Neuropathies

Vasculitic neuropathy pathology can be classified on size of involved vessels; large arterioles include small arteries and large arterioles (75–300 μm in diameter), and microvessels include the smallest arterioles, endoneurial capillaries, and venules (<40 μm in diameter) (Gwathmey et al., 2014). Nerve biopsy, frequently supplemented with biopsy of neighboring muscle, is necessary to document vasculitic pathology.

Microvasculitis

A microvasculitis pathology may be common to a number of clinically disparate plexopathies, including brachial and lumbosacral plexopathies (associated with or without diabetes or impaired glucose tolerance, and with or without pain), idiopathic or spontaneous brachial plexopathy (Parsonage-Turner syndrome), and hereditary brachial plexopathy (Dyck and Windebank, 2002; van Alfen, 2011; Massie et al., 2012). Nerve roots and peripheral nerves are frequently involved, leading to the establishment of the terms cervical or lumbosacral radiculoplexus neuropathies (Gwathmey and Burns, 2014). Idiopathic and hereditary plexopathies likely have an autoimmune trigger with possible components of biomechanical stress (van Alfen, 2011). Hereditary forms are associated with SEPT9 mutations and a predisposition to the above triggers and a similar inflammatory pathology.

Pathologic findings include perivascular and vessel wall inflammation, hemosiderin deposition, leading to occlusion of vessels, with resultant axonal degeneration. Muscle biopsy may also show vessel wall inflammation, and concurrent biopsy of nerve and neighboring muscle may increase diagnostic yield (Figure 2.7). There is variable axonal loss, and nerve fascicles may be affected to different degrees (Figure 2.5) (Gwathmey and Burns, 2014).

Recent investigations describe hourglass-like fascicular constrictions of peripheral nerves at one or more sites in a symptomatic nerve (mononeuropathy) or when the clinical features suggest a plexopathy (Parsonage-Turner syndrome) (Sunagawa et al., 2017; Pan et al., 2011). The constrictions are evident during

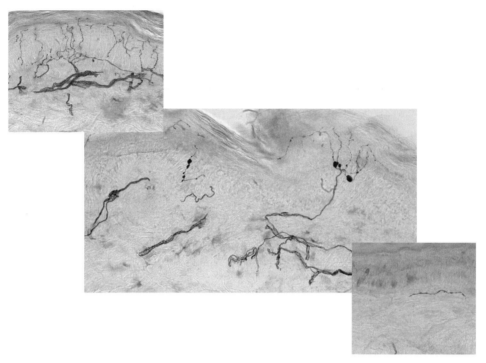

Figure 2.6 Skin biopsy of unmyellinated intraepidermal nerve fibers. Central photomicrograph showing reduced density of fibers with swellings. Upper left photomicrograph shows normal fiber density. Lower right photomicrograph shows markedly reduced fiber density. See also Figure 1.7.
University of Utah Cutaneous Pathology Laboratory, with permission.

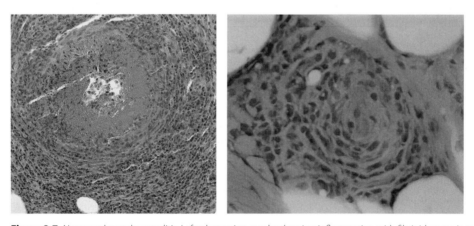

Figure 2.7 Nerve and muscle vasculitis. Left: photomicrographs showing inflammation with fibrioid necrosis and partial occlusion of small vessel in nerve. Right: photomicrograph showing inflammation and occlusion of small vessel in muscle.
Photomicrographs from A. Pestronk, MD, and Y. Harati, MD, with permission.

surgery or can be viewed with ultrasound. Underlying pathology is speculative but includes local inflammatory reaction resulting in focal edema and vascular compromise, but mechanisms of actual nerve (axonal) damage are not clear (Lundborg, 2003).

Primary Demyelinating Polyneuropathy

Demyelinating neuropathies are felt to involve a primary immune-mediated attack on myelin, with secondary damage to axons. The immune-mediated

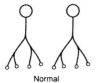 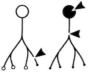

Normal   Neuropathic denervation   Collateral reinnervation

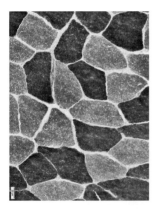 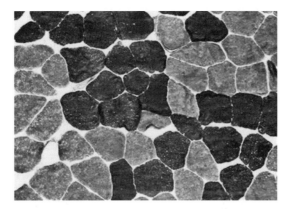

Figure 2.8 Diagram of collateral reinnervation of muscle fibers following axonal loss. Motor unit remodeling leads to fiber-type grouping on muscle biopsy (left photomicrograph normal muscle; right photograph marked fiber-type grouping). Photomicrographs from A. Pestronk, MD, with permission.

pathology includes humoral factors, and nerve roots and peripheral nerves of all lengths are vulnerable. This causes diffusely distributed symptoms and signs (proximal and distal), but there is a greater pathologic burden on distal nerves.

There are pathologic similarities among immune-mediated polyneuropathies, with humoral and cellular factors in various combinations, including complement-fixing antibodies, macrophages, and T cells activation (Dalakas, 2014). Immune targets on nerves are known for a limited number of neuropathies, and there is evidence for molecular mimicry between antibody and structural epitopes shared with pathogenic organisms. Microscopic pathologic changes are perivascular and endoneurial inflammatory infiltrates, and segmental demyelination mediated by macrophages. In some neuropathies, there can be a primary attack on axons and nodes of Ranvier (Franssen and Straver, 2013; 2014).

Collateral Reinnervation

Loss of motor nerve fibers results in an intrinsic compensatory process whereby terminal branches from surviving motor units sprout processes to reinnervate denervated muscle fibers. The process of collateral reinnervation is visible on muscle biopsy as a fiber-type grouping (Figure 2.8). The process slows the rate of loss of CMAP amplitude and is detected on needle EMG by abnormal spontaneous activity, reduced motor unit recruitment, and enlarged and complex motor units. The degree of collateral reinnervation is limited in extent by physical boundaries in muscles (fascicular boundaries).

References

Arnold R, Kwai NC, Krishnan AV. Mechanisms of axonal dysfunction in diabetic and uraemic neuropathies. *Clin Neurophysiol.* 2013;124:2079–90.

Bennett DL, Woods CG. Painful and painless channelopathies. *Lancet Neurol.* 2014;13:587–99.

Campbell WW. Evaluation and management of peripheral nerve injury. *Clin Neurophysiol.* 2008;119:1951–65.

Chan AC, Wilder-Smith EP. Small fiber neuropathy: Getting bigger! *Muscle Nerve.* 2016;53:671–82.

Chaudhry V, Cornblath DR. Wallerian degeneration in human nerves: serial electrophysiological studies. *Muscle Nerve.* 1992;15:687–93.

Chen ZL, Yu WM, Strickland S. Peripheral regeneration. *Annu Rev Neurosci.* 2007;30:209–33.

Dalakas MC. Pathogenesis of immune-mediated neuropathies. *Biochim Biophys Acta.* 2014.

Dyck PJ, Herrmann DN, Staff NP. Assessing decreased sensation and increased sensory phenomena in diabetic polyneuropathies. *Diabetes.* 2013;62:3677–86.

Dyck PJ, Windebank AJ. Diabetic and nondiabetic lumbosacral radiculoplexus neuropathies: new insights into pathophysiology and treatment. *Muscle Nerve.* 2002;25:477–91.

Farrar MA, Park SB, Krishnan AV, Kiernan MC, Lin CS. Axonal dysfunction, dysmyelination, and conduction failure in hereditary neuropathy with liability to pressure palsies. *Muscle Nerve.* 2014;49:858–65.

Franssen H. The node of Ranvier in multifocal motor neuropathy. *J Clin Immunol.* 2014;34 Suppl 1:S105–11.

Franssen H, Straver DC. Pathophysiology of immune-mediated demyelinating neuropathies-part I: neuroscience. *Muscle Nerve.* 2013;48:851–64.

Franssen H, Straver DC. Pathophysiology of immune-mediated demyelinating neuropathies – Part II: Neurology. *Muscle Nerve.* 2014;49:4–20.

Gaudet AD, Popovich PG, Ramer MS. Wallerian degeneration: gaining perspective on inflammatory events after peripheral nerve injury. *J Neuroinflammation.* 2011;8:110.

Gwathmey KG, Burns TM, Collins MP, Dyck PJ. Vasculitic neuropathies. *Lancet Neurol.* 2014;13:67–82.

Lundborg G. Commentary: hourglass-like fascicular nerve compressions. *J Hand Surg Am.* 2003;28:212–14.

Massie R, Mauermann ML, Staff NP, Amrami KK, Mandrekar JN, Dyck PJ, et al. Diabetic cervical radiculoplexus neuropathy: a distinct syndrome expanding the spectrum of diabetic radiculoplexus neuropathies. *Brain.* 2012;135:3074–88.

Mellgren SI, Nolano M, Sommer C. The cutaneous nerve biopsy: technical aspects, indications, and contribution. *Handb Clin Neurol.* 2013;115:171–88.

Pan YW, Wang S, Tian G, Li C, Tian W, Tian M. Typical brachial neuritis (Parsonage-Turner syndrome) with hourglass-like constrictions in the affected nerves. *J Hand Surg Am.* 2011;36:1197–203.

Robinson LR. How electrodiagnosis predicts clinical outcome of focal peripheral nerve lesions. *Muscle Nerve.* 2015;52:321–33.

Slater RR, Jr. Carpal tunnel syndrome: current concepts. *J South Orthop Assoc.* 1999;8:203–13.

Sunagawa T, Nakashima Y, Shinomiya R, Kurumadani H, Adachi N, Ochi M. Correlation between "hourglass-like fascicular constriction" and idiopathic anterior interosseous nerve palsy. *Muscle Nerve.* 2017;55:508–12.

Uncini A, Kuwabara S. Nodopathies of the peripheral nerve: an emerging concept. *J Neurol Neurosurg Psychiatry.* 2015;86:1186–95.

van Alfen N. Clinical and pathophysiological concepts of neuralgic amyotrophy. *Nat Rev Neurol.* 2011;7:315–22.

Clinical Evaluation

Chapter 3

Introduction

This chapter presents a series of steps to aid in obtaining a detailed evaluation based on questions with "yes" or "no" answers. The steps progress through clinical history, neurologic examination, and electrodiagnostic testing (Chapter 4). A full understanding of the clinical history should be as if the clinician has experienced what the patient has experienced. With a thorough characterization of symptoms, signs from the neurologic examination should be predictable or confirmatory. The electrodiagnostic study can verify lesion localization and estimate underlying pathology.

Clinical History

The clinical history is the most important step, and at the conclusion the type of neuropathy is usually evident.

Preliminary Question: Within the peripheral nervous system: to exclude cortical and spinal sites, and psychogenic factors?

Not all sensory and motor symptoms localize to the peripheral nervous system. Symptoms of numbness, paresthesias, pain, weakness and fatigue, and associated signs must be consistent in the context of anatomy, physiology, and pathology of the peripheral nervous system. Patterns of abnormalities may represent central rather than peripheral sites of pathology.

When symptoms and signs do not localize to lesions in either the central or peripheral nervous systems, the question of a psychogenic cause (somatoform disorder) arises. A frank discussion and questions about other non-physical factors is appropriate.

It will be assumed that the answer to the Preliminary Question is "yes," with localization in the peripheral nervous system.

Step 1: What part of the peripheral nervous system is involved: root, plexus, single nerves, multiple nerves, diffuse peripheral nerves?

A series of deductive questions can include or exclude sites in the peripheral nervous system

Table 3.1 Questions to Address When Evaluating Peripheral Neuropathies

Step 1: What is the distribution?	Mononeuropathy
	Mononeuropathy multiplex
	Distal-predominant polyneuropathy
	Distal and proximal polyneuropathy
	Plexopathy
	Radiculopathy
	Asymmetric, unusual
Step 2: What nerve fibers are involved?	Somatic: motor, sensory, both
	Autonomic
Step 3: What is the time course?	Acute
	Subacute
	Chronic
	Very chronic
Step 4: Are there other features?	Physical features: high arches, hammer toes
	Social conditions: alcohol, diets
	Medical conditions: comorbid diseases
	Medications
	Family history

(Table 3.1). The sites can be considered in a distal to proximal order, or vice versa, to aid in forming questions. Mononeuropathies are common, and mononeuritis multiplex may involve different nerves in different limbs. Mononeuropathies and mononeuritis multiplex usually cause sensory loss and weakness in the distribution of the nerve(s). Peripheral polyneuropathies are roughly symmetric and sensory symptoms may predominate over weakness (or vice versa), and follow a length-dependent pattern with onset in the feet and slow progression of symptoms in a stocking-glove distribution, but there are exceptions to this pattern. Plexus-level disorders are diffuse and cannot be localized to single nerves, are usually unilateral (within a limb), painful, and include sensory loss and weakness. Root-level disorders are usually

17

Table 3.2 Examples of Positive and Negative Sensory and Motor Symptoms

	Sensory Symptoms	Motor Symptoms
Positive	Paresthesias	Fasciculations
	Pain	Cramps
	-burning	
	-squeezing or tightness	
	-electric-like	
	-hyper sensitivity	
Negative	Numbness	Weakness
	Reduced or absent sensation	Atrophy
	Postural instability	

unilateral and frequently involve radiating pain and, less commonly, weakness.

Step 2: What types of nerve fibers are involved: sensory, motor, autonomic nerves?

Patients are more attuned to sensory than motor symptoms, and autonomic dysfunction may not be apparent to the patient (Table 3.1). Symptoms may be considered positive or negative in nature (Table 3.2) (Dyck et al., 2013). Positive sensory symptoms such as burning, lancinating pain, and hyperpathic sensations suggest involvement of small diameter nerve somatic or unmyelinated somatic fibers. Negative sensory symptoms such as numbness and inability to feel touch suggest involvement of large-diameter somatic fibers. Unsteadiness with eyes closed also suggests the involvement of large fibers that subserve proprioception.

Cramps of new onset or a worsening pattern in distal leg and foot can be considered a positive motor symptom. Weakness is a negative motor symptom, and occurs late in a neuropathy because collateral reinnervation compensates for mild to moderate motor nerve fiber loss, and the weakness of intrinsic foot muscles may go unnoticed. The apparent absence of motor symptoms does not exclude subclinical motor involvement, and the needle EMG is more sensitive to mild motor fiber loss. Motor symptoms, positive or negative, are due to large-diameter somatic nerve involvement.

Inquiry into the symptoms of autonomic nerve involvement can be helpful, and include lack of pedal sweating (dry socks), cracked skin about the heel, impotence in men, and frequent orthostatic dizziness.

Step 3: What is the time course: acute, subacute, chronic progressive, chronic very slow progressive?

Every disease has a temporal course (acute, subacute, chronic) and a momentum (rapidly progressive, slow progressive, very slow progressive) (Table 3.1). Traditionally in neurology, acute is over hours to a day, but few neuropathies are truly acute (mononeuropathy multiplex neuropathies may have a sudden onset). More commonly, acute polyneuropathies worsen over weeks, and the Guillain-Barré syndrome has an acute time course of progression of up to four weeks. Subacute, in the context of neuropathies, is four to eight weeks. Chronic slow progressive is eight weeks to years. Chronic very slow progressive denotes symptoms that may have an insidious onset with progression over years, and, if over decades, raises the possibility of a hereditary neuropathy.

Most neuropathies are progressive, and rarely do neuropathies follow a clear stepwise pattern of progression (mononeuropathies in mononeuritis multiplex are an exception). Natural remissions and relapses are very rare, and remissions usually reflect the effects of treatment while relapses reflect the consequences of treatment withdrawal.

Step 4: Other pertinent features: medical history, medications, social factors, family history?

To complete an evaluation, other factors should be sought. Comorbid diseases such as collagen vascular diseases are associated with mononeuritis multiplex, and diabetes frequently leads to peripheral neuropathies. A number of medications have neurotoxic properties. Excessive alcohol consumption (to a marked degree) or a very restrictive diet raises the question of excesses or deficiencies. A family history of a neuropathy may not be apparent, and specific inquiries should be made about family members who may have unsuspected symptoms or findings (Table 3.3).

Clinical Examination

The examination steps parallel those in the clinical history and verify the distribution and nature of nerve involvement.

Step 5: Within the peripheral nervous system: exclude cortical, spinal, psychogenic sites?

This step allows for confirmation that signs are consistent with a disorder of peripheral nerves, and assures exclusion of signs localized to the central nervous system, such as spasticity and hyperreflexia.

Step 6: What types of nerve fibers are involved: sensory, motor, autonomic nerves?

Table 3.3 Questions to Ask About Family Members to Support a Hereditary Neuropathy

Historical features

    Difficulty with running, sports, or military activities due to foot/ankle issues

    Arthritic foot troubles (representing incorrect diagnoses of arthritis or poliomyelitis)

    Use of braces/orthotic devices

    Foot troubles due to pressure or sores

    Foot surgeries

Physical features

    High arches

    Hammer or curled toes

    Claw hands

    Wasting of distal muscles (thin feet, legs, and hands)

    Heel cord shortening (inability to dorsiflex ankle to <90 degrees)

    Difficulty walking on heels (reduced elevation of toes)

    Difficulty rising from a kneeling position

Note: Photographs can be taken of family members (legs and feet) for review by the clinician.

Sensory and motor nerve functions can be tested separately. Sensory perception can be roughly divided into modalities served by nerve fibers of different diameters (Gilman, 2002). With bedside sensory testing, the following distinctions are commonly made: large-diameter fibers are assessed by light touch, vibration, and joint position sense, and also tendon reflexes; small-diameter fibers are assessed by sharp pin and cold perception. Motor function is served by large-diameter fibers.

Sensory nerve assessment, except for tendon reflexes, represents a patient's interpretation of how an applied stimulus is perceived, and it is essential that the patient understands the desired degree of attention to the stimulus. Another point is to ensure that the patient accurately registers the stimulus when applied to an uninvolved or less-involved site before testing the region of involvement.

The sensory examination serves another purpose in that a patient may not appreciate the degree of sensory impairment, especially if progression has been slow. This is most important with diabetic neuropathies where alteration in peripheral vasculature increases the risk of skin ulcerations in the foot due to unappreciated trauma.

A: Light-touch perception can be assessed by the examiner touching the skin with the lightest possible tactile finger pressure; normally the stimulus should be immediately detectable.

A distal–proximal gradient can be confirmed if light touch is reduced or absent at the dorsum of the foot by touching at more proximal sites along the shin until it is perceived.

B: Vibration can be tested with a 128-Hz tuning fork applied to a joint; normally it should extinguish about the same time for the patient as for the examiner holding the tuning fork. A distal–proximal gradient can be confirmed if vibration perception extinguishes early or is absent at the great toe (but may not be pathologic in patients >70 years old) by applying the end of the fork at more proximal bony sites (malleoli, knee) until it is perceived. The degree of loss can be approximated by the number of seconds the vibration is perceived by the examiner. A calibrated tuning fork is available (Pestronk et al., 2004).

C: Joint position sense can be assessed by moving a toe or finger up or down at the distal phalangeal joint. Slow movement (over one to two seconds) rather than rapid movement is more sensitive for an abnormality. Normal sensitivity is ≤1 degree at the finger and 3 degrees at the toe (Gilman, 2002).

D: Tendon reflexes are mediated by a reflex arc that is more vulnerable to afferent (sensory) nerve fiber loss than efferent (motor) fiber loss. Testing does not require patient interpretation, and thus represents an objective assessment of sensory nerves: an absent reflex supports large-fiber sensory nerve loss.

E: Mildly noxious stimulus perception can be assessed by gently applying the pokey (pointed) end of a safety pin; normally a patient can distinguish between the pokey versus the dull end of the pin, but several touches must be made in a small area because some areas of skin may be less sensitive. A distal–proximal gradient can be confirmed, if the patient is unable to perceive the pokey end at the dorsum of the foot, by touching at more proximal sites along the shin until it is perceived.

A new safety pin should be used with each patient.

F: Temperature sensation testing is difficult because "hot" is 40–45°C and "cold" is 5–10°C, and suitable probes are rarely available. The circular disks on the 128-Hz tuning fork can be applied to the patient's skin and should be perceived by the patient as cool, but consistency of tuning fork temperature is poor.

G: Testing with a 10-g monofilament on the sole of the foot, with insensitivity to touch to several applications (one out of three sites) is a strong risk factor for foot ulcers in patients with diabetes (Abbott et al., 2002).

Quantitative vibration and temperature threshold testing instruments are available, but instruments are expensive and testing algorithms complex and not practical for routine clinical evaluations.

Motor nerve involvement is assessed by the presence of muscle atrophy and weakness. In the lower extremity, assessment of extensor digitorum brevis muscle bulk is helpful, but may be reduced in healthy people over the age of 70 years. Manual strength testing of lesser toe extension (extensor digitorum brevis muscle) and great toe extension (extensor hallucis longus) is useful as mild weakness can be better appreciated in these muscles than from more proximal muscles (anterior tibialis muscle). The ability of a patient to elevate their toes when standing on their heels is more sensitive for mild weakness than testing ankle dorsiflexion by manual muscle testing. Plantar flexion weakness must be profound to be detected by manual muscle testing, and is found only in severe neuropathies. Mild weakness can be better appreciated having the patient stand on their toes.

Autonomic testing at the bedside is challenging. Measurement of orthostatic blood pressure changes can be helpful if symptoms of such are elicited. An absence of sweating assessed by finding dry socks during the examination, and the presence of dry and cracked skin of the foot, is supportive. Quantitative autonomic testing instruments are available, but instruments are expensive and testing algorithms complex and not practical for routine clinical evaluations.

Step 7: What part of the peripheral nervous system: root, plexus, single nerves, multiple nerves, diffuse peripheral nerves?

Acute radiculopathies from disk disease are usually painful and frequently have clinically apparent weakness and sensory findings in the distribution of the affected root. Chronic radiculopathies are frequently associated with spine (neck, lower back) pain and some radicular-like pain, but may have no or equivocal clinical findings of sensory disturbance or weakness. For all radiculopathies, tendon reflexes may be reduced in the root distribution compared to the other side.

Plexopathies vary in the extent of nerve damage within the plexus, and thus clinical features vary. Acute plexopathies include traumatic and non-traumatic causes, while chronic and progressive plexopathies have a variety of causes. Plexopathies involve both sensory and motor nerves proximal to the formation of named nerves, and clues are that abnormalities of sensory loss and weakness cannot be readily explained by the involvement of a distal nerve. Tendon reflexes are usually reduced or absent in the affected limb.

Most polyneuropathies follow a length-dependent pattern of involvement such that, over time, as sensory disturbances advance from the foot to the knee (as a stocking is unrolled), the length of nerve is the same as from the neck to the hand, and with further progression can advance up the arm (as a glove is unrolled). In the extreme, the involved nerve lengths are equal to that of thoracic nerves, and a shield distribution of sensory loss can be demonstrated along the anterior trunk.

Mononeuropathies are readily identified based on the distribution of sensory and motor signs to an individual nerve, or multiple individual nerves (mononeuropathy multiplex). The most common mononeuropathies are the median nerve at the wrist (carpal tunnel syndrome), ulnar nerve at the elbow, and lateral femoral cutaneous nerve (meralgia paresthetica). Mononeuropathy multiplex can involve different combinations of nerves.

Step 8: What is the time course: acute, chronic slowly progressive, chronic very slowly progressive?

Certain clinical examination features suggest slow progression (months to years), such as marked muscle atrophy, finger flexion tendon contractures (claw hand), tight Achilles tendon (straight angle between shin and foot), and high arches and hammer toes.

Electrodiagnostic Evaluation

The electrodiagnostic examination is an extension of the neurologic examination, and general aspects of its role in the overall evaluation are presented here because it can verify and clarify answers from the clinical and examination questions above (Bromberg and Brownell, 2012). Details of electrodiagnostic testing are given in Chapter 4.

Step 9: What types of nerve fibers are involved: sensory, motor nerves?

Sensory nerve studies are more sensitive to the effects of axonal loss (low-amplitude/absent SNAP) because with motor nerve fiber loss, collateral reinnervation preserves CMAP amplitude. In neuropathies with mild degrees of motor nerve fiber loss the CMAP may be normal, and needle EMG of distal muscles is necessary to demonstrate loss. Of note, many neuropathies are named by the predominant symptom, and "primary sensory neuropathies" may also have mild motor nerve involvement. Most neuropathies involve sensory fibers, and testing the longest sensory nerves (sural, superficial fibular/peroneal nerves) is appropriate (England et al., 2005). Nerve conduction testing of medial and lateral plantar nerves has technical difficulties, and false positive abnormalities are possible without experience testing these nerves.

Step 10: What is the underlying pathology: primary axonal, primary demyelinating, conduction block?

This is the most important role of electrodiagnosis in peripheral neuropathies, but also the most challenging. Primary axonal neuropathies are much more common than primary demyelinating neuropathies, but identification of the latter has implications for possible treatment. Sensory nerve fiber loss frequently leads to absent SNAPs, and it is more practical to use motor nerves to assess for underlying pathology (primary demyelinating, primary axonal). Sets of diagnostic criteria for nerve conduction metrics are available to distinguish primary demyelination from the effects of slowed conduction due to axonal loss and are discussed in Chapter 4.

Focal conduction block represents blockage of nerve impulses in a sufficient number of nerve fibers to reduce the CMAP or SNAP amplitude across the site. Apparent or false focal conduction block can occur in the setting where there is only slowing of conduction across the site. Diagnostic criteria are available to help ensure true conduction block pathology, and are discussed in Chapter 4.

Step 11: What is the extent of denervation: mononeuropathy, plexopathy, length-dependent?

The clinical examination can largely define the distribution and extent of nerve involvement, but the clinical examination is less sensitive for mild degrees of damage or slow loss. The involvement of individual nerves can be assessed by nerve conduction studies and needle EMG.

Step 12: What is the time course of denervation: active, chronic, very chronic?

Most neuropathies follow a chronic time course, but some progress very slowly and have an insidious onset and are of longer duration than the patient believes. In these situations, there may be marked axonal loss and distal sensory and motor responses may be absent. An electrodiagnostic hint for the very chronic nature, and hence possible hereditary neuropathy, is a markedly reduced number of motor units recorded with needle EMG, and motor unit waveforms that are of very high amplitude but of simple waveform shapes.

Epidemiologic Considerations

Step 13: Epidemiologic features: gender distributions, age at onset, occupation/avocation, incidence rates?

The list of potential causes of nerve damage is large and can be reduced by the above steps. Further refinement can be achieved by consideration of epidemiologic factors to estimate likelihoods and probabilities with the particular patient.

Neuropathies do not have marked gender predilections, but some have age distributions (hereditary in young individuals, associated with adult-onset comorbidities in older individuals), and such features can shift likelihoods of cause. Occupation and avocation activities can provide clues. The probability of an unusual variant of a common condition is much more likely than a rare type of neuropathy. When the final differential diagnosis is reached it is economic to list possible underlying or causative disorder in order of probabilities, and order tests accordingly.

Clinical and Electrodiagnostic Reports

A full evaluation should result in written clinical and electrodiagnostic reports. It is crucial that both be convincing to the referring physician and impart clear and useful information. The clinical report should conclude with a concise summary of the history and clinical features that led to localization and the differential diagnosis. Recommendations should be given for further electrodiagnostic and laboratory tests, and for treatment and management.

The electrodiagnostic study report should include summary tables of nerve conduction and needle EMG data, as when presented only in prose these data are difficult to read. Consideration should be given for including waveforms. The electrodiagnostic report should be able to stand alone, and consist of an electrodiagnostic conclusion and an overall clinical conclusion. Thus, the report should have a very brief history and pertinent examination findings that will be used to support the clinical conclusion (Jablecki et al., 2005).

References

Abbott CA, Carrington AL, Ashe H, Bath S, Every LC, Griffiths J, et al. The North-West Diabetes Foot Care Study: incidence of, and risk factors for, new diabetic foot ulceration in a community-based patient cohort. *Diabet Med.* 2002;19:377–84.

Bromberg M, Brownell A. *Role of electrodiagnosis in the evaluation of peripheral neuropathies.* In: Donofrio P, ed. *Textbook of Peripheral Neuropathy.* New York: demosMedical, 2012, p. 117–29.

Dyck PJ, Herrmann DN, Staff NP. Assessing decreased sensation and increased sensory phenomena in diabetic polyneuropathies. *Diabetes.* 2013;62:3677–86.

England JD, Gronseth GS, Franklin G, Miller RG, Asbury AK, Carter GT, et al. Distal symmetric polyneuropathy: a definition for clinical research: report of the American Academy of Neurology, the American Association of Electrodiagnostic Medicine, and the American Academy of Physical Medicine and Rehabilitation. *Neurology.* 2005;64:199–207.

Gilman S. Joint position sense and vibration sense: anatomical organisation and assessment. *J Neurol Neurosurg Psychiatry.* 2002;73:473–7.

Jablecki CK, Andary MT, Di Benedetto M, Horowitz SH, Marino RJ, Rosenbaum RB, et al. American Association of Electrodiagnostic Medicine guidelines for outcome studies in electrodiagnostic medicine. *Muscle Nerve.* 1996;19:1626–35.

Jablecki CK, Busis NA, Brandstater MA, Krivickas LS, Miller RG, Robinton JE. Reporting the results of needle EMG and nerve conduction studies: an educational report. *Muscle Nerve.* 2005;32:682–5.

Pestronk A, Florence J, Levine T, Al-Lozi MT, Lopate G, Miller T, et al. Sensory exam with a quantitative tuning fork: rapid, sensitive and predictive of SNAP amplitude. *Neurology.* 2004;62:461–4.

Electrodiagnostic Evaluation

Introduction

Electrodiagnostic studies verify and augment clinical and examination findings, help localize lesion sites, and provide an estimate of underlying nerve pathology. Studies consist of nerve conduction tests and needle EMG, usually performed in that order. Of the two, nerve conduction studies are the most informative in evaluating peripheral neuropathies.

Testing Strategies

A spectrum of nerves and muscles are available for electrodiagnostic study, and their selection can be based on set protocols or individually designed for each patient to assess features determined by the above clinical steps (Jablecki et al., 1996). There are a limited number of nerves and muscles to study amongst the types of neuropathies, and while both approaches will include similar nerves, the approaches differ fundamentally. With protocol studies, analysis frequently occurs after all data are gathered; with designed studies, the results of each test are analyzed to determine if they are technically adequate and if the electrodiagnostic interpretation makes clinical sense. With the former, incongruities may not come to light when the patient is available; with the latter, incongruities can be addressed as the study proceeds.

There are a limited number of electrodiagnostic tests for autonomic nerve dysfunction that can be performed on standard EMG machines, but they are generally less informative than those that can be performed in a full autonomic testing laboratory (see Chapter 5).

This section reviews basic principles of nerve conduction and EMG studies, and how nerve pathology is detected by these studies. Common nerve conduction pitfalls and interpretation cautions are also presented. Specific electrodiagnostic findings are presented in chapters on individual neuropathies.

Nerve Conduction Tests

Most somatic nerves contain sensory and motor nerve fibers, which can be separated for individual study by placement of recording electrodes over cutaneous or motor branches, respectively. Nerves are electrically excited at supramaximal intensities to ensure all fibers are activated. Myelinated fibers are studied and impulses move along axons by saltatory conduction. Nerves can be stimulated anywhere along their length, and impulses move away from the stimulating electrode in both directions. Sensory nerve recordings can be made from conduction in orthodromic or antidromic directions, with the latter more common and yielding a larger amplitude response (Wilbourn, 1994). Motor nerve responses result from conduction in the orthodromic direction, but antidromic conduction contributes to F-wave responses (Falck and Stalberg, 1995).

The sensory nerve response is the SNAP, and the motor nerve response is the CMAP. The range of conduction velocities in normal nerves is 40–70 m/s for sensory nerves and 41–65 m/s for motor nerves (Table 4.1) (Kimura et al., 1986). The SNAP represents summed responses of individual nerve fiber action potentials in a nerve, and the CMAP represents summed responses of individual muscle fiber action potentials in a motor unit (Wilbourn, 1994). The number of fibers in a normal sensory nerve is in the thousands and their action potentials are of relatively low voltage and short duration, and thus the SNAP is in microvolts (μV). The number of nerve fibers in a normal motor nerve is in the hundreds but each motor axon branches hundreds of times in a muscle, and thus the number of muscle fiber action potentials making up the CMAP is in the hundreds of thousands. Further, muscle fiber action potentials are of larger amplitude and longer duration than sensory nerve potentials, and the CMAP is in millivolts (mV).

Both sensory nerve action potentials and muscle fiber motor unit action potentials are biphasic,

Table 4.1 Anatomic and Physiologic Features of Peripheral Nerve Fibers and Nerves

	Number of Fibers in a Nerve	Number of Action Potentials from a Nerve	Single Action Potential Duration	Conduction Velocity Range of a Nerve
Sensory	4,000–6,000	4,000–6,000	1 msec	40–70 m/s
Motor	100–200+	20,000–40,000+	6 msec	41–65 m/s

Milliseconds (msec), meters per second (m/s).

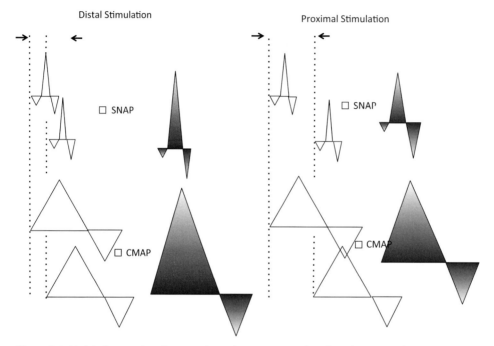

Figure 4.1 Model of summation of nerve and muscle action potentials to form the SNAP and CMAP, illustrating normal phase cancellation. Upright and inverted triangles represent negative and positive components of the fastest and slowest single sensory nerve fiber or motor unit action potentials. Effects of phase cancellation are accentuated with longer conduction distances.

initially negative followed by a lesser positive waveform component (the SNAP waveform may have an initial small positive component, and thus can be triphasic) (Figure 4.1). In the algebraic summation of arriving action potentials (sensory or motor), later-arriving negative phases are partially canceled by earlier-arriving positive phases. Sensory nerve action potentials are very brief (~1 msec) and the phase cancellation effect is great; motor unit action potentials are much longer (~6 msec) and the phase cancellation effect is lower. With longer conduction distances the range of nerve fiber conduction velocities leads to greater temporal spread (dispersion) of arriving action potentials under the recording electrode between the fastest and slowest fibers.

SNAP and CMAP conduction metrics can be divided into those related to the number of axons and those related to the integrity of myelin (Table 4.2). For both sensory and motor responses, amplitude is usually measured by the height of the negative peak of the waveform (Figure 4.2). For the CMAP, the negative peak area is also a useful metric (see below). Amplitude and area are proportional to the number of axons, but only an approximation as an accurate predication cannot be made for motor axon number due to collateral reinnervation, and for sensory nerves because responses may be unrecordable when ~20% of fibers remain.

The integrity of myelin is represented by nerve conduction timing metrics (Table 4.2). Timing

Table 4.2 SNAP and CMAP Nerve Conduction Metrics

Axonal Loss

SNAP: negative peak amplitude (μV) – LLN

CMAP: negative peak amplitude (mV) or area (mV*ms) – LLN

Myelin Integrity

SNAP: distal latency (msec) – ULN

CMAP: distal latency (msec) – ULN

SNAP: distal and segmental conduction velocities (m/s) – LLN

CMAP: segmental conduction velocities (m/s) – LLN

SNAP: temporal dispersion: negative peak duration (msec) – ULN

CMAP: temporal dispersion: negative peak duration (msec) – ULN

F-wave: distal latency; minimum, median (msec) – ULN

Microvolts (μV); millivolts (mV); area (mV*msec), milliseconds (msec); meters per second (m/s). Lower limits of normal (LLN); upper limits of normal (ULN).

measures for both SNAP and CMAP include distal latency (conduction time over standard nerve lengths), and segmental conduction velocities. Most timing measures are for the fastest fibers reaching the recording electrodes. Note that a conduction velocity can be obtained for sensory nerves based on the distal latency and conduction distance, but for motor nerves there is an incalculable delay across the neuromuscular junctions incorporated in the distal latency, and thus motor conduction velocities are calculated along segments of the nerve (Figure 4.2). The effect of the spread of arrival times that make up the summed SNAP and CMAP potentials can be measured by the duration of the waveform's negative peak. The F-wave is based on antidromic motor nerve action potentials subsequently eliciting an orthodromic response back to the muscle, but only 1%–3% of antidromic fiber action potentials result in an orthodromic response. F-wave metrics are the minimum latency, maximum latency, and dispersion of latencies recorded from a set number of responses (10–32) (Nobrega et al., 1999).

Nerve conduction metrics are expressed as limits of upper or lower limits of normal (ULN or LLN, respectively) (Table 4.2). Methods for gathering normal data and the statistical method to determine ULN and LLN are important but rarely known or discussed as most limiting values are passed along from one laboratory to another. For normal nerves, there is a small degree of variability in nerve conduction metric values based on subject height (relative nerve length), age, and gender, and lesser effects on body habitus (greater distance

between sensory nerves and the skin where recording electrodes are placed due to adipose tissue, and digital circumstances for ring electrodes). An important statistical concept is that there are distributions of normal data for all nerve conduction metrics, and a specific patient's nerve conduction value may be close to the limit for that metric, and therefore not strictly abnormal, but should be interpreted as perhaps closer to the abnormal limit than it is predicted to be, and thus possibly pathologic.

Assessing Nerve Pathology

Three pathologic states can be assessed by electrodiagnostic tests:

- primary axonal loss
- primary demyelination
- primary focal conduction block

It is not uncommon for there to be combinations of pathology in a nerve, making data interpretation challenging, and that is why the term "primary" is emphasized. Assessment of pathologic states is made primarily from nerve conduction studies, as needle EMG can verify axonal loss but cannot identify the site of pathology, whether primary or secondary axonal loss, or quantitatively determine the amount of axonal loss.

When interpreting nerve conduction studies, it is important to appreciate that descriptions of pathology and associated effects on nerve conduction metrics are based on models and frequently from *in vitro* data on single nerve fibers. However, nerves *in situ* function in an environment where many nerve fibers are clustered together and nerve conduction (normal or pathologic) may be affected by ionic current factors (ephaptic effects) and expected nerve conduction values may not be as predicted from models (McComas, 2016).

Primary Axonal Loss

Sensory nerve responses are affected to a greater degree by axonal loss than are motor nerve responses, and hence are more sensitive to detecting mild axonal neuropathies. SNAP amplitude is correlated with myelinated fiber density on nerve biopsy, and when the fiber density falls to <20%, SNAP amplitude is below the LLN (Perkins and Bril, 2014). With motor nerves, collateral reinnervation tends to reduce the fall in the CMAP with progressive axon loss. A CMAP amplitude may remain above the LLN until >50% of fibers are lost, and in the extreme a response can be

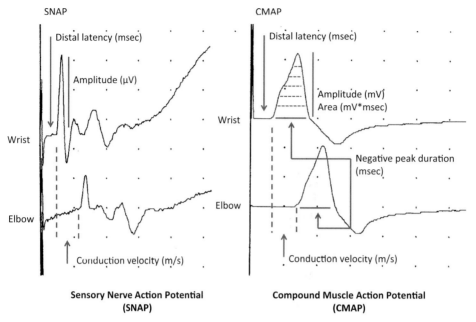

Figure 4.2 SNAP and CMAP metrics.

recorded from a single remaining motor nerve fiber (Herrmann et al., 1999).

Most neuropathies involve damage to sensory and motor fibers, although the proportion varies with the type of neuropathy. Accordingly, in planning nerve conduction studies it is advantageous to first test a sensory nerve. A length-dependent pattern can be verified by testing a distal leg nerve; if the SNAP is absent, testing a more proximal sensory nerve in the hand (digital nerve) can document a response, and, if also absent, testing the superficial radial nerve as a more proximal nerve. Motor nerve involvement can be measured by testing a nerve of the same length as the sensory nerve, such as the fibular/peroneal or tibial nerve; if absent, testing motor nerves to hand muscles can provide information. It is important to keep in mind that an absent response suggests severe axonal loss, but does not provide information as to primary or secondary axonal loss. For a mononeuropathy, testing a neighboring but unaffected nerve can isolate the involved nerve. If a condition is unilateral, testing the same nerve on the other side isolates the pathology.

Primary Demyelination

The pathology of primary demyelinating neuropathies is felt to be loss or damage to myelin at multiple sites along nerve fibers (multifocal demyelination). This results in slowed conduction documented by some combination of prolonged distal latency, slowed segmental conduction velocity, prolonged F-wave latency, and abnormal temporal dispersion. Focal conduction block of some nerve fibers may be present if a sufficient number of consecutive myelin segments are damaged, or if there is functional block at nodes of Ranvier (see below). The distribution of myelin damage can vary along the nerve, with greater degrees at very distal or proximal sites. Further, the numbers of fibers affected will vary among nerves and during the clinical course of the neuropathy. If a primary demyelinating neuropathy is suspected, testing nerve conduction over longer nerve lengths is helpful to optimize inclusion of more involved segments (the ulnar nerve is suitable with lengths from the axilla to the wrist).

Neuropathies can include both primary demyelinating and secondary axonal pathology. Since sensory nerve involvement results in low or absent SNAP amplitudes, most nerve conduction studies to assess for primary demyelination rely on testing of motor nerves. An important factor to consider is that axonal loss usually includes some of the largest and fastest-conducting fibers, and the remaining nerve fibers will conduct at slower (but normal) velocities. Thus, the first issue in assessing whether there is primary

Table 4.3 Electrodiagnostic "Guidelines" for Primary Demyelination of Motor Nerves (Greater Slowing than Expected for the Degree of Axonal Loss)

CMAP distal latency:

>125% of ULN

CMAP conduction velocity:

<75% of LLN

F-wave latency:

>125% of ULN

CMAP negative peak duration (measured as return of baseline of last negative peak):

median nerve >6.6 msec

ulnar nerve >6.7 msec

peroneal nerve >7.6 msec

tibial nerve >8.8 msec

CMAP proximal–distal negative peak duration:

>30%

Notes: Based on findings from patients with amyotrophic lateral sclerosis, with the addition of negative peak duration. Guidelines applied to motor nerves (CMAP); lower limit of normal (LLN); upper limit of normal (ULN). Modified from Cornblath et al. (1992) and Isose et al. (2009).

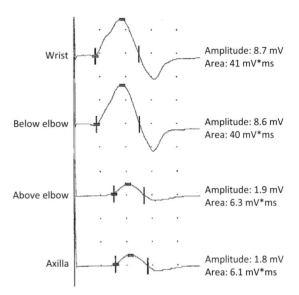

Wrist — Amplitude: 8.7 mV / Area: 41 mV*ms

Below elbow — Amplitude: 8.6 mV / Area: 40 mV*ms

Above elbow — Amplitude: 1.9 mV / Area: 6.3 mV*ms

Axilla — Amplitude: 1.8 mV / Area: 6.1 mV*ms

Figure 4.3 Conduction block showing reduction of the CMAP waveforms at focal site in the forearm (between below and above the elbow).

demyelination is to factor in effects of axonal loss on conduction velocity metrics. One approach to determining the limits of the effect of axonal loss is to study a neuropathy with only axonal loss. Data from patients with amyotrophic lateral sclerosis show that axonal loss slows conduction to limited degrees: distal latency <125% ULN, segmental conduction velocity <75% LLN, and F-wave distal latency <125% ULN (Cornblath et al., 1992).

To show evidence for primary demyelination, nerve conduction metrics must be slower than can be attributed to axonal loss, and such abnormalities must be documented in more than one nerve to ensure that the findings are distributed and not isolated. A number of criteria are available for the diagnosis of acute and chronic demyelinating neuropathies in the form of tables listing limiting nerve conduction values that need to be met (Alam et al., 1998; Bromberg, 2011). Diagnostic sensitivity of the various criteria, as tested on patients with clinical diagnoses of demyelinating neuropathies, ranges from ~40% to ~90%. This range emphasizes that the degree and distribution of demyelination varies among patients, and nerve conduction values must be combined with clinical feature when making a diagnosis of primary demyelinating neuropathies. A set of conduction values have been offered as a "guideline" for when

to consider primary demyelination (Table 4.3), at which time fulfillment of formal criteria can be considered (Bromberg, 2011). Formal criteria for primary demyelination for acute and chronic immune neuropathies are given in Chapters 19 and 24, respectively.

It is recognized that some primary axonal neuropathies, such as diabetic neuropathies, include a degree of slowing, but a distinction should be made between mild slowing and that supporting primary demyelination.

Primary Focal Conduction Block

With focal conduction block, nerve conduction is normal over segments proximal to and distal to the block. Focal conduction block can be demonstrated by showing that CMAP area or amplitude to stimulation proximal to the block is reduced relative to the CMAP from stimulation distal to the block (Figure 4.3). Impulse blocking can be due to functional changes (antibodies affecting ion channels at the node of Ranvier) or structural (loss or damage to several contiguous myelin segments at a focal area). It is not known how many fibers need to be blocked in order to document block with nerve conduction studies.

Primary focal conduction block pathology is the most challenging to confirm as adherence to technical issues is essential (see below) and elements of primary demyelination frequently coexist and must be

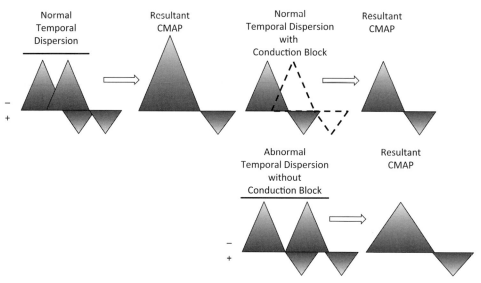

Figure 4.4 Model of true conduction block (top series) and apparent conduction block (bottom series) due to the effects of abnormal temporal dispersion. Upright and inverted triangles represent negative and positive components of the fastest and slowest single motor unit action potentials. The effects of phase cancellation leading to apparent conduction block are accentuated with greater temporal between the fastest- and slowest-conducting fibers.

taken into consideration to ensure that there is true conduction block (Bromberg and Franssen, 2015). When there is demyelination of some fibers at a focal site, there may be apparent conduction block due to slowing of conduction across the segment that results in a greater degree of temporal dispersion and phase cancellation that reduces CMAP area or amplitude to proximal stimulation (Figure 4.4).

The uncertainty of knowing how many fibers are truly blocked and how many are only slowed (apparent conduction block) has led to the classification of conduction block as Definite Block and Probable Block (Table 4.4) (Olney and Hanson, 1988; Olney et al., 2003). The degrees of certainty represent balances between the percentage reduction in CMAP area or amplitude and the increase in negative peak duration (degree of abnormal temporal dispersion) between stimulation proximal and distal to the proposed focal site. CMAP negative peak area is more sensitive than amplitude, and is the preferred metric when considering conduction block. There are two useful numbers to keep in mind: If the distal CMAP amplitude is <1 mV, it is not possible to accurately define conduction block as normal temporal dispersion of the few remaining fibers can reduce proximal CMAP size. If the distal CMAP amplitude is >1 mv and there is a 50% drop in CMAP size to proximal stimulation there is definite block (Bromberg and Franssen, 2015).

The tibial nerve cannot be used for evidence of focal conduction block between knee and ankle because in normal individuals there is a marked drop (~66%) in CMAP size stimulating at the popliteal fossa compared to stimulating at the ankle. This is attributed to volume conduction from different muscles activated at the different stimulation sites, and it is difficult to distinguish normal from pathologic changes in CMAP size (Barkhaus et al., 2011).

In the setting of an acute focal primary axonal lesion, nerve conduction studies within the first two days after the lesion may have features of conduction block (reduced CMAP size to proximal stimulation and normal to distal stimulation) because it requires several days for the distal axons to lose their ability to conduct (Chaudhry and Cornblath, 1992). In these circumstances, repeating or performing nerve conduction studies four to five days after the lesion will be more informative.

Focal conduction block occurs most commonly at sites of entrapment: the median nerve at the wrist, the ulnar nerve at the elbow, and the fibular/peroneal nerve at the fibular head. If conduction block is suspected after stimulation at a proximal site, it is strengthened by showing that the CMAP area or amplitude remains low when stimulating at a second, more proximal site (Figure 4.3). However, if the amplitude is higher at the second site, then

Table 4.4 Criteria for Focal Motor Nerve Conduction Block (CB). CMAP Responses from Proximal Stimulation Compared to Distal Stimulation

	CMAP Area	CMAP Amplitude	CMAP Negative Peak Duration
Definite CB	Reduced by >40%	Reduced by >50%	Increased by <30%
Probable CB	Reduced by >30%	Reduced by >40%	Increased by <30%
Possible CB	Reduced by >40%	Reduced by >50%	Increased by 31–60%

Note: Applies to median and ulnar nerves for stimulation distally at the wrist compared to proximally up to axilla.

Source: Modified from Olney et al. (2003).

Median SNAP

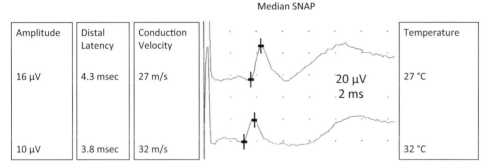

Amplitude	Distal Latency	Conduction Velocity		Temperature
16 µV	4.3 msec	27 m/s	20 µV .2 ms	27 °C
10 µV	3.8 msec	32 m/s		32 °C

Figure 4.5 Effects of low temperature on SNAP metrics.

stimulation at the first proximal site was likely submaximal.

In the setting of polyneuropathies, conduction block occurs mostly in immune neuropathies, and it is important to distinguish block at sites away from entrapment sites. Potential very proximal sites of block are most challenging as nerves lie deep in proximal limb segments, and adequate electrical stimulation is problematic. Given the challenges in accurately documenting conduction block away from entrapment sites, it is conservative to test the involved nerve twice to be sure, as, not infrequently, block is not reproducible on the second test, and thus initially reflected a technical issue. Further, a number of acute immune neuropathies may have reversible conduction block, and it may not be apparent that there was block until it is shown to have resolved on a second study (see Chapter 18) (Kuwabara et al., 1998).

Nerve Conduction Pitfalls and Cautions in Interpretation

There are technical issues that must be considered when performing nerve conduction studies, especially in the diagnosis of primary demyelinating and focal conduction block neuropathies.

Temperature

Nerve temperature has a linear effect on nerve conduction velocities, and cool limb temperatures prolong distal latency and slow conduction velocity, and also increase SNAP amplitude due to prolongation of nerve fiber action potentials and subsequent reduced degree of phase cancellation (Figure 4.5) (Wilbourn, 1994; Falck and Stalberg, 1995). Temperature correction factors are available, but are not recommended as a substitute for adequate warming of a limb to >30°C. Once warmed, a limb will cool down rapidly, and since cool temperatures have a greater effect on sensory nerve studies, it is recommended that sensory studies be conducted before motor nerve studies. Cool temperatures can also obscure conduction block, which may not be apparent at limb temperatures <37°C (Franssen et al., 1999).

Recording Electrode Position

CMAP amplitude may not be maximal when the active recording electrode position is placed by relying on anatomic landmarks, as there can be marked differences in CMAP amplitude among waveforms recorded at different sites over the muscle, even when all waveforms have initial negative onsets (Figure 4.6). Finding the maximal CMAP requires empirically

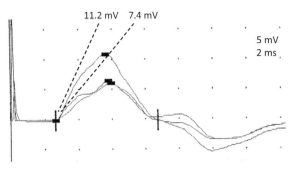

Figure 4.6 Effects of changes in position of active recording electrode on CMAP amplitude. Electrode moved short distances (several millimeters). Note steeper slope of the initial negative deflections associated with higher amplitudes.

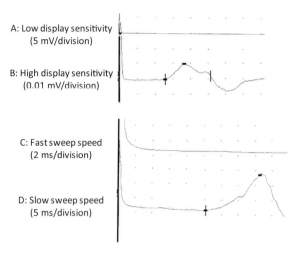

Figure 4.7 Possibility of missing low amplitude or prolonged CMAP responses. A and B: low amplitude CMAP missed with default nerve conduction settings of 5 mV/division amplitude. C and D: slowly conducted CMAP missed with default nerve conducting settings of 2 ms/division duration.

moving the active recording electrode over the muscle in small increments (Bromberg and Spiegelberg, 1997). Finding the electrode site that yields the maximal amplitude is essential when nerve conduction studies may need to be repeated during the course of a neuropathy to avoid misinterpreting subsequent CMAP values that are higher or lower than the first values.

Measurement Errors

Distal latency and conduction velocity values rely upon accurate measurement of nerve length. Three types of errors are encountered; measuring distances carelessly (which can be minimized by attention to detail) (Landau et al., 2002), measuring over rounded body contours (which cannot be adjusted for) (Landau et al., 2005), and measuring over flexed joints (which should be performed in a consistent manner) (Landau et al., 2002).

Under- and Over-Stimulation

Under-stimulation can be an issue when the stimulating electrode is not over the nerve: an optimal stimulating electrode position can be determined by applying a submaximal current and moving the electrode medially and laterally over the nerve to achieve the highest response, and then increasing the intensity at that site to achieve a maximal response (Bromberg and Franssen, 2015). Understimulation is a major factor when assessing for conduction block at proximal stimulation sites when nerves lie deep. Maximal stimulator output (100 mA or 300 V) and stimulation duration (up to 1.0 ms) may not be sufficient.

Overstimulation of the median nerve at the wrist in patients with thin distal body habitus or at the axilla can activate the ulnar nerve and artificially contribute to the median CMAP, recognized by an alteration of the waveform by the added components. Excessive stimulating currents (>120% of that which achieves a maximal CMAP) can activate the nerve at more distant nodes of Ranvier, resulting in shorter distal latency or faster conduction velocity, or a jump over (or reduction) at a site of focal conduction block.

Very Slow or Low CMAP Potentials

Missing a very low motor response associated with marked axonal loss can occur when the screen display sensitivity is at the common default setting of 5 mV/div. Before a motor response is listed as absent, assessment at 0.1 mV/div may reveal a response (Figure 4.7). Missing a very prolonged motor distal latency or slowed response associated with a primary demyelinating neuropathy can occur when the display sweep speed is short (2 ms/div). If such a neuropathy is suspected, assessment at 5 ms/div can reveal a late response (Figure 4.7).

Low SNAPs

The intrinsic noise level in sensory nerve conduction studies is ~2–3 microV, and low-amplitude SNAPs can be artificially increased or decreases depending upon their juxtaposition on background signal noise. With SNAP amplitudes <5 μV, it is appropriate to average four or more responses to achieve a more accurate amplitude.

Mismarked SNAP and CMAP Waveforms

EMG machines use built-in algorithms for determining waveform latency and amplitude, and metrics are automatically transferred to data tables. While the markers are generally placed accurately, errors occur and appear as incorrect data in the tables. It is important to verify marker placement in the waveforms before closing a study.

Needle EMG

EMG is more sensitive in detecting mild axonal loss than is CMAP amplitude due to collateral reinnervation preserving CMAP amplitude. Denervation is detected with needle EMG by the presence of fibrillation potentials and positive sharp waves; however, the degree of axonal loss can be gauged only qualitatively as mild, moderate, or severe based on the degree of reduced motor unit recruitment and amplitude. EMG may not be able to determine the site of a denervating lesion, but for focal neuropathies it may be possible to assess for unaffected muscles proximal to a lesion site, and for proximal processes (plexopathies and radiculopathies) it may be possible to localize lesion(s) by assessing muscles innervated by unaffected nerves or roots.

Electrodiagnostic Report and Interpretation

The electrodiagnostic report is unique among laboratory tests because it represents the results of a consultation by a physician who has taken a history, performed a neurologic examination, conducted a set of electrodiagnostic tests, and then combined all elements to form an interpretation. Guidelines have been formulated for what should be in a report: history and examination sections, tables of nerve conduction and needle data, summary of issues and findings not included in the tables, and a two-part conclusion of electrodiagnostic findings and an overall clinical interpretation (Jablecki et al., 2005). The history should include items that will be used to support the clinical interpretation. The summary should include key electrodiagnostic features that will be used in the interpretation, and also technical issues that influence the data and unique features of the data such as

waveform characteristics. The electrodiagnostic interpretation should summarize the findings that lead to conclusions about underlying pathology. The clinical interpretation combines all data into a clinical diagnosis. If uncertainty exists, suggestions for further testing can be included. This summary can include suggestions for further treatment or management, but be cautious about making firm recommendations that the referring physician may not want follow.

Is an Electrodiagnostic Evaluation Required for Every Polyneuropathy?

This is an important question for healthcare utilization in terms of time, costs, achieving a refined diagnosis, and management decisions. There are data supporting clarification of diagnosis in >40% of patients based on electrodiagnostic evaluation, and also data supporting only a 1% clarification, and the differences likely represent conclusions based on different sets of patients (Bodofsky et al., 2017). In the setting of a patient with known diabetes mellitus or with the metabolic syndrome who presents with typical symptoms of distal pain and numbness, an electrodiagnostic evaluation is not likely to add to the clinical diagnosis; however, for most patients an electrodiagnostic evaluation is worthwhile as it may change a diagnosis, provide evidence for severity, and help with management and prognosis (England et al., 2005)

References

Alam TA, Chaudhry V, Cornblath DR. Electrophysiological studies in the Guillain-Barre syndrome: distinguishing subtypes by published criteria. *Muscle Nerve.* 1998;21:1275–9.

Barkhaus PE, Kincaid JC, Nandedkar SD. Tibial motor nerve conduction studies: an investigation into the mechanism for amplitude drop of the proximal evoked response. *Muscle Nerve.* 2011;44:776–82.

Bodofsky EB, Carter GT, England JD. Is electrodiagnostic testing for polyneuropathy overutilized? *Muscle Neuropathy.* 2017;55:301–4.

Bromberg MB. Review of the evolution of electrodiagnostic criteria for chronic inflammatory demyelinating polyradicoloneuropathy. *Muscle Nerve.* 2011;43:780–94.

Bromberg MB, Franssen H. Practical rules for electrodiagnosis in suspected multifocal motor neuropathy. *J Clin Neuromuscul Dis.* 2015;16:141–52.

Bromberg MB, Spiegelberg T. The influence of active electrode placement on CMAP amplitude. *Electroencephalogr Clin Neurophysiol.* 1997;105:385–9.

Chaudhry V, Cornblath DR. Wallerian degeneration in human nerves: serial electrophysiological studies. *Muscle Nerve.* 1992;15:687–93.

Cornblath DR, Kuncl RW, Mellits ED, Quaskey SA, Clawson L, Pestronk A, et al. Nerve conduction studies in amyotrophic lateral sclerosis. *Muscle Nerve.* 1992;15:1111–15.

England JD, Gronseth GS, Franklin G, Miller RG, Asbury AK, Carter GT, et al. Distal symmetric polyneuropathy: a definition for clinical research, report of the AAN, AAEM and AAPM&R. *Neurology.* 2005;64:199–207.

Falck B, Stalberg E. Motor nerve conduction studies: measurement principles and interpretation of findings. *J Clin Neurophysiol.* 1995;12:254–79.

Franssen H, Wieneke GH, Wokke JH. The influence of temperature on conduction block. *Muscle Nerve.* 1999;22:166–73.

Herrmann DN, Griffin JW, Hauer P, Cornblath DR, McArthur JC. Epidermal nerve fiber density and sural nerve morphometry in peripheral neuropathies. *Neurology.* 1999;53:1634–40.

Isose S, Kuwabara S, Kokubun N, Sato Y, Mori M, Shibuya K, et al. Utility of the distal compound muscle action potential duration for diagnosis of demyelinating neuropathies. *J Peripher Nerv Syst.* 2009;14:151–8.

Jablecki CK, Busis NA, Brandstater MA, Krivickas LS, Miller RG, Robinton JE. Reporting the results of needle EMG and nerve conduction studies: an educational report. *Muscle Nerve.* 2005;32:682–5.

Kimura J, Machida M, Ishida T, Yamada T, Rodnitzky RL, Kudo Y, et al. Relation between size of compound sensory or muscle action potentials, and length of nerve segment. *Neurology.* 1986;36:647–52.

Kuwabara S, Yuki N, Koga M, Hattori T, Matsuura D, Miyake M, et al. IgG anti-GM1 antibody is associated with reversible conduction failure and axonal degeneration in Guillain-Barre syndrome. *Ann Neurol.* 1998;44:202–8.

Landau ME, Barner KC, Campbell WW. Effect of body mass index on ulnar nerve conduction velocity, ulnar neuropathy at the elbow, and carpal tunnel syndrome. *Muscle Nerve.* 2005;32:360–3.

Landau ME, Diaz MI, Barner KC, Campbell WW. Changes in nerve conduction velocity across the elbow due to experimental error. *Muscle Nerve.* 2002;26:838–40.

McComas A. Can cross-talk occur in human myelinated nerve fibers? *Muscle Nerve.* 2016;54:361–5.

Nobrega JA, Manzano GM, Novo NF, Monteagudo PT. Sample size and the study of F waves. *Muscle Nerve.* 1999;22:1275–8.

Olney RK, Hanson M. AAEE case report #15: ulnar neuropathy at or distal to the wrist. *Muscle Nerve.* 1988;11:828–32.

Olney RK, Lewis RA, Putnam TD, Campellone JV, Jr. Consensus criteria for the diagnosis of multifocal motor neuropathy. *Muscle Nerve.* 2003;27:117–21.

Perkins B, Bril V. Electrophysiologic testing in diabetic neuropathy. *Handb Clin Neurol.* 2014;126:235–48.

Wilbourn AJ. Sensory nerve conduction studies. *J Clin Neurophysiol.* 1994;11:584–601.

Diagnostic Testing

Chapter 5

Introduction

Laboratory tests for the evaluation of neuropathies can be divided into two groups; one to assess underlying pathology, and the other to assess underlying causes (Table 5.1). For the first group, electrodiagnostic studies (nerve conduction studies and needle EMG) are the most important as they are readily available and can provide information on axon and myelin integrity. Autonomic nerve tests can assess for cardiovascular involvement, but are not readily available outside of large medical centers. Ultrasound and MRI are noninvasive imaging tests that assess nerve structure. There are also invasive studies such as skin and nerve biopsies that directly provide information about pathology. In the second group, laboratory tests can identify comorbid disorders associated with peripheral neuropathies, and include more specific tests on serum and cerebrospinal fluid for biomarkers of neuropathies.

Electrodiagnostic Studies

General principles of nerve conduction and EMG and how pathologic changes are detected are reviewed in Chapter 4, and specific changes are discussed in chapters on individual neuropathies.

Autonomic Tests

Nerve fibers in the autonomic system are greater in number than those in the somatic system, and many neuropathies involve both systems, but symptoms from somatic nerve dysfunction usually surpass those from autonomic nerve dysfunction. Except for rare disorders where symptoms of dysautonomia are the main peripheral nerve symptoms, autonomic testing is not commonly helpful in the evaluation of neuropathies.

The autonomic nervous system is not assessable to direct testing, and tests measure end-organ responses to physiological and pharmacological perturbations

Table 5.1 Laboratory Tests to Aid in Establishing Causes of Polyneuropathies

Assessment of Underlying Pathology	Assessment of Underlying Causes
Noninvasive	Basic screening tests
• Electrophysiologic nerve conduction/EMG studies	• serum vitamin B12/ methylmalonic acid
• Imaging MRI nerve/muscle ultrasound nerve/ muscle	• two-hour glucose tolerance
Invasive	Tests based on clinical/ electrodiagnostic findings
• nerve biopsy	• cerebral spinal fluid for protein/cells
• skin biopsy	• serum/urine immunoelectrophoresis
	• serum antibody tests
	• genetic tests

Table 5.2 Autonomic Nerve Testing

Cardiovagal Function
　　Heart rate variability to deep breathing
　　Heart rate response to valsalva maneuver
　　Heart rate response to postural change
Sympathetic Adrenal Function
　　Blood pressure response to postural change
　　Blood pressure response to valsalva maneuver
　　Blood pressure response to isometric exercise
　　Cold pressor test
Pseudomotor Function
　　Axon reflex-mediated sweat test
　　Thermoregulatory sweat test
　　Electrodermal test

Source: Modified from Freeman and Chapleau (2013).

(Table 5.2) (Freeman and Chapleau, 2013). A battery of tests provides more information than single tests, and tests include changes in blood pressure and heart rate with upright posture (tilt table test), changes in blood pressure to valsalva maneuver, the quantitative sweat test (QSART), and total body sweat production to elevated temperature (thermoregulatory sweat test). Many of these tests require special equipment and are available at selected academic institutions. However, some tests of the autonomic nervous system can be performed on routine EMG machines, such as beat-to-beat heart rate variability with respiration and electrodermal changes due to insensible perspiration (sudomotor function), but these tests are not generally helpful in the evaluation of neuropathies.

Nerve and Muscle Imaging

Peripheral nerves and muscles can be imaged using high-resolution ultrasound and MR neurography, and both techniques provide a degree of spatial resolution of lesions within the peripheral nervous system that is not available from electrodiagnostic studies. For both techniques, there are continuing improvements in signal processing, and there are efforts at quantification of images. Clinical uses of imaging include assessing disorders affecting proximal nerves (roots and plexus), entrapment neuropathies (at proximal and distal sites, and at common and unexpected sites), and assessment of traumatic causes. Comparisons between ultrasound and MR techniques show that both are accurate for entrapment localization (Pham et al., 2014).

Ultrasound

Ultrasound studies can be performed rapidly and are noninvasive. Studies require specific ultrasound machines and an operator with training and experience. Peripheral nerves can be viewed in cross and longitudinal sections, including those as small as digital nerves (Yalcin et al., 2013), deep in the brachial plexus (Lapegue et al., 2014), and nerve roots (Zhu et al., 2014). Ultrasound images can be viewed as dynamic (real-time) or as still images. Metrics include quantitative nerve cross-sectional area measurements and nerve echogenicity (Hobson-Webb, 2013). With some machines, nerve vascularity (and pathologic change in vascularity) can be viewed by Doppler imaging.

Ultrasound imaging can be used in conjunction with electrodiagnostic studies in the same laboratory sitting, and can provide supporting evidence for nerve conduction findings or unique information. In many cases ultrasound can localize the site of a lesion along a nerve more easily than by nerve conduction studies. In one laboratory's experience, ultrasound was helpful in refining the diagnosis and treatment in a quarter of patients and was confirmatory in another quarter

(Padua et al., 2007). Ultrasound can detect enlarged nerves in the setting of acute and chronic immune neuropathies (Grimm et al., 2016a; Kerasnoudis et al., 2016) and hereditary neuropathies (Grimm et al., 2016b).

Magnetic Resonance Neurography

MR neurography is noninvasive, and MRI machines are readily available and interpretations are not operator-dependent, but studies are costly. Imaging sequences are evolving, and include T2-weighting and diffuse weighting (Pham et al., 2014; Eppenberger et al., 2014). MR neurography can visualize nerves at proximal and distal levels, and compared to ultrasound affords better three-dimensional visualization of surrounding structures (including neighboring muscles) and can better delineate nerves in proximal structures. Image contrast levels can be adjusted during viewing, and data can be reprocessed at later times.

Laboratory Testing

After the clinical diagnosis and electrodiagnostic characterization of a polyneuropathy comes the question of underlying cause. This endeavor is challenging, and can be divided into two tiers, screening tests (mostly blood studies) and specific tests based on the unique clinical and electrodiagnostic features (blood, spinal fluid, and biopsy studies) (Table 5.1). Among the spectrum of screening tests commonly ordered to determine cause, many are inappropriate, such as structural or bony imaging (MRI of brain and spine), and many have no objective data to support their specificity for cause (Callaghan et al., 2012). An analysis of testing practices by neurologists for length-dependent neuropathies indicates that most diagnostic information comes from the history and a limited number of informative diagnostic tests (Callaghan et al., 2014).

Screening Laboratory Tests

Commonly considered blood tests (complete blood count, erythrocyte sedimentation rate, random blood glucose, renal function, liver function, thyroid functions, folate levels) reflect an assessment of general metabolic status, and any abnormalities are rarely directly related to an underlying metabolic cause for a neuropathy. An evidence-based literature review of the utility of laboratory tests for length-dependent polyneuropathies found that tests of glucose, vitamin B12, and serum protein electrophoresis/immunofixation have the highest yield (England et al., 2009b).

Diabetes and Metabolic Syndrome

The metabolic syndrome is a cluster of five elements; obesity, insulin resistance, hypertension, hypertriglyceridemia, and dyslipidemia, and for the last four elements, independent of whether they are treated (Alberti et al., 2009). Prevalence of the metabolic syndrome rises with age, up to 15% of the population >40 years of age. Prediabetes and diabetes are the two elements most strongly associated with peripheral neuropathy, but the other elements of the syndrome are frequently overlooked because they are being treated (Callaghan and Feldman, 2013). Given the high prevalence of diabetes, there is high-level evidence for performing a two-hour glucose tolerance test when other tests of diabetes (hemoglobin A1c, fasting glucose) are normal in the setting of painful sensory length-dependent neuropathies. (Singleton et al., 2001; Smith, 2012).

B12 and Metabolites

The role of cyanocobalmin (vitamin B12) deficiency as a cause of peripheral neuropathy in the absence of myelopathic features (subacute combined degeneration) is controversial, including what serum B12 levels are critical. There is the possibility of subclinical B12 deficiency contributing to a peripheral neuropathy when B12 levels are in the low normal range (<~350 ng/L) (Kumar, 2010). Cases of peripheral neuropathy attributed to B12 deficiency are rare and from small patient series. The utility of testing levels of metabolites (methylmalonic acid and homocysteine) is not clear (Saperstein et al., 2003). Elevated methylmalonic acid is more specific for B12 deficiency than is elevated homocysteine (Kumar, 2010; Saperstein et al., 2003). However, low normal levels with normal metabolites are encountered in the elderly, as are neuropathies, and the association may not imply causation.

Immunoglobulin Testing

Monoclonal proteins of uncertain significance (MGUS) increase with age (~5–7% of the population >70 years of age), and may be encountered more commonly (5%) in patients with chronic polyneuropathies than in the general population (Kelly et al., 1981;

Kyle et al., 2006). Testing for a monoclonal protein is important in the setting of a chronic immune or inflammatory neuropathy (discussed in Chapters 24 and 25). The method of testing determines sensitivity, and when screening for MGUS, serum protein electrophoresis and serum free light chain testing have high sensitivity, with a small additional percentage detected with the addition of serum immunofixation (Katzmann et al., 2009). The presence of a monoclonal protein should lead to determination of whether it is of uncertain significance, by testing for quantitative immunoglobulin and by a skeletal x-ray survey for lytic lesions. Long-term surveillance is required as there is a 1% per year conversion of MGUS to a dyscrasia, which may or may not involve peripheral nerves (Kyle et al., 2006).

Special Laboratory Tests

For a limited number of neuropathies with unique features suspected by the clinical history and electrodiagnostic evaluation, special laboratory tests can provide support for underlying causes, and are discussed in chapters on individual neuropathies. However, as screening tests the following tests have low sensitivity and specificity, and are costly.

Thyroid Function Tests

Studies of thyroid dysfunction as a cause of polyneuropathy are not rigorous. Among patients with untreated thyroid disease, distal sensory complains have been reported in 29% who were found to be hypothyroid and in 14% found to be hyperthyroid, but clinical findings were minimal (reduced ankle reflexes) and nerve conduction studies were unremarkable for both groups (Duyff et al., 2000). Thyroid treatment had no significant effect on symptoms. The prevalence of abnormal thyroid function tests among patients with polyneuropathy is similar to that among healthy individuals in the general population (Gallagher et al., 2013).

Rheumatologic Tests

Rheumatologic tests frequently ordered to diagnose the cause of a neuropathy include erythrocyte sedimentation rate (ESR), C-reactive protein (CRP), antinuclear antibody (ANA), antineutrophil cytoplasmic antibodies (ANCA), anti-double-stranded DNA (dsDNA), rheumatoid factor (RF), anti-Ro (anti-SSA), and anti-La (anti-SSB) or extractable nuclear antigen antibodies. Data on the diagnostic yield of rheumatologic tests for a relationship to a neuropathy, and a confirmatory response to treatment, are sparse. Among patients with polyneuropathies, elevated ESR and CRP are encountered in approximately one-third, and are more commonly abnormal than ANA and ANCA (Gallagher et al., 2013). However, the frequency of abnormalities is similar to that among healthy individuals. In the clinical setting of a possible vasculitic neuropathy (mononeuritis multiplex), rheumatologic tests are reasonable, and reviewed in Chapter 23. Tests of anti-Ro and anti-La for Sjögren syndrome are appropriate in the setting of sensory small-fiber neuropathy and sicca syndrome (see Chapter 38)

Renal Failure and Creatinine Level

Peripheral neuropathy occurs only when renal function is markedly compromised, with glomerular function <12 ml/min and creatinine levels >4 mgms/ml (Krishnan and Kiernan, 2007). These values represent end stage renal disease.

Folate Deficiency

Given the metabolic interactions of folate with B12, a folate deficiency could cause a polyneuropathy in the setting of B12 deficiency, but for unclear reasons does not do so, except when there is a marked nutritional deficiency (Kumar, 2010; Koike et al., 2015). Furthermore, a deficiency rarely occurs as an isolated laboratory finding.

Vitamin B6 Excess

Pyridoxine (vitamin B6) hypervitaminosis can cause a sensory polyneuropathy, likely due to toxicity at the dorsal root ganglia (Schaumburg et al., 1983). The severity of the neuropathy is dose-dependent and can occur with excess vitamin supplementation, and is discussed further in Chapter 33.

Hepatic Function Tests

Polyneuropathy occurs in patients with chronic liver disease, but the literature is sparse (Chaudhry et al., 1999). Symptoms are of a length-dependent neuropathy of mild degree. Hepatic function test values of concern are not clear, but liver disease is usually sufficiently severe to warrant liver transplantation.

Spinal Fluid Analysis

Cerebral spinal fluid analysis for white cell count and elevated protein has a low diagnostic yield, except

when considering primary immune (demyelinating) neuropathies (discussed in Chapters 18 and 24].

Ganglioside Antibody Tests

Antibodies (mostly IgM) to epitopes in myelin and axons (glycoproteins and glycolipids) are associated with acute immune neuropathies and rare forms of chronic immune neuropathies. Commonly considered antibodies are to myelin-associated glycoprotein (anti-MAG), GM-1/GM-2, GD1a/GD1b, and sulfatide. In acute immune neuropathies, the role of anti-ganglioside antibodies has provided insight to underlying pathology (molecular mimicry), but given the acute time course and turn-about time for the laboratory result, the diagnostic utility of such testing is not clear, and is reviewed in Chapter 18. In the setting of a chronic immune neuropathies and the presence of an IgM monoclonal gammopathy, high titers of anti-MAG antibodies have the highest sensitivity for identifying a specific type of neuropathy (Nobile-Orazio et al., 2008). However, such antibodies may be present in individuals without neuropathy, although usually at low titers. In the setting of multifocal motor neuropathy with conduction block, elevated titers of GM1 ganglioside antibodies may be high, but are normal in about half of cases. The threshold for clinically significant titer levels is not always clear, and methods of testing (and titer levels) vary among laboratories (Nobile-Orazio and Giannotta, 2011).

Genetic Testing for Hereditary Neuropathies

Genetic tests for mutations can establish an unequivocal diagnosis when there is a high suspicion for a hereditary neuropathy. A genetic mutation can be considered when there is strong evidence for a very long-standing neuropathy, but a family history may be vague or lacking as *de novo* mutations are rare but do occur. Over 40 genes have thus far been found associated with familial neuropathies and clinical algorithms are available to guide efficient testing (see Chapter 42) (Saporta et al., 2011). The first step is to assess motor nerve conduction velocities in the arm to separate the neuropathy into type 1, with velocities <38 m/s, and type 2, with normal or near-normal velocities (Miller et al., 2011). An evidence-based literature review for the utility of gene testing showed good evidence for genetic testing when the clinical findings support the likelihood of a hereditary neuropathy, and the selection of gene tests should be guided by electrodiagnostic features (type 1 or 2) and the relative prevalence of specific gene mutations (England et al., 2009b). The role of genetic testing for length-dependent polyneuropathies without clinical suspicion for a hereditary neuropathy is of low yield (Murphy et al., 2012). Finally, methodologies for gene testing are evolving rapidly, and panels that test known genes are becoming reasonable in cost. When such testing is uninformative, whole gene sequencing is possible, but there are challenges when a mutation of unknown significance is found.

Nerve and Skin Biopsies

Underlying nerve pathology can only be obtained from direct microscopic inspection. Pathologic features of the whole nerve and surrounding tissue can be observed from nerve biopsies, commonly from the sural or superficial fibular/peroneal sensory nerves. Pathologic abnormalities of small-diameter sensory fibers can be observed in skin biopsies. Clinical conditions dictate which tissue to biopsy: nerve biopsies are helpful in diagnosing suspected vasculitis of peripheral nerves, and skin biopsies can be helpful in diagnosing sensory predominant and painful neuropathies (Sommer et al., 2010; King and Ginsberg, 2013).

Nerve Biopsy

Whole-nerve biopsies are usually performed when an underlying small vessel vasculitis is clinically suspected. It is common to include muscle in the biopsy procedure, as the additional tissue increases the yield of finding vessel pathology (Agadi et al., 2012).

A nerve biopsy is an invasive procedure, with removal of a nerve segment, leaving a permanent deficit. For this reason, most biopsies are of distal segments of sensory nerves because in length-dependent neuropathies there is frequently distal sensory loss, and further loss from the biopsy is less of an issue for the patient. However, distal nerves in the leg may be markedly involved, with few fibers remaining for analysis, and biopsy of involved arm nerves may be indicated. Under rare conditions, biopsy of a motor nerve (fascicular biopsy) may be considered.

Routine studies include paraffin, frozen and methacrylate preparations, and the use of a variety of histologic stains. Tissue is analyzed in cross and longitudinal sections. Special studies include electron microscopy, nerve fiber morphometry, and teased fiber preparations where individual fibers are separated and analyzed (technically difficult and performed at selected institutions).

Skin Biopsies

Intraepidermal nerve endings are viewed from 3-mm punch biopsies or from excised raised skin blisters produced by suction applied to the skin (Mellgren et al., 2013). Both procedures are easily performed and minimally invasive. Comparisons are made of intraepidermal fiber densities and nerve morphology from distal (ankle-level) and proximal (thigh-level) sites. Biopsy sites along the limb must match similar levels used to obtain normal data. Local laboratories can be established in departments of pathology, and commercial laboratories are available.

Intraepidermal nerve fiber density reflects both unmyelinated and small myelinated fibers as seen in the sural nerve biopsies (Herrmann et al., 1999; Mellgren et al., 2013). While both fiber types are viewed in nerve biopsies, the assessment of intraepidermal nerve fibers has greatest utility in small-fiber neuropathies, when sensory nerve studies are within normal limits (Herrmann et al., 1999). Figures of normal and abnormal intraepidermal nerve terminals are in Chapters 1 and 2.

Biopsies for Amyloid

When amyloidosis is suspected, the diagnosis is confirmed by demonstrating amyloid protein in tissue. Selection of tissue for biopsy is important, and while nerve (sural) appears reasonable, involvement may be patchy and missed (overall yield 0–83%) (Lam et al., 2015). Addition of muscle tissue can increase the yield. An alternative biopsy site with high yield and little morbidity is an aspirate of abdominal fat (van Gameren et al., 2006).

Utility of Autonomic Testing, Nerve, and Skin Biopsy

An evidence-based literature review for the utility of autonomic testing, nerve biopsy, and skin biopsy for the diagnosis of length-dependent polyneuropathies found varying levels of support: Autonomic testing can document autonomic involvement in autonomic neuropathies (fair scientific evidence) and small-fiber sensory neuropathies (fair scientific evidence, but less certain benefit). Nerve biopsy is useful for suspected amyloid neuropathy, mononeuropathy multiplex due to vasculitis or with atypical demyelinating neuropathies (accepted) but uncertain for evaluation of length dependent neuropathies (uncertain evidence). Skin biopsy can assess intraepidermal fiber density for small-fiber neuropathies (uncertain evidence) (England et al., 2009a).

Overall Diagnostic Test Yield

It is to be appreciated that despite extensive evaluations, >20% of patients with length-dependent polyneuropathies will have no demonstrable cause despite extensive laboratory testing (Dyck et al., 1981; Lubec et al., 1999), and that repeat testing over time is unlikely to yield a diagnosis (Notermans et al., 1994).

References

Agadi JB, Raghav G, Mahadevan A, Shankar SK. Usefulness of superficial peroneal nerve/peroneus brevis muscle biopsy in the diagnosis of vasculitic neuropathy. *J Clin Neurosci.* 2012;19:1392–6.

Alberti KG, Eckel RH, Grundy SM, Zimmet PZ, Cleeman JI, Donato KA, et al. Harmonizing the metabolic syndrome: a joint interim statement of the International Diabetes Federation Task Force on Epidemiology and Prevention; National Heart, Lung, and Blood Institute; American Heart Association; World Heart Federation; International Atherosclerosis Society; and International Association for the Study of Obesity. *Circulation.* 2009;120:1640–5.

Callaghan B, Feldman E. The metabolic syndrome and neuropathy: therapeutic challenges and opportunities. *Ann Neurol.* 2013;74:397–403.

Callaghan B, McCammon R, Kerber K, Xu X, Langa KM, Feldman E. Tests and expenditures in the initial evaluation of peripheral neuropathy. *Arch Intern Med.* 2012;172:127–32.

Callaghan BC, Kerber KA, Lisabeth LL, Morgenstern LB, Longoria R, Rodgers A, et al. Role of neurologists and diagnostic tests on the management of distal symmetric polyneuropathy. *JAMA Neurol.* 2014;71:1143–9.

Chaudhry V, Corse AM, O'Brian R, Cornblath DR, Klein AS, Thuluvath PJ. Autonomic and peripheral (sensorimotor) neuropathy in chronic liver disease: a clinical and electrophysiologic study. *Hepatology.* 1999;29:1698–703.

Duyff RF, Van den Bosch J, Laman DM, van Loon BJ, Linssen WH. Neuromuscular findings in thyroid dysfunction: a prospective clinical and electrodiagnostic study. *J Neurol Neurosurg Psychiatry.* 2000;68:750–5.

Dyck PJ, Oviatt KF, Lambert EH. Intensive evaluation of referred unclassified neuropathies yields improved diagnosis. *Ann Neurol.* 1981;10:222–6.

England JD, Gronseth GS, Franklin G, Carter GT, Kinsella LJ, Cohen JA, et al. Practice Parameter: evaluation of distal symmetric polyneuropathy: role of autonomic testing, nerve biopsy, and skin biopsy (an evidence-based review). Report of the American Academy of Neurology, American Association of Neuromuscular and Electrodiagnostic Medicine, and American Academy of Physical Medicine and Rehabilitation. *Neurology.* 2009a;72:177–84.

England JD, Gronseth GS, Franklin G, Carter GT, Kinsella LJ, Cohen JA, et al. Practice Parameter: evaluation of distal symmetric polyneuropathy: role of laboratory and genetic testing (an evidence-based review). Report of the American Academy of Neurology, American Association of Neuromuscular and Electrodiagnostic Medicine, and American Academy of Physical Medicine and Rehabilitation. *Neurology.* 2009b;72:185–92.

Eppenberger P, Andreisek G, Chhabra A. Magnetic resonance neurography: diffusion tensor imaging and future directions. *Neuroimaging Clin N Am.* 2014;24:245–56.

Freeman R, Chapleau MW. Testing the autonomic nervous system. *Handb Clin Neurol.* 2013;115:115–36.

Gallagher G, Rabquer A, Kerber K, Calabek B, Callaghan B. Value of thyroid and rheumatologic studies in the evaluation of peripheral neuropathy. *Neurol Clin Pract.* 2013;3:90–8.

Grimm A, Decard BF, Schramm A, Probstel AK, Rasenack M, Axer H, et al. Ultrasound and electrophysiologic findings in patients with Guillain-Barre syndrome at disease onset and over a period of six months. *Clin Neurophysiol.* 2016a;127:1657–63.

Grimm A, Vittore D, Schubert V, Lipski C, Heiling B, Decard BF, et al. Ultrasound pattern sum score, homogeneity score and regional nerve enlargement index for differentiation of demyelinating inflammatory and hereditary neuropathies. *Clin Neurophysiol.* 2016b;127:2618–24.

Herrmann DN, Griffin JW, Hauer P, Cornblath DR, McArthur JC. Epidermal nerve fiber density and sural nerve morphometry in peripheral neuropathies. *Neurology.* 1999;53:1634–40.

Hobson-Webb LD. Neuromuscular ultrasound in polyneuropathies and motor neuron disease. *Muscle Nerve.* 2013;47:790–804.

Katzmann JA, Kyle RA, Benson J, Larson DR, Snyder MR, Lust JA, et al. Screening panels for detection of monoclonal gammopathies. *Clin Chem.* 2009;55:1517–22.

Kelly JJ, Jr., Kyle RA, O'Brien PC, Dyck PJ. Prevalence of monoclonal protein in peripheral neuropathy. *Neurology*. 1981;31:1480–3.

Kerasnoudis A, Pitarokoili K, Haghikia A, Gold R, Yoon MS. Nerve ultrasound protocol in differentiating chronic immune-mediated neuropathies. *Muscle Nerve*. 2016;54:864–71.

King R, Ginsberg L. The nerve biopsy: indications, technical aspects, and contribution. *Handb Clin Neurol*. 2013;115:155–70.

Koike H, Takahashi M, Ohyama K, Hashimoto R, Kawagashira Y, Iijima M, et al. Clinicopathologic features of folate-deficiency neuropathy. *Neurology*. 2015;84:1026–33.

Krishnan AV, Kiernan MC. Uremic neuropathy: clinical features and new pathophysiological insights. *Muscle Nerve*. 2007;35:273–90.

Kumar N. Neurologic presentations of nutritional deficiencies. *Neurol Clin*. 2010;28:107–70.

Kyle RA, Therneau TM, Rajkumar SV, Larson DR, Plevak MF, Offord JR, et al. Prevalence of monoclonal gammopathy of undetermined significance. *N Engl J Med*. 2006;354:1362–9.

Lam L, Margeta M, Layzer R. Amyloid polyneuropathy caused by wild-type transthyretin. *Muscle Nerve*. 2015;52:146–9.

Lapegue F, Faruch-Bilfeld M, Demondion X, Apredoaei C, Bayol MA, Artico H, et al. Ultrasonography of the brachial plexus, normal appearance and practical applications. *Diagn Interv Imaging*. 2014;95:259–75.

Lubec D, Mullbacher W, Finsterer J, Mamoli B. Diagnostic work-up in peripheral neuropathy: an analysis of 171 cases. *Postgrad Med J*. 1999;75:723–7.

Mellgren SI, Nolano M, Sommer C. The cutaneous nerve biopsy: technical aspects, indications, and contribution. *Handb Clin Neurol*. 2013;115:171–88.

Miller LJ, Saporta AS, Sottile SL, Siskind CE, Feely SM, Shy ME. Strategy for genetic testing in Charcot-Marie-disease. *Acta Myol*. 2011;30:109–16.

Murphy SM, Laura M, Fawcett K, Pandraud A, Liu YT, Davidson GL, et al. Charcot-Marie-Tooth disease: frequency of genetic subtypes and guidelines for genetic testing. *J Neurol Neurosurg Psychiatry*. 2012;83:706–10.

Nobile-Orazio E, Gallia F, Terenghi F, Allaria S, Giannotta C, Carpo M. How useful are anti-neural IgM antibodies in the diagnosis of chronic immune-mediated neuropathies? *J Neurol Sci*. 2008;266:156–63.

Nobile-Orazio E, Giannotta C. Testing for anti-glycolipid IgM antibodies in chronic immune-mediated demyelinating neuropathies. *J Peripher Nerv Syst*. 2011;16(Suppl 1):18–23.

Notermans NC, Wokke JH, van der Graaf Y, Franssen H, van Dijk GW, Jennekens FG. Chronic idiopathic axonal polyneuropathy: a five year follow up. *J Neurol Neurosurg Psychiatry*. 1994;57:1525–7.

Padua L, Aprile I, Pazzaglia C, Frasca G, Caliandro P, Tonali P, et al. Contribution of ultrasound in a neurophysiological lab in diagnosing nerve impairment: A one-year systematic assessment. *Clin Neurophysiol*. 2007;118:1410–16.

Pham M, Baumer T, Bendszus M. Peripheral nerves and plexus: imaging by MR-neurography and high-resolution ultrasound. *Curr Opin Neurol*. 2014;27:370–9.

Saperstein DS, Wolfe GI, Gronseth GS, Nations SP, Herbelin LL, Bryan WW, et al. Challenges in the identification of cobalamin-deficiency polyneuropathy. *Arch Neurol*. 2003;60:1296–301.

Saporta AS, Sottile SL, Miller LJ, Feely SM, Siskind CE, Shy ME. Charcot-Marie-Tooth disease subtypes and genetic testing strategies. *Ann Neurol*. 2011;69:22–33.

Schaumburg H, Kaplan J, Windebank A, Vick N, Rasmus S, Pleasure D, et al. Sensory neuropathy from pyridoxine abuse. A new megavitamin syndrome. *N Engl J Med*. 1983;309:445–8.

Singleton JR, Smith AG, Bromberg MB. Increased prevalence of impaired glucose tolerance in patients with painful sensory neuropathy. *Diabetes Care*. 2001;24:1448–53.

Smith AG. Impaired glucose tolerance and metabolic syndrome in idiopathic neuropathy. *J Peripher Nerv Syst*. 2012;17(Suppl 2):15–21.

van Gameren II, Hazenberg BP, Bijzet J, van Rijswijk MH. Diagnostic accuracy of subcutaneous abdominal fat tissue aspiration for detecting systemic amyloidosis and its utility in clinical practice. *Arthritis Rheum*. 2006;54:2015–21.

Yalcin E, Akyuz M, Onder B. Early radial digital neuropathy of the thumb due to flexor pollicis longus tendinitis: value of ultrasound in an uncommon mild neuropathy. *Muscle Nerve*. 2013;47:772–5.

Zhu YS, Mu NN, Zheng MJ, Zhang YC, Feng H, Cong R, et al. High-resolution ultrasonography for the diagnosis of brachial plexus root lesions. *Ultrasound Med Biol*. 2014;40:1420–6.

Section 2

Proximal Neuropathies

Pathology of proximal elements, nerve roots, and plexuses, can be considered neuropathies, and are also frequently considered in the differential diagnosis of more distal nerve pathology. Bony spine pain (neck and back) and diffuse limb pain are common symptoms that lead to the consideration of proximal neuropathies. Pain syndromes are difficult to assess electrodiagnostically as they infrequently cause measureable sensory or motor nerve loss. The evaluation of spine pain commonly includes spine imaging, and with the high frequency of age-related bony changes, one role for electrodiagnostic testing is to lend support for proximal nerve damage, and ultimately for or against a surgically correctable cause.

Chapter 6

Radiculopathies

Introduction

Radiculopathy refers to symptoms and signs due to pressure on a nerve root as it exits through the spinal foramen narrowed by vertebral bone overgrowth and disk protrusions or as part of spinal canal stenosis. The term "sciatica" is applied to a variety of painful back and leg conditions, and evaluation most commonly discloses a lumbar radiculopathy (Ropper and Zafonte, 2015). Radiculopathies are not strictly considered to be a peripheral neuropathy, but the question of a radiculopathy can be erroneously considered in the evaluation of a peripheral neuropathy due to inaccurate localization leading to an inappropriately ordered MRI scan that shows likely age-related abnormalities in the spine, which further complicates making the appropriate diagnosis (Boden et al., 1990; Matsumoto et al., 2010). Nerve root involvement occurs in polyradiculoneuropathies, but does not account for the chief symptoms. Coexistent subclinical radiculopathies in the setting of symptomatic distal entrapment neuropathies have been considered as contributing to the "double-crush syndrome," but there is no objective evidence to support this entity. Bilateral lumbosacral root compression from central disk protrusion with leg weakness and bowel and bladder dysfunction raises concern for a cauda equina syndrome, which is a neurologic emergency.

Anatomy

Root anatomy follows an orderly regional numbering pattern (Figures 1.4 and 1.5). Of note, there are eight cervical roots and seven vertebrae, and thus root numbers C1–C7 lie above the corresponding numbered vertebra, while roots C8–S2 lie below the corresponding numbered vertebrae. A myotome is the group of muscles innervated by a single root, but a muscle commonly receives innervation from several roots, and root innervation of a muscle can vary among individuals. Tables 6.1 and 6.2 list cervical and lumbosacral innervation patters, respectively, while thoracic patterns have lesser localization importance. A dermatome is the area of skin innervated by a single root, but dermatomes territories overlap to a degree, and areas of skin supplied by a root can vary among individuals, and dermatomal maps are not exact.

Pathology

Root compression results from protruding disks, hypertrophic bone growth, and spinal ligament hypertrophy that narrows spinal foramina at lumbosacral levels. The degree of resultant nerve pathology varies from mild and reversible to axonal and severe. The frequency of symptomatic radiculopathies varies by root level (Table 6.3) (Wilbourn and Aminoff, 1998). Sensory nerve damage causes radicular pain and is the most common symptom, but motor root damage is more important in the diagnosis as it causes muscle denervation detected by needle EMG.

Peripheral neuropathies commonly have a length-dependent pathology, and may also include involvement of posterior myotomes (polyradiculoneuropathy), but the mechanism is less clear why short nerve segments are affected in length-dependent neuropathies. Immune-mediated polyneuropathies involve pathology along both long and short nerve segments and roots, and a polyradiculoneuropathy pattern is common. Thoracic roots can be affected in the setting of diabetes and with reactivation of herpes zoster (shingles) (Stewart, 1989).

Clinical Features

Radiating pain from the neck or lower back down the limb is a common symptom, but weakness is less common. Most radiculopathies are asymmetric, but lumbosacral spinal stenosis and the cauda equina

43

Table 6.1 Muscle, Nerve, and Root Innervation, Cervical Region

Muscle – Nerve	Root Innervation
Proximal Nerves	
Romboid – dorsal scapular	C5
Supraspinatus – suprascapular	C5, C6
Infraspinatus – supascapular	C5, C6
Deltoid – axillary	C5, C6
Biceps brachii – musculocutaneous	C5, C6
Brachialis – musculocutaneous	C5, C6
Radial Nerve	
Triceps	C6, C7
Anconeus	C6, C7
Brachioradialis	C5, C6
Extensor carpi radialis	C6, C7
Extensor pollicis brevis	C8
Extensor indicis proprius	C8
Median Nerve	
Pronator teres	C6, C7
Flexor carpi radialis	C6, C7
Flexor pollicis longus	C8, T1
Pronator quadratus	C8, T1
Abductor pollicis breavis	C8, T1
Ulnar Nerve	
Flexor carpi ulnaris	C7, C8
Flexor digitorum profundus (med)	C8, T1
Abductor digit minimi	C8, T1
Adductor pollicis	C8, T1
First dorsal interosseous	C8, T1

Underlined roots represent greatest root contribution to muscle.

Table 6.2 Muscle, Nerve, and Root Innervation, Lumbosacral Region

Muscle–Nerve	Root Innervation
Proximal Nerves	
Iliacus – lumbar plexus	L2, L3, L4
Adductor longus – obturator	L2, L3, L4
Tensor fascia lata – gluteal	L5
Gluteus medius – gluteal	L5
Gluteus maximal – gluteal	L5, S1
Femoral Nerve	
Vastus medialis/lateralis	L2, L3, L4
Rectus femoris	L2, L3, L4
Fibular/Peroneal Nerve	
Biceps – short head	L5, S1
Anterior tibialis	L4, L5
Extensor hallucis	L5, S1
Peroneal longus	L5, S1
Extensor digitorum brevis	L5, S1
Tibial Nerve	
Semitendinosis – sciatic	L5, S1
Semimembranosis – sciatic	L5, S1
Biceps femoris – long head – sciatic	L5, S1
Posterior tibial	L5, S1
Flexor digitorum longus	L5, S1
Gastrocnemius lateral head	S1
Gastrocnemius medial head	L5, S1, S2
Soleus	S1, S2
Abductor hallucis	S1, S2
Abductor digiti quniti pedis	S1, S2

Underlined roots represent greatest root contribution to muscle.

syndrome can cause bilateral symptoms. It may be difficult to elicit a clear history of radicular symptoms, and radiculopathies can exist without classic radicular pain. Sensory signs follow a dermatomal distribution, but dermatomal outlines may be vague due to the degree of root damage and overlap of unaffected roots contributing to a dermatome. Loss of the tendon reflex in the same root distribution is supportive, but reflexes may be symmetric. A chronic pattern is common, but acute radiculopathies occur, more often in the lumbosacral region. Thoracic radiculopathies with both motor and sensory involvement are frequently associated with diabetes (see Chapter 28), while sensory radiculopathies are associated with herpes infection (shingles).

Diagnostic Evaluation

Imaging Evaluation

MRI studies have to some extent replaced electrodiagnostic studies for the diagnosis of radiculopathies, but the high frequency of imaging abnormalities in adults that are not clinically significant supports a role for electrodiagnosis to confirm root impingement and not relying entirely on imaging.

Electrodiagnostic Evaluation

Distal nerve conduction studies are usually normal because sensory nerve damage is preganglionic and does not reduce SNAP amplitude, and motor

Table 6.3 Frequency of Cervical, Thoracic, and Lumbosacral Radiculopathies Based on Electrodiagnostic Findings

Level	Roots	Frequency	Overall
Cervical			~10–15%
	C5	~2%	
	C6	~20%	
	C7	~70%	
	C8	~8%	
Thoracic	T1 – T12		~2%
Lumbosacral			~70–80%
	L2 – L4	~10%	
	L5	~50%	
	S1	~40%	

Source: Modified from Wilbourn and Aminoff (1998).

nerve damage is mild and also does not reduced the CMAP amplitude. F-waves and H-waves may have prolonged latencies and are supportive, but it is questionable as to whether such abnormalities can stand alone to document a radiculopathy. Needle EMG is the most informative study and is considered positive and supportive when findings of denervation in the form of positive waves and fibrillation potentials are found in two or more muscles innervated by the same root, and preferably innervated by different nerves, and abnormalities are not detected in muscles innervated by uninvolved roots adjacent to the involved root (Wilbourn and Aminoff, 1998). Motor unit changes are usually mild and subjective interpretation leads to over-interpretation. EMG study of paraspinal muscles is less specific because they are innervated by posterior rami with overlapping root innervation. Among lumbosacral paraspinal muscles, the multifidus muscle layer is generally considered to have monosegmental innervation, but there is also evidence for multiple root innervation (Lalive et al., 2004). A needle mapping protocol using surface landmarks and distances has been developed to optimize exploration of the multifidus layer to aid localization, and while the premise of single-root innervation is not verified, mapping can narrow the root distribution (Haig, 1997). Thoracic radiculopathies are difficult to study with needle EMG, especially to document involvement of a single root because intercostal muscles are thin with concern for puncturing a lung, and respiratory motor unit activity obscures the signals. The rectus abdominis muscle has multiple root innervations and may be used as a substitute.

Root innervation patterns can differ among individuals, and published myotome charts vary in root and muscle assignments (Tables 6.1 and 6.2). Myotomes have been verified at time of surgery, which confirms clinical experience and highlights individual variations (Levin et al., 1996; Wilbourn and Aminoff, 1998; Levin, 2002).

Double-Crush Syndrome

The concept of the double-crush syndrome is based on an initial mild (commonly subclinical) proximal nerve compression (radiculopathy) that compromises axonal transport along the nerve, and impairs the nerve's ability to resist the effects of a second mild focal compression (entrapment) at a distal site, and thus lowers the threshold for a symptomatic distal mononeuropathy (Upton and McComas, 1973). While the presenting distal entrapment syndromes can be demonstrable electrodiagnostically, not all proximal lesions are diagnostically secure, and some are based on the presence of neck pain or on bony abnormalities observed in imaging studies. The syndrome initially was proposed for upper extremity roots and nerve entrapment disorders, but has been extended to lower extremity mononeuropathies. The concept has led to the recommendation to perform a needle EMG "root screen" as part of the evaluation for a distal entrapment mononeuropathy, searching for subclinical proximal denervation, with consideration for surgical intervention at the proximal site.

There are issues with the concept. The syndrome focuses on sensory nerves, and critical review of the proposed pathophysiology points out that a proximal lesion would not impede axoplasmic flow along a sensory nerve because the spinal root segment affected by any cervical compression would be at a preganglionic location. Further, the majority of distal focal mononeuropathies are caused by alterations of myelin (focal slowing or conduction block) and not by axonal pathology (Wilbourn and Gilliatt, 1997). Epidemiologically, neck (and lower back) pain and cervical (and lumbosacral) bony disease are common and increase with age; at the same time distal entrapment neuropathies (carpal tunnel syndrome) occur more frequently with age (Richardson et al., 1999; Lo et al., 2012), and a coincidence is more likely than causation. There are data showing EMG findings in proximal muscles in patients with carpal tunnel syndrome, but with no clinical or electrodiagnostic correlations between findings at the two sites (Kwon et al., 2006). Given the lack of clear a pathophysiologic linkage between the two lesions, routine needle EMG root screens do not appear clinically useful. The concept of double-crush has also been raised for thoracic outlet syndrome, and is discussed in Chapter 7.

Management

The prime question is whether symptoms and signs can be relieved by surgical decompression. The answer is dependent upon the sum of clinical, electrodiagnostic, and imaging features. Consultation with a thoughtful surgeon is appropriate, and a conservative therapeutic approach is reasonable when clinical and testing data are equivocal.

References

Boden SD, Davis DO, Dina TS, Patronas NJ, Wiesel SW. Abnormal magnetic-resonance scans of the lumbar spine in asymptomatic subjects. A prospective investigation. *J Bone Joint Surg Am*. 1990;72:403–8.

Haig AJ. Clinical experience with paraspinal mapping. II: A simplified technique that eliminates three-fourths of needle insertions. *Arch Phys Med Rehabil*. 1997;78:1185–90.

Kwon HK, Hwang M, Yoon DW. Frequency and severity of carpal tunnel syndrome according to level of cervical radiculopathy: double crush syndrome? *Clin Neurophysiol*. 2006;117:1256–9.

Lalive PH, Truffert A, Magistris MR. Lombosacral radiculopathy (L3-S1) and specificity of multifidus EMG. *Neurophysiol Clin*. 2004;34:41–7.

Levin KH. Electrodiagnostic approach to the patient with suspected radiculopathy. *Neurol Clin*. 2002;20:397–421, vi.

Levin KH, Maggiano HJ, Wilbourn AJ. Cervical radiculopathies: comparison of surgical and EMG localization of single-root lesions. *Neurology*. 1996;46:1022–5.

Lo SF, Chou LW, Meng NH, Chen FF, Juan TT, Ho WC, et al. Clinical characteristics and electrodiagnostic features in patients with carpal tunnel syndrome, double crush syndrome, and cervical radiculopathy. *Rheumatol Int*. 2012;32:1257–63.

Matsumoto M, Okada E, Ichihara D, Watanabe K, Chiba K, Toyama Y, et al. Age-related changes of thoracic and cervical intervertebral discs in asymptomatic subjects. *Spine (Phila Pa 1976)*. 2010;35:1359–64.

Richardson JK, Forman GM, Riley B. An electrophysiological exploration of the double crush hypothesis. *Muscle Nerve*. 1999;22:71–7.

Ropper AH, Zafonte RD. Sciatica. *N Engl J Med*. 2015;372:1240–8.

Stewart JD. Diabetic truncal neuropathy: topography of the sensory deficit. *Ann Neurol*. 1989;25:233–8.

Upton AR, McComas AJ. The double crush in nerve entrapment syndromes. *Lancet*. 1973;2:359–62.

Wilbourn AJ, Aminoff MJ. AAEM minimonograph 32: the electrodiagnostic examination in patients with radiculopathies. American Association of Electrodiagnostic Medicine. *Muscle Nerve*. 1998;21:1612–31.

Wilbourn AJ, Gilliatt RW. Double-crush syndrome: a critical analysis. *Neurology*. 1997;49:21–9.

Plexopathies

Introduction

Brachial and lumbosacral plexuses are a "plaiting" or interweaving of multiple strands of nerve fibers between nerve roots and named nerves. Consideration for a plexopathy arises when symptoms and signs cannot be localized to roots or individual nerves. Causes of plexopathies vary, and the complex interweaving of nerves makes challenging the identification of which segments in the plexus are involved (Table 7.1). Electrodiagnostic tests are useful to sort out involved components, and imaging modalities can be helpful.

Anatomy

The brachial plexus is formed from nerve roots C5–T1 (Table 7.2, Figure 1.4). Ventral portions of roots form three trunks: C5–C6 the upper trunk, C7 the middle trunk, and C8–T1 the lower trunk. Each trunk divides into anterior and posterior divisions: anterior divisions of the upper trunk form the lateral cord, anterior division of the lower trunk form the medial cord, and posterior divisions of the three trunks form the posterior cord. Named nerves emerge from cords: the lateral cord gives rise to the musculocutaneous nerve and then joins the medial cord to form the median nerve; the posterior cord gives rise to the axillary nerve, the upper and lower subscapular nerves, and the thoracodorsal nerve before it forms the radial nerve; the medial cord gives rise to the medial cutaneous nerves of the arm and forearm before forming the ulnar nerve and distally joining the lateral cord to contribute to the median nerve. Proximally, C5–C7 roots immediately give rise to the long thoracic nerve. The dorsal scapular and suprascapular nerves rise from proximal portions of the lateral cord. The medial and lateral pectoral nerves rise from the lateral and medial cords.

The lumbosacral plexus is formed from roots T12–S4 (Table 7.3, Figure 1.5). The lumbar portion derives from roots T12 (small contribution)–L4, and forms the plexus within the psoas major muscle. The femoral nerve is formed from anterior divisions of roots L2–L4, and the obturator nerve from posterior divisions of roots L2–L4. Other nerves given off include sensory nerves; lateral femoral cutaneous (L2–L3), iliohypogastric, ilioinguinal, and genitofemoral (collectively called inguinal nerves, from L1); and motor nerves to the psoas and iliacus muscles. The sacral portion derives from roots S1–S4. The anterior division with contributions from L4–L5 roots makes up the lateral portion of the sciatic nerve (fibular/peroneal nerve), and the posterior division with contributions from S1–S4 roots makes up the medial portion of the sciatic nerve (tibial nerve). The lumbosacral trunk joins the two plexuses with fibers from L4 and L5 roots.

Pathology

Blunt trauma from accidents (motorcycle and automobile) frequently includes injury to a plexus and surrounding nerve structures, while penetrating wounds and surgery are associated with more focal injury to the plexus (Table 7.1). Plexus nerve damage usually represents stretching injuries, with combinations of axon rupture and damage to the basal membrane, endoneurium, perineurium, and epineurium (van Alfen and Malessy, 2013). Severe stretching can also cause nerve root evulsion from the spinal cord. Nerve damage leads to Wallerian degeneration of distal axon segments. If basal lamina tubes remain intact, regenerating axons have the potential to reach target muscles, but the process is slow with anatomic barriers along the way, and reinnervation rarely restores lost function. Cancer invasion is mostly from breast or lung metastases, and Pancost tumors classically include a Horner syndrome. Radiation-induced plexus damage may occur in close proximity or decades after treatment, and is associated with microvascular changes and fibrosis in the nerve. Heavy

Table 7.1 Sites, Mechanisms, and Causes of Injury to Brachial and Lumbosacral Plexuses

Site	Anatomy	Pathology	Causes
Brachial Plexus			
Upper trunk	Normal	Focal pressure	Motor vehicle seat belts
			Burners/stingers
			Rucksack palsy
		Medical	Tumor
			Neuralgic amyotrophy
			Post-radiation
		Trauma	Motorcycle accidents
			Obstretical (Erb palsy)
Lower trunk		Focal pressure	Neurogenic thoracic outlet syndrome
		Trauma	Sternotomy
		Medical	Cancer (Pancost tumor)
			Obstretical (Klumpke palsy)
Pan plexus		Medical	Cancer
			Post-radiation
			Nerve tumor
		Trauma	Penetrating wounds
Lumbosacral Plexus			
Lumbar and sacral	Normal	Focal pressure	Hematoma
			Post-radiation
			Nerve tumors
			Malignant tumors
			Microvasculitic
		Trauma	Motor vehicles
			Surgical

backpacks (rucksacks) can exert downward pressure on the upper trunk. Stingers and burners from contact sports represent trauma to the upper trunk. Both of these causes have favorable outcomes.

Thoracic Outlet Syndrome

The term refers to a group of disorders that compromise nerves or vessels traversing the region between the clavicle and first rib, and frequently attributed to a cervical rib from C7 to T1, but also considered when there is no evidence for a fibrous band or other bony or muscle anomaly (Ferrante, 2012). The syndrome can be considered in four categories based on underlying pathology: neural, nonspecific, vascular, and a combination of vascular and neural. There is controversy over the boundary between neural and nonspecific forms, while vascular and trauma causes are exceedingly rare.

True neurologic thoracic outlet syndrome is very rare, and when the incidence of a cervical rib is considered (0.5–2% of the population), only 1 in 20,000–80,000 with such a rib anomaly experiences nerve compression in the thoracic outlet. Compression involves the T1 root more than the C8 root, leading to greater atrophy and weakness of thenar eminence muscles compared to hypothenar eminence muscles and the first dorsal interosseous muscle.

Nonspecific thoracic outlet syndrome is entertained when symptoms (mostly sensory in the hands and arms) are associated with little or no electrodiagnostic findings, and diagnosis frequently relies upon a spectrum of provocative maneuvers that have questionable pathophysiological bases. Vascular causes are due to compression of the subclavian artery or vein with nerve damage secondary to ischemia or thrombus.

Table 7.2 Innervation Pattern of Roots, Trunks, Cords, and Nerves for the Brachial Plexus

Upper Trunk		Middle Trunk		Lower Trunk	
Muscle – Nerve Roots	**Sensory Nerves**	**Muscle – Nerve Roots**	**Sensory Nerves**	**Muscle – Nerve Roots**	**Sensory Nerves**
Supraspinatus: C5, C6	Lateral antibrachial cutaneous: 100%	Pronator teres: C6, C7	Median (digit II, III): 75%	Abductor pollicis brevis: C8, T1	Ulnar (digit II): 100%
Infraspinatus: C5, C6	Median (digit I): 100%	Flexor carpi radialis: C6, C7		Flexor pollicis longus: C8, T1	Medial antibrachial cutaneous: 100%
Biceps brachii: C5, C6	Superficial radial : 60%	Triceps: C6, C7		Pronator quadratus: C8, T1	
Deltoid: C5, C6		Anconeus: C6, C7		Extensor indicis proprius: C6, C7, C8	
Teres minor: C5, C6		Extensor carpi radialis: C6, C7		Extensor pollicis brevis: C8	
Triceps: C6, C7		Extensor digitorum communis: C5, C6, C7		Extensor carpi ulnarus: C6, C7, C8	
Pronator teres: C6, C7				First dorsal interosseous: C8, T1	
Flexor carpi radalis: C6, C7				Abductor digiti minimi: C8, T1	
Brachioradialis: C5, C6				Adductor pollicis: C8, T1	
Extensor carpi radialis: C6, C7				Flexor digitorum profundus IV, V: C6, C7, C8	
Brachialis: C5, C6				Flexor carpi ulnaris: C7, C8	

Lateral Cord		Posterior Cord		Medial Cord	
Muscle – Nerve Roots	**Sensory Nerves**	**Muscle – Nerve Roots**	**Sensory Nerves**	**Muscle – Nerve Roots**	**Sensory Nerves**
Biceps brachii: C5, C6	Lateral antibrachial cutaneous: 100%	Latissimus dorsi	Superficial radial: 100%	Abductor pollicis brevis: C8, T1	Ulnar (digit V): 100%
Brachialis: C5, C6	Medial antibrachial cutaneous: 100%	Deltoid: C5, C6		Oppones pollicis: C5, C6, C7, C8	Medial antibrachial cutaneous: 100%
Pronator teres: C6, C7		Teres minor: C5, C6		Flexor pollicis longus: C8, T1	
Flexor carpi radialis: C6, C7		Triceps: C6, C7		First dorsal interosseous: C8, T1	
		Anconeus: C6, C7		Adductor pollicis: C8, T1	
		Brachioradialis: C5, C6		Abductor digit minimi: C8, Ti	

(continued)

Table 7.2 (continued)

Lateral Cord		Posterior Cord		Medial Cord	
Muscle – Nerve Roots	**Sensory Nerves**	**Muscle – Nerve Roots**	**Sensory Nerves**	**Muscle – Nerve Roots**	**Sensory Nerves**
		Extensor carpi radialis: C6, C7		Flexor carpi ulnaris: C6, C7, C8	
		Extensor digitorum communis: C5, C6, C7		Flexor digitorum profundus IV, V: C6, C7, C8	
		Extensor pollicis brevis: C7, C8			
		Extensor carpi radialis: C6, C7			
		Extensor indicis proprius: C6, C7, C8			

Underlined roots represent greatest root contribution to muscle.

Idiopathic Microvasculitis

A microvasculitis of nerve vessels may be common to a number of clinically disparate plexopathies, including cervical and lumbosacral plexopathies (associated with or without diabetes or impaired glucose tolerance, and with or without pain), those considered idiopathic or spontaneous (Parsonage-Turner syndrome or neuralgic amyotrophy), and hereditary forms (Dyck and Windebank, 2002; van Alfen, 2011; Massie et al., 2012). Pathologic findings may be axonal degeneration, multifocal fiber loss, injury neuromas, and hemosiderin deposition, and perivascular and vessel wall inflammation.

There is recent evidence in the clinical setting of typical Parsonage-Turner for hourglass-like constrictions of individual nerves demonstrated at time of surgery or by ultrasound that are not anatomically within the plexus (Pan et al., 2011). The pathological significance is not clear, but hypothesized to represent inflammation around the nerve, resulting in local edema, and vascular compromise (Lundborg, 2003). Similar findings are encountered in mononeuropathies (Sunagawa et al., 2017).

Nerve roots and peripheral nerves are also frequently involved together, leading to the terms "cervical or lumbosacral radiculoplexus neuropathies." They occur spontaneously, but a significant portion of patients describes recent vaccinations or surgery. Marked pain at onset is common, but damage to sensory nerves is much less apparent than to motor nerves.

Hereditary brachial plexopathy has similar clinical and pathologic features with non-hereditary (idiopathic) forms, but follows an autosomal dominant pattern with variable penetrance (van Alfen, 2011). Mutations or duplication of the septin-9 (SEPT9) gene on chromosome 17 have been detected in 50% of familial cases. Some families have dysmorphic features, including short stature, hypotelorism, epicanthic folds, and dysmorphic ears.

Clinical Evaluation

In the setting of trauma to the proximal arm or pelvis, neurologic symptoms are weakness and sensory loss that cannot be attributed to involvement of single nerves. Nerve root evulsion is associated by marked sensory loss in the root dermatome.

Idiopathic plexopathies present with sudden onset of pain in a focal region followed shortly thereafter (days to weeks) by weakness of muscles in the same region, but with little sensory loss compared to weakness. Most plexopathies are predominantly unilateral in distribution, but mild symptoms and needle EMG abnormalities can be found in contralateral muscles. Idiopathic brachial plexopathies frequently also involve distal individual nerves, particularly weakness in the distribution of the anterior interosseous nerve (England and Sumner, 1987). Diabetic plexopathies more commonly involve the lumbosacral compared to the cervical plexus, and those in the lumbosacral region are frequently associated with a length-dependent polyneuropathy. Clinical features of lumbosacral plexopathies can overlap with those of radiculopathies and sciatic nerve pathologies. Plexopathies related to cancer and radiation therapy usually have an insidious onset of weakness and sensory loss with or without pain, and the course is chronic (van

Table 7.3 Innervation Pattern of Roots, Trunks, Cords, and Nerves for the Lumbosacral Plexus

Femoral Nerve		Obturator Nerve	Femoral Nerve
Muscle – Roots	**Sensory Nerves**	**Muscle – Roots**	**Muscle – Roots**
Iliopsoas: L1, L2, L3, L4	Ilio-inguinal, -hypogastric, Genitofemoral: L1	Adductor magnus: L2, L3, L4	Biceps femoris: – short head: L5, S1, S2
Rectus femoris: L2, L3, L4	Lateral femoral cutaneous: L2, L3	Adductor longus: L2, L3, L4	Anterior tibial: L4, L5
Vastus lateralis: L 2, L3, L4	Saphanous: L2, L3, L4	Adductor brevis: L2, L3, L4	Fibular/peroneal longus: L4, L5
Vastus medialis: L2, L3, L4			Fibular/peroneal brevis: L5, S1
Vastus intermedius: L2, L3, L4			Fibular/peroneal tertius: L5, S1
Pectineus: L2, L3, L4			
Sartorius: L2, L3, L4			

Fibular/Peroneal Nerve	Tibial Nerve	Pudendal Nerve
Muscle – Roots	**Muscle – Roots**	
Extensor digitorum longus: L5, S1	Adductor magnus: L2, L3, L4	External urethreal sphincter: S2, S3, S4
Extensory hallucis longus: L5, S1	Biceps femoris – long head: L4, L5, S1	External anal sphincter: S2, S3, S4
Extensor digitorum brevis: L5, S1	Gastrocnimus – medial & lateral heads: S1, S2	
	Solius	
	Posterior tibial: L5, S1	**Gluteal Nerve**
	Flexor digitorum longus: L5, S1, S2	Gluteal medius: L4, L5, S1
	Flexor hallucis longus: L5, S1, S2	Gluteal minimus: L4. L5, S1
	Abductor hallucis: S1, S2	Gluteus maximus: L5, S1, S2
	Flexor digitorum breavis: S1, S2	
	Flexor hallucis brevis: S1, S2	
	Abductor digiti minimi: S1, S2	
	Flexor digiti minim: S1, S2i	
	Adductor hallucis: S1, S2	
	Interossei: S1, S2	

Underlined roots represent greatest root contribution to muscle.

Alfen and Malessy, 2013). Sacral plexopathies most commonly are cancer-related (Tavee et al., 2007). Recurrent plexopathies are rare, but are associated with hereditary or idiopathic causes, and those associated with diabetes.

Birth injuries most commonly involve the upper trunk, but may also involve the middle and lower trunks and root avulsions. While many are associated with difficult deliveries they also occur with uncomplicated births. Overall, plexopathies are characterized by symptoms of weakness greater than those of sensory loss.

Signs include muscle atrophy and weakness, which may be marked in degree, and weakness can extend beyond proximal muscles and involve nerves innervating distal muscles. Sensory perception abnormalities may be mild. Tendon reflexes are frequently absent in weak muscles.

Diagnostic Evaluation

Electrodiagnostic Evaluation

Electrodiagnostic studies can determine which elements of the plexus are involved, and the strategy to localizing to the plexus is documentation of nerve damage in two or more nerves or root distribution, and sparing paraspinal muscles (Tables 7.2 and 7.3). However, a plexopathy may include damage to nerve roots (radiculoplexopathy) (Laughlin and Dyck, 2013). Sensory nerve conduction studies are more sensitive to postganglionic sensory loss than motor nerve conduction studies. In the brachial plexus, sensory nerve conduction studies can support which elements of the plexus are involved based on their dermatomes, and side-to-side comparisons (as most plexopathies are unilateral) are useful if axonal loss is mild (Ferrante, 2004). In the lumbosacral plexus, fewer sensory nerves are available for study. The needle EMG study can document the distribution of denervation, and is particularly useful for studying proximal muscles (Ferrante, 2004).

Electrodiagnostic studies are used to diagnose true neurogenic thoracic outlet syndromes (neural or vascular) based on documenting highly characteristic findings. In sensory nerve conduction studies, there is loss of SNAP amplitude (absolute or relative to the uninvolved side) from the medial antibrachial cutaneous and ulnar sensory nerves. In motor nerve conduction studies, there is loss of CMAP amplitude from median > ulnar motor nerves, and on needle EMG study chronic denervation in T1 > C8-innervated muscles (Tsao et al., 2014).

In the setting of idiopathic plexopathies, denervation may be very regional within a muscle, supporting damage to distal (intramuscular) nerve segments (England and Sumner, 1987).

The challenge in the electrodiagnosis of lumbosacral plexopathies is distinguishing between lesions to the roots, plexus, and sciatic nerve (Tavee et al., 2007). While the absence of denervation in paraspinal muscles supports a plexopathy and presence of sensory responses supports a radiculopathy, clinical experience indicates that in the elderly and those with concurrent diabetes scattered denervation in paraspinal muscles is common and sensory responses may also be low or absent.

Imaging Evaluation

MRI imaging can be helpful to document diffuse distribution of signal changes in plexus and muscle (Massie et al., 2012). Findings include increased T2 signal in nerves, revealing greater extent of nerve involvement in the plexus and also nerve roots. Signal changes in muscle could distinguish subacute changes (edema) to chronic fatty atrophy.

Management

Management of traumatic brachial plexopathies is based on underlying cause and factors, and can involve nerve repairs or grafts and tendon transfers to enhance remaining function (Limthongthang et al., 2013). Idiopathic brachial plexopathies include pain and weakness, but an evidence-based literature review found no randomized trials to guide treatment, but retrospective series suggests that oral prednisone given early may shorten the duration of pain and lead to earlier recovery (van Alfen et al., 2009). With the finding of hourglass-like constrictions, the degree of recovery may depend upon the extent of constriction, not changed by surgical intervention (Pan et al., 2011).

Obstetrical brachial plexopathies include a range of severities of nerve injury (Romana and Rogier, 2013). Upper trunk plexopathies more often have complete recovery without treatment, and a 3–4 months period of observation is reasonable. Limb deformities may result from muscle imbalance and co-contractions leading to bone deformities. Surgical interventions are reasonable if there is no recovery or limited recovery after six months, and include nerve grafting and tendon transfers.

Management strategies for thoracic outlet syndrome are not clear due to controversies in the over diagnoses of neurogenic versus nonspecific types. Management of true neurogenic thoracic outlet syndromes is surgery to section the fibrous band. In the setting of vague symptoms and tests and lack of clear diagnostic findings, surgery has resulted in iatrogenic nerve damage, making it hard to interpret outcomes (Wilbourn, 1988). An evidence-based literature review found one randomized study comparing transaxillary first rib resection with subclavicular neuroplasty that favored the former due to less pain; a second study compared scalene muscle botulinum toxin versus saline injections and found no difference in pain relief but did find less paresthesias with botulinum (Povlsen et al., 2014),

Management of diabetic lumbosacral radiculoplexus neuropathies is unclear as there are no randomized trials available, but some degree of spontaneous improvement occurs (Chan et al., 2012).

Overall, the extent and rate of motor nerve recovery varies, based on the nature of axonal loss, distance between the lesion and target, and patient age. Root avulsions result in permanent sensory and motor loss. Neurotmesis is challenging to overcome because the basement lamina is disrupted and nerve outgrowth limited due to loss of neural tubular guidance and scar tissue. Lengths greater than 50 cm to the target muscle are not amenable to reinnervation and nerve grafting may be appropriate. Neurapraxia lesions can resolve rapidly or undergo remyelination over weeks. In the setting of idiopathic brachial plexopathy, there is usually improvement; with diabetic/non-diabetic cervical and lumbosacral plexopathies weakness may worsen, remain stable, or improve.

Sensory symptoms can be clinically significant issues, especially when pain is intractable to analgesics. Other modalities can be used, including transcutaneous nerve stimulation, nerve and ganglion blocks. With a flail limb that is damaged due to lack of sensory perception, amputation has been considered.

References

Chan YC, Lo YL, Chan ES. Immunotherapy for diabetic amyotrophy. *Cochrane Database Syst Rev.* 2012;6:CD006521.

Dyck PJ, Windebank AJ. Diabetic and nondiabetic lumbosacral radiculoplexus neuropathies: new insights into pathophysiology and treatment. *Muscle Nerve.* 2002;25:477–91.

England JD, Sumner AJ. Neuralgic amyotrophy: an increasingly diverse entity. *Muscle Nerve.* 1987;10:60–8.

Ferrante MA. Brachial plexopathies: classification, causes, and consequences. *Muscle Nerve.* 2004;30:547–68.

Ferrante MA. The thoracic outlet syndromes. *Muscle Nerve.* 2012;45:780–95.

Laughlin RS, Dyck PJ. Electrodiagnostic testing in lumbosacral plexopathies. *Phys Med Rehabil Clin N Am.* 2013;24:93–105.

Limthongthang R, Bachoura A, Songcharoen P, Osterman AL. Adult brachial plexus injury: evaluation and management. *Orthop Clin North Am.* 2013;44:591–603.

Lundborg G. Commentary: hourglass-like fascicular nerve compressions. *J Hand Surg Am.* 2003;28:212–14.

Massie R, Mauermann ML, Staff NP, Amrami KK, Mandrekar JN, Dyck PJ, et al. Diabetic cervical radiculoplexus neuropathy: a distinct syndrome expanding the spectrum of diabetic radiculoplexus neuropathies. *Brain.* 2012;135:3074–88.

Pan YW, Wang S, Tian G, Li C, Tian W, Tian M. Typical brachial neuritis (Parsonage-Turner syndrome) with hourglass-like constrictions in the affected nerves. *J Hand Surg Am.* 2011;36:1197–203.

Povlsen B, Hansson T, Povlsen SD. Treatment for thoracic outlet syndrome. *Cochrane Database Syst Rev.* 2014;11:CD007218.

Romana MC, Rogier A. Obstetrical brachial plexus palsy. *Handb Clin Neurol.* 2013;112:921–8.

Sunagawa T, Nakashima Y, Shinomiya R, Kurumadani H, Adachi N, Ochi M. Correlation between "hourglass-like fascicular constriction" and idiopathic anterior interosseous nerve palsy. *Muscle Nerve.* 2017;55:508–12.

Tavee J, Mays M, Wilbourn AJ. Pitfalls in the electrodiagnostic studies of sacral plexopathies. *Muscle Nerve.* 2007;35:725–9.

Tsao BE, Ferrante MA, Wilbourn AJ, Shields RW. Electrodiagnostic features of true neurogenic thoracic outlet syndrome. *Muscle Nerve.* 2014;49:724–7.

van Alfen N. Clinical and pathophysiological concepts of neuralgic amyotrophy. *Nat Rev Neurol.* 2011;7:315–22.

van Alfen N, Malessy MJ. Diagnosis of brachial and lumbosacral plexus lesions. *Handb Clin Neurol.* 2013;115:293–310.

van Alfen N, van Engelen BG, Hughes RA. Treatment for idiopathic and hereditary neuralgic amyotrophy (brachial neuritis). *Cochrane Database Syst Rev.* 2009:CD006976.

Wilbourn AJ. Thoracic outlet syndrome surgery causing severe brachial plexopathy. *Muscle Nerve.* 1988;11:66–74.

Mononeuropathies

Mononeuropathies are common, and while the anatomy of single nerves is simple as represented in diagrams, anatomic variations and other challenges can make it difficult to identify lesion sites. Underlying pathology is frequently inferred, as there are few situations where nerves are biopsied. Because of these difficulties, a number of disorders considered to be mononeuropathies are treated with surgical release procedures, and the literature on management is thusly focused. However, evidence-based literature reviews reveal few well-controlled trials to unequivocally support surgical release over conservative management. Further, given difficulties with accurate diagnosis and localization, many may not be true entrapment neuropathies, and may represent other medical issues (Campbell and Landau, 2008). Suspected (not true neurogenic) forms are the thoracic outlet syndrome (see Chapter 7), radial tunnel syndrome, ulnar nerve entrapment at the arcade of Struthers, piriformis syndrome, and tarsal tunnel syndrome (each considered in specific chapters). Other mononeuropathies, such as anterior interosseous neuropathy, may represent proximal ischemia of nerve fascicles (England and Sumner, 1987), and may also be associated with hourglass-like constrictions of nerve (Sunagawa et al., 2017).

Many true mononeuropathies represent focal lesions at sites of anatomical narrowing of supportive structures or sites of focal external pressure (entrapment sites). For most focal lesions, electrodiagnostic testing with nerve conduction studies are used to show nerve slowing or conduction block across the site, with normal conduction along distal and proximal nerve segments. Needle EMG can only document whether there is axonal loss, but cannot localize the site. For mononeuropathies that are located distally along a nerve, it is difficult to assess and show normal conduction in more distal segments. Thus, it is common to rely upon comparisons with parallel or contralateral uninvolved nerves or by differences from normal values. Imaging studies, ultrasound, and MR neurography are being used to aid in identification of the lesion site and suggest cause, and to add to the diagnosis and management of unusual mononeuropathies.

During the assessment of mononeuropathies, testing the asymptomatic side may reveal subclinical nerve involvement. This may raise the question of a hereditary neuropathy with predisposition to pressure (HNPP), and further testing of other nerves remote from the nerve in question may be informative (see Chapter 42).

References

Campbell WW, Landau ME. Controversial entrapment neuropathies. *Neurosurg Clin N Am*. 2008;19:597–608, vi–vii.

England JD, Sumner AJ. Neuralgic amyotrophy: an increasingly diverse entity. *Muscle Nerve*. 1987;10:60–8.

Sunagawa T, Nakashima Y, Shinomiya R, Kurumadani H, Adachi N, Ochi M. Correlation between "hourglass-like fascicular constriction" and idiopathic anterior interosseous nerve palsy. *Muscle Nerve*. 2017;55:508–12.

Median Nerve Neuropathies

Chapter

8

Introduction

The median nerve is the most common mono-neuropathy, with involvement most frequently at the wrist (carpal tunnel syndrome), while sites in the hand are infrequent, sites in the forearm controversial, and more proximal sites very rare (case reports). Nerve conduction studies, and recently ultrasound studies, are used to verify the lesion site, and ultrasound can provide information on underlying pathologic causes, especially if symptoms and electrodiagnostic findings are unusual. Much effort has been expended to nerve conduction testing protocols to improve sensitivity for detecting pathology at the wrist, but there is no "gold standard" test for carpal tunnel syndrome. Sites in the forearm (pronator teres and anterior interosseous syndromes) are less likely due to nerve entrapment and more likely due to fascicular infarctions from microvasculitis or other causes of constriction at more proximal sites along the nerve.

Anatomy

The median nerve is formed from sensory nerve fibers that enter the cord mostly over C5–C6 roots and travel in the upper trunks and lateral cord, with some contribution from the C7 root traveling in the middle trunk. Motor nerve fibers leave from roots C5–T1, but most from C8–T1 roots, and travel through the lower trunk and medial cord (Figure 8.1, Table 8.1). In the axilla and arm the median nerve lies close to the ulnar and radial nerves.

At the elbow, the nerve is medial to the biceps tendon. Its nerve passes between the superficial and deep heads of the pronator teres muscle, but there are variations in the relationships of the nerve to the pronator teres and flexor digitorum superficialis muscles. In the forearm, the anterior interosseous nerve branches after leaving the pronator teres muscle and innervates the radial portion of the flexor digitorum profundus muscle and the flexor pollicis longus and

pronator quadratus muscles. The palmar cutaneous branch leaves the median nerve above the wrist and innervates skin of the palm.

The median nerve continues through the carpal tunnel, and in the hand the recurrent motor branch innervates the abductor pollicis brevis, opponens pollicis, and a portion of the flexor pollicis brevis muscles, and other branches innervate the first and second lumbrical muscles. Sensory nerves innervate the medial portion of digit I, all of digits II and III, and the radial portion of digit IV, plus portions of the palm.

There are anomalous innervation patterns of motor nerves (Martin Gruber) and variations in branching patterns in the hand (Riche-Cannieu) (discussed in Chapter 1). Median sensory nerves innervate both sides of digit IV in about 4% of individuals, and the ulnar nerve innervates both sides in about 14% of individuals.

Pathology

Median mononeuropathies result from a variety of causes and different pathologies (Table 8.2). External pressure results in greater sensory than motor symptoms and signs, which usually represent neurapraxic pathology with good recovery. Direct trauma from humoral fractures, stab and gunshot wounds, and other forces can damage axons. The degree of damage is variable, and ultrasound may be helpful to assess the nature and distribution of damage (Padua et al., 2013). Pressure on the nerve in the carpal tunnel is usually transient and intermittent and affects myelin, but over time can cause axonal damage.

Microvasculitis involving median nerve fascicules at proximal sites, as postulated for the Parsonage-Turner syndrome, is the more likely cause of insidious weakness traditionally considered to be entrapment of the anterior interosseous nerve (anterior interosseous syndromes) (Pham et al., 2014). Patients frequently describe arm or forearm pain at the onset, similar to that with classic Parsonage-Turner syndrome. Further,

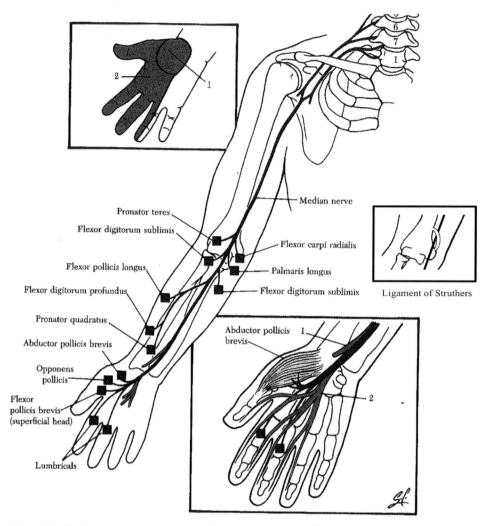

Figure 8.1 Median nerve anatomy. Inset top left: cutaneous innervation (1 = palmar cutaneous branch, 2 = main median cutaneous branches). Inset middle right: rare ligament of Struthers with entrapped nerve.
From S Oh, MD, with permission.

in the classic syndrome there is frequent involvement of median innervated muscles in the forearm, in addition to shoulder weakness (England and Sumner, 1987). Recent findings of hourglass-like constrictions in nerves in Parsonage-Turner syndrome and anterior interosseous syndrome suggest an inflammatory-vascular comprise pathology (Sunagawa et al., 2017).

Axilla

Clinical Features

Sensory loss and weakness attributed to the median nerve may be combined with that from the ulnar and radial nerves as they are in close proximity. When only the median nerve is involved, there is sensory loss in the palm and along digits I–III, and weakness of flexion of digits I and II.

Diagnostic Evaluation

Electrodiagnostic studies cannot localize the lesion site to the axilla, as stimulation proximal to the site of the lesion for nerve conduction cannot be performed reliably. Needle EMG studies can document the degree of denervation, and determine if more than the median nerve is involved. Imaging by x-ray, ultrasound or MRI can help define structural issues and causes.

Table 8.1 Predominant Root Innervation of Muscles Supplied by the Median Nerve

Muscle	Root Innervation
Pronator teres	C7
Flexor carpi radialis	C6 – C7
Flexor digitorum sublimis	C6 – C7
Palmaris longus	C7 – C8
Flexor pollicis longus (anterior interosseous nerve)	C7 – C8
Flexor digitorum sublimis/superficialis	C7 – C8 – T1
Flexor digitorum profundus (anterior interosseous nerve) (digits II – III)	C7- C8
Pronator quadratus (anterior interosseous nerve)	C7 – C8 – T1
Abductor pollicis brevis	C8 – T1
Opponnens pollicis	C8 – T1
Flexor pollicis brevis (superficial head)	C8 – T1
Lumbricals (digits II – III)	C8 – T1

Management

Pressure palsies from the abnormal use of crutches and from sleep positions resolve without intervention. Nerve damage from trauma is variable and can include axonal damage. Surgical consultation may be warranted.

Arm

Clinical Features

Sensory and motor loss is similar to that for injuries in the axilla, and the clinical circumstances help to differentiate between the two sites.

Diagnostic Evaluation

Needle EMG can define the distribution of nerve involvement. Imaging studies can help define underlying structural issues.

Management

Management is similar to that for injuries in the axilla.

Elbow

A supracondylar fibrous process or bony ligament (ligament of Struthers), from the distal humerus to the medial epicondyle (Figure 8.1) occurs in 2% of the population, but a median nerve entrapment at this site is exceedingly rare (case reports) (Suranyi, 1983).

Clinical Features

Sensory loss and weakness in the median nerve distribution can be accompanied by pain, and follows a chronic time course.

Diagnostic Evaluation

Motor nerve conduction studies can localize the lesion to above the elbow if there is an element of conduction block by stimulating above the block showing a reduction of the CMAP size compared to stimulating below the block. Needle EMG can verify axonal loss in the median nerve distribution, but not the specific site. Imaging studies can determine if there is a causative skeletal variation, but a fibrous band may not be apparent on imaging.

Management

Surgical confirmation and release is appropriate.

Forearm

Two median nerve syndromes are described in the forearm, the pronator teres syndrome and the anterior interosseous syndrome. There is controversy as to whether their frequent diagnoses represent true nerve entrapment syndromes or other causes such as tendonitis, compartment syndromes (Dalton et al., 2014), the consequences of hourglass-like constrictions, or microvasculis at more proximal nerve segments (England and Sumner, 1987; Sunagawa et al., 2017).

Table 8.2 Sites, Mechanisms, and Causes of Injury to the Median Nerve

Site	Anatomy	Pathology	Causes
Axilla	Normal	Focal pressure	Crutch
			Sleep position
			Compartment syndrome
		Trauma	Fracture
			Penetrating wound
			Hematoma
Arm	Normal	Focal pressure	Sleep palsy
			Tourniquet
			Compartment syndrome
		Trauma	Fracture
			Penetrating wounds
			Fistulas
			Vessel cannulation
Elbow	Normal	Trauma	Fracture
			Venipuncture
	Anatomic variant (ligament of Struthers)	Focal pressure	Supracondylar spur
Forearm	Normal	Trauma	Fracture
			Fistula
		Microvasculitis	Variant Parsonage-Turner
		Focal pressure	Pronator teres syndrome
			Anterior interosseous syndrome
Wrist	Normal	Focal pressure	Idiopathic
			Work-related
			Pregnancy
			Rheumatoid arthritis
			Diabetes mellitus
			Hereditary neuropathy/pressure palsies
Hand	Normal	Focal pressure	Work-related
	Anatomic variant (recurrent median nerve)	Focal pressure	Work-related

Pronator Teres Syndrome

The median nerve passes between two parts of the pronator teres muscle. A variety of symptoms are described under pronator teres syndrome, and the syndrome can be divided based on likely pathology. A true neurogenic syndrome, with surgical confirmation, has sensory loss in median innervated digits and palm and weakness of median innervated forearm (excluding the pronator teres muscle) and hand muscles is extraordinarily rare (Morris and Peters, 1976). A nonspecific pronator teres syndrome based on non-localizing pain exacerbated by movements but with no electrodiagnostic localization is more common.

Diagnosis is by electrodiagnostic studies; primarily needle EMG that localizes the lesion distal to the pronator teres muscle. Ultrasound studies may be helpful to identify or confirm focal nerve changes.

Therapy for true pronator teres syndrome is surgical exploration, but surgery for nonspecific pronator teres syndrome is likely over-performed when a focal lesion cannot be demonstrated, and conservative following is appropriate.

Anterior Interosseous Syndrome

The anterior interosseous nerve branch contains only motor fibers, and passes through the anterior interosseous membrane and innervates the flexor pollicis longus, flexor digitorum profundus (radial portion), and the pronator quadratus muscles. Symptoms attributed to entrapment at this site are the inability to pinch (make a circle with the thumb and index finger). Obvious causes include midshaft radius fractures, but proximal radius and supracondylar fractures may mimic localization to the forearm. The most common clinical situation is idiopathic weakness without obvious cause. Entrapment neuropathy is likely rare, and a microvasculitis involving median nerve fascicules at more proximal sites, as postulated for Parsonage-Turner syndrome, is more likely (Pham et al., 2014). In support are the finding that many patients describe pain in the arm at onset, as in classic Parsonage-Turner syndrome, and median innervated muscles are frequently also involved in the classic syndrome (England and Sumner, 1987).

Diagnosis is aided by a history of acute or subacute pain, and electrodiagnostic studies, primarily needle EMG, that localizes the lesion to the median nerve, but the distribution of denervation may be partial as only a few fasciculations may be involved. Ultrasound may be helpful in defining hourglass-like constrictions.

Therapy is usually conservative and improvement in strength is common. Recent studies describe hourglass-like constrictions that can involve both nerves (and other nerves), and while the pathology is not clear, surgical intervention (neurolysis) may not result in clinical improvement (Sunagawa et al., 2017)

Wrist

The median nerve, along with nine flexor tendons and the median artery, pass through the carpal tunnel. Ultrasound studies show marked changes of position of the median nerve with respect to the tendons with normal flexion and extension movements at the wrist. Acroparesthesias were recognized in the late 1800s, and the utility of nerve conduction studies for diagnosis began to be investigated in the mid-1900s. Testing initially relied on motor nerve conduction metrics, but efforts now rely on a combination of sensory and motor conduction studies, and variations continue to be developed. A distinction to be made is symptomatic median mononeuropathy at the wrist (carpal tunnel syndrome) versus asymptomatic nerve conduction

Table 8.3 Relative Risk Factors for Development of Carpal Tunnel Syndrome

Work-related Risk Factors
Repetition
Force
Repetition + force
Posture + force
Associations
Female gender
Elevated body mass index
Co-morbidities
Diabetes mellitus
Rheumatoid arthritis
Pregnancy

Source: Modified from Werner (2006).

abnormalities found during electrodiagnostic evaluation for other issues. Carpal tunnel syndrome is common, and a number of risk factors and comorbidities are identified (Werner, 2006) (Table 8.3).

Clinical Features

A constellation of symptoms includes numbness, tingling, and burning pain in the distribution of the median nerve, but patients frequently mention involvement of the fifth digit. The distribution of symptoms can extend proximally, but a site of pathology at the wrist becomes less likely when symptoms extend to the shoulder and neck (Stevens et al., 1999). Thenar muscle atrophy and weakness of thumb abduction occurs as a late finding.

Clinical assessment includes inspection for thenar muscle atrophy, assessment for thumb abduction weakness, and testing of sensory perception abnormalities, such as light-touch and two-point discrimination, to demarcate the distribution of involvement to the median nerve. Hand diagrams filled in by the patient for their overall symptom experience are available. Provocative maneuvers such as Phalen sign, reverse Phalen sign, light percussion over the nerve (Tinel sign) or deep pressure to the volar wrist are described to bring out symptoms, but an evidence-based review revealed few well-designed studies and a wide range of sensitivity (0.04–0.80) and specificity (0.25–0.95) (Keith et al., 2009). Verification of a median neuropathy at the wrist relies upon nerve conduction studies, and lately ultrasound studies, but there is no gold standard as symptoms may be episodic and nerve conduction studies normal.

Diagnostic Evaluation

Electrodiagnostic Studies

Pathology is thought to be due to increased pressure on the nerve at the carpal tunnel, initially affecting myelin. Electrodiagnostic studies of sensory nerves are more sensitive than motor nerves because the major symptoms are sensory, and sensory nerve fibers are of the largest diameter and more sensitive to conduction slowing. Motor studies are supportive, and essential when the SNAP is absent. Assessing changes in conduction timing over short nerve segments (~8–10 cm) is more sensitive than over long segments because the region of pathology at the wrist is restricted in length, and the normal conduction over flanking proximal and distal segments dilutes the magnitude of slowing over traditional distances (~14 cm). However, distance measurement errors become an issue when segments are very short (1–4 cm).

Both antidromic and orthodromic sensory nerve studies measurements are used and are equivalent, but antidromic responses may be of higher amplitude and easier to assess. Sensory distal latency measurements from the peak of the waveform are more accurately identified than from the onset. However, calculating conduction velocities from peak latencies is not a true velocity of the fastest fibers. Conduction velocities across proximal segments of the median nerve (wrist to elbow) may be mildly slowed, attributed to retrograde axonal atrophy (Chang et al., 2002).

Sensory and motor response amplitude values reflect axonal integrity, but values vary due to technical issues and the shape of patient's fingers (low compared to high circumference values), and are less sensitive markers of axonal pathology. However, focal block at the wrist is supported when the SNAP amplitude from stimulation in the palm is double that from stimulating proximal to the carpal tunnel (Lesser et al., 1995).

A variety of electrode placement arrangements for stimulation and recording sensory and motor nerve responses are available to document median nerve slowing across the wrist (Table 8.4, Figures 8.2–8.11)

Table 8.4 Sensory and Motor Nerve Conduction Studies to Aid in the Diagnosis of Median Nerve Entrapment at the Wrist

Figures	Nerve Studies	Conduction	Distances	Significant Distal Latency Differences
	Sensory Nerves			
8.2	Median (digit II) vs ulnar (digit IV)	Antidromic	~14 cm	≥0.5 ms
8.3	Median (digit IV) vs ulnar (digit IV)	Orthodromic	~14 cm	≥0.3 ms–≥0.4 ms
8.4	Median (digit I) vs radial (digit I)	Antidromic	~10 cm	≥0.4 ms–≥0.5 ms
8.5	Median (palm) vs ulnar (palm)	Antidromic	~8 cm	≥0.2 ms–≥0.3 ms
8.6	Median (digit II) vs median (digit II)	Antidromic	~14 cm vs ~7 cm	≥0.5 ms
8.7	Median (digit II)	Antidromic	~1 cm	≥0.4 ms–≥0.5 ms
8.8	Sensory Index (sum of differences)			
	• Median (digit IV) vs ulnar (digit IV)	Orthodromic	~8 cm	≥0.3 ms
	• Median (digit IV) vs ulnar (digit IV)	Antidromic	~14 cm	≥0.4 ms
	• Median (digit I) vs radial (digit I)	Antidromic		≥0.5
				Sum of differences ≥0.9 ms
	Motor Nerves			
8.9	Median (thenar) vs ulnar (hypothenar)	Orthodromic	~7 cm	≥1.5 ms
8.10	Median (thenar) vs ulnar (thenar)	Orthodromic	~7 cm median vs ~7 cm ulnar	≥0.8 ms
8.11	Median (lumbrical) vs ulnar (interossi)	Orthodromic	~10 cm	≥0.8 ms

Notes: Stimulating and recording electrode arrangement, including direction of conduction, distances, and timing differences: referenced to Figures 8.2–8.11, which illustrate electrode arrangements.

Source: Adapted from (Werner and Andary, 2011).

Median Sensory (II) vs Ulnar Sensory (V) – Antidromic

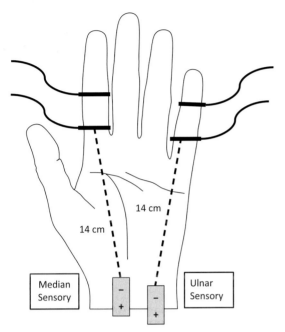

Figure 8.2 Diagram of stimulating and recording electrodes to document median mononeuropathy at the wrist. Antidromic median sensory response from wrist to digit II vs ulnar sensory response from wrist to digit V.
Adapted and redrawn from Werner and Andary (2011).
See Table 8.4.

Median Sensory (IV) vs Ulnar Sensory (IV) – Antidromic

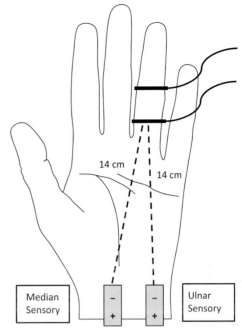

Figure 8.3 Diagram of stimulating and recording electrodes to document median mononeuropathy at the wrist. Antidromic median sensory response from wrist to digit IV vs ulnar sensory response from wrist to digit IV.
Adapted and redrawn from Werner and Andary (2011).
See Table 8.4.

(Werner and Andary, 2011). Most tests rely on comparisons (differences) between the timing of sensory responses of median nerve conduction through the carpal tunnel with ulnar or radial nerve conduction passing external to the tunnel, showing slowed conduction with the former and normal with the latter.

When sensory responses using conventional techniques are absent, electrodiagnostic conformation commonly relies upon motor nerve studies. However, in the setting of extreme median nerve pathology a sensory response can frequently be recorded with an amplitude in the ~1–2 microV range, requiring averaging of up to 250 responses (Seror and Seror, 2015). When the sensory response is absent, the motor response recording from the second lumbrical muscle is better preserved than that from the abductor pollicis brevis muscle (Yates et al., 1981).

An evidence-based literature review supports an electrodiagnostic algorithm in the setting of clinically suspected carpal tunnel syndrome: two complementary tests (both normal or both abnormal) should suffice to refute or make the diagnosis, but if the initial tests are normal and clinical suspicion remains high, additional tests are recommended (Table 8.4, Figures 8.2–8.11) (Jablecki et al., 2002). Pooled sensitivities using this algorithm are 0.65–0.85 and specificities are 0.97–0.98.

A nerve conduction "index" has been proposed that combines the sum of differences values from three sensory nerve conduction tests: palm difference (median vs ulnar across palm difference) + ring finger difference (median vs ulnar to digit IV difference) + thumb difference (median vs radial to digit I difference), with normal values ≤0.9 ms (Table 8.4). Sensitivity and specificity are 0.83 and 0.97, respectively (Robinson et al., 1998). Arguments for an index derived from multiple tests are: a single nerve conduction test result could be erroneous due to technical issues; a single nerve conduction test result could be falsely positive or negative; and it is easier to consider

Median Sensory (I) vs Radial Sensory (I) – Antidromic

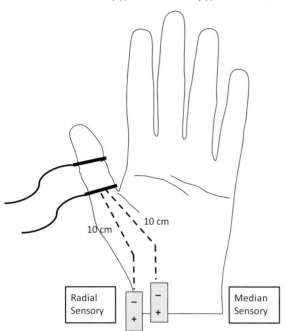

Figure 8.4 Diagram of stimulating and recording electrodes to document median mononeuropathy at the wrist. Antidromic median sensory response from wrist to digit I vs radial sensory response from wrist to digit I.
Adapted and redrawn from (Werner and Andary (2011). See Table 8.4.

Median Sensory Palm vs Ulnar Sensory Palm – Orthodromic

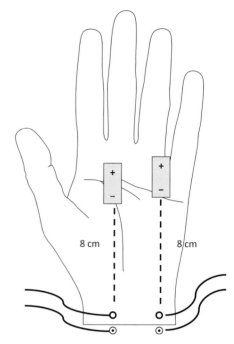

Figure 8.5 Diagram of stimulating and recording electrodes to document median mononeuropathy at the wrist. Orthodromic median sensory response from palm to wrist vs ulnar sensory response from palm to wrist.
Adapted and redrawn from Werner and Andary (2011). See Table 8.4.

a single index number than keeping track of individual results from several tests. The index cannot be used when median sensory conduction is severely affected and the SNAP response in one or more nerves is absent.

Not all patients who meet clinical criteria for carpal tunnel syndrome have abnormal nerve conduction studies. Conservative therapy leads to similar percentages of improvement compared to patients who have nerve conduction abnormalities. Those who do not have nerve conduction abnormalities tend to be of younger age and more lean stature (Witt et al., 2004).

Needle EMG has a lesser role, and confirms axonal loss in the abductor pollicis brevis muscle. It can also assess for more widespread abnormalities that support a different or concurrent diagnosis (length-dependent polyneuropathy, plexopathy, radiculopathy). Needle EMG has been advocated to search for a concurrent radiculopathy, as in the double-crush syndrome (see Chapter 6).

Median-ulnar Nerve Anastomoses and Carpal Tunnel Syndrome

Median-ulnar nerve anastomoses (Martin-Gruber) may be present in the setting of carpal tunnel syndrome, resulting in unusual nerve conduction findings (Rubin and Dimberg, 2010). One anastomosis pattern includes ulnar nerve fibers accompanying median nerve fibers at the elbow, with the ulnar fibers leaving to join the main ulnar nerve in the forearm. When this pattern is present in the setting of carpal tunnel syndrome there is the expected slowing of the motor median nerve response recorded from thenar muscles to wrist stimulation; however, stimulation over the median nerve at the elbow activates both median and ulnar fibers, and the latter arrive early at ulnar innervated thenar muscles (portion of the flexor pollicis brevis muscle). Depending upon the degree of slowing at the wrist, the short latency of the ulnar response to elbow stimulation may result in a non-physiologic conduction velocity (>100 m/s), and

Median Sensory (II) vs Median Sensory (II) – Antidromic

Median Sensory (II) - Antidromic

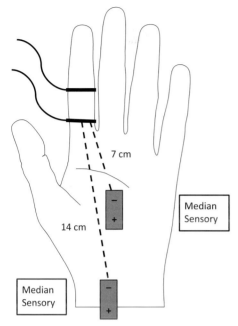

7 cm

14 cm

Median
Sensory

−
+

Median
Sensory

−
+

Figure 8.6 Diagram of stimulating and recording electrodes to document median mononeuropathy at the wrist. Antidromic median sensory response from wrist to digit II response vs median sensory response from palm to digit II.
Adapted and redrawn from Werner and Andary (2011). See Table 8.4.

the waveform may include separate negative humps (Figure 8.12).

Ultrasound Imaging

Ultrasound can provide useful information to aid (or make) the diagnosis, provide anatomical information helpful to a surgeon if a release is indicated, provide an alternative diagnosis when electrodiagnostic studies are not supportive of pathology at the wrist, or discover anatomic abnormalities mimicking the syndrome (Cartwright and Walker, 2013).

Ultrasound diagnosis is based on documenting a large median nerve cross-sectional area in the carpal tunnel. A diagnostic variation is showing an enlargement of the nerve in the carpal tunnel relative to values at a more proximal site along the median nerve (wrist-to-forearm ratio >1.4). An evidence-based literature review of ultrasound in patients with electrodiagnostic abnormalities supports confirmation of the diagnosis of carpal tunnel syndrome

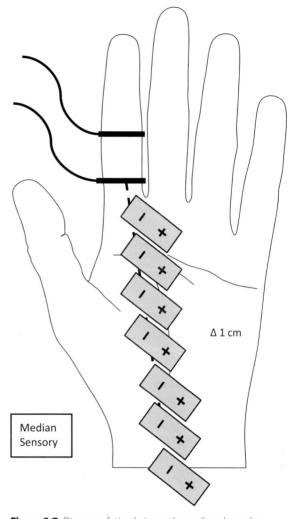

Median
Sensory

Δ 1 cm

Figure 8.7 Diagram of stimulating and recording electrodes to document median mononeuropathy at the wrist. Antidromic median sensory response wrist to digit II in 1-cm distance increments.
Adapted and redrawn from Werner and Andary (2011). See Table 8.4.

with sensitivity of 0.82–0.97 and specificity of 0.73–0.98 when the cross-sectional area is >8.5–10 mm² (Cartwright et al., 2012).

Unsuspected anatomic variants in the carpal tunnel include bifid median nerves at the wrist (10–15%), and persistent median artery (5–10%). Alternate pathology to explain symptoms has been found, including neuromas, Schwannomas, ganglion cysts, and arthritic conditions (Cartwright et al., 2012).

Index: Median-Ulnar Sensory +
Median-Ulnar (IV) +
Median-Radial (I)

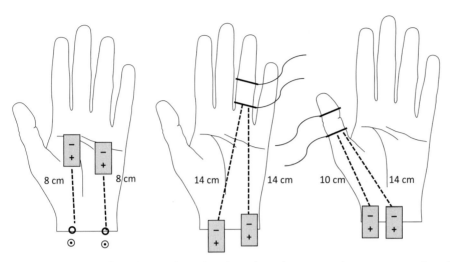

Figure 8.8 Diagram of stimulating and recording electrodes to document median mononeuropathy at the wrist. Index based on sum of differences for: (1) orthodromic median sensory response from palm to wrist vs ulnar sensory response from palm to wrist; (2) antidromic median sensory response from wrist to digit IV vs ulnar sensory response from wrist to digit IV; (3) antidromic median sensory response from wrist to digit I vs radial sensory response from wrist to digit I.
Adapted and redrawn from Werner and Andary (2011). See Table 8.4.

Median Motor vs Ulnar Motor – Orthodromic

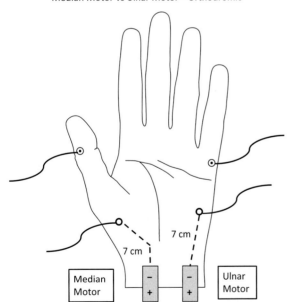

Figure 8.9 Diagram of stimulating and recording electrodes to document median mononeuropathy at the wrist. Orthodromic median motor response from wrist to thenar eminence vs ulnar motor response from wrist to hypothenar eminence.
Adapted and redrawn from Werner and Andary (2011). See Table 8.4.

Management

Carpal tunnel syndrome severity can be staged based on electrodiagnostic findings (Padua et al., 1997):

- mild: prolonged sensory responses with or without reduced sensory nerve action potential amplitude
- moderate: sensory nerve abnormalities as for "mild" but also prolonged median motor responses
- severe: reduced thenar compound muscle action potential and evidence for denervation on needle EMG (fibrillation potentials, reduced recruitment with increased motor unit action amplitude) (Stevens, 1997)

A spectrum of management options is available, but controlled trials are lacking to make objective recommendations. An evidence-based literature review for management includes:

- relative rest
- workplace modifications (O'Connor et al., 2012)
- exercise and immobilization by a splint (Page et al., 2012b; Page et al., 2012a)
- nonsteroidal anti-inflammatory drugs, oral or injected steroids (Marshall et al., 2007)
- therapeutic ultrasound (Page et al., 2013)

Median Motor vs Ulnar Motor – Orthodromic

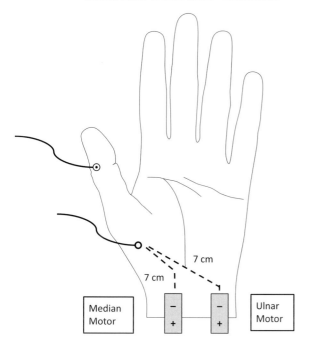

Figure 8.10 Diagram of stimulating and recording electrodes to document median mononeuropathy at the wrist. Orthodromic median motor response from wrist to thenar eminence vs ulnar motor response from wrist to thenar eminence.

Adapted and redrawn from Werner and Andary (2011). See Table 8.4.

Median Motor vs Ulnar Motor – Orthodromic

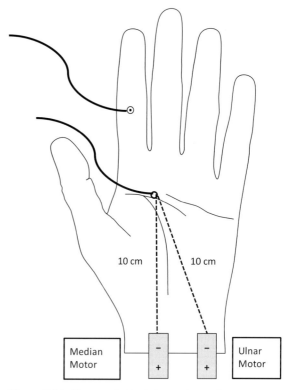

Figure 8.11 Diagram of stimulating and recording electrodes to document median mononeuropathy at the wrist. Orthodromic median motor response from wrist to interosseous muscles vs ulnar motor response from wrist to interosseous muscles.

Adapted and redrawn from Werner and Andary (2011). See Table 8.4.

- surgical release either by open surgery (Scholten et al., 2007) or endoscopic surgery (Vasiliadis et al., 2014)

An evidence-based literature review and resultant consensus statement supports electrodiagnostic confirmation before surgical release is contemplated (Sandin et al., 2010). Recommendations for surgical release include:

- evidence for median nerve denervation or significant degree of functional impairment
- continued symptoms after initial course of non-operative treatment
- second, non-operative treatment fails to resolve symptoms within 2–7 weeks

In the setting of concurrent medical conditions (diabetes mellitus, rheumatoid arthritis, pregnancy, radiculopathy) there is insufficient evidence for recommendations, and management (non-surgical or surgical) depends upon clinical judgment.

Hand

Clinical Features

Variations in the course of distal motor branch to thenar muscles occurs and lesions can cause weakness of abduction of digit I without sensory abnormalities (Bennett and Crouch, 1982). Causes include focal pressure associated with work activities and configuration of tools held in the palm.

Diagnostic Evaluation

Diagnosis is by normal sensory nerve conduction studies and abnormal needle EMG documenting denervation in thenar muscles.

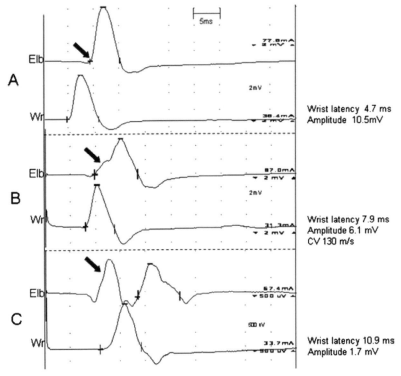

Figure 8.12 CMAP waveforms from patients with Martin-Gruber anastomosis and median entrapment neuropathy at the wrist: A: pair of traces from patient with mild neuropathy showing normal CMAP to wrist stimulation (Wr) and mild initial positive deflection to stimulation at the elbow (Elb) due to ulnar nerve fibers at the wrist and reaching the thenar eminence before median fibers (which are slowed across the wrist). B: pair of traces from patient with moderately severe median neuropathy showing more marked positive deflection and late-arriving median response riding on early-arriving ulnar response. C: pair of traces from patient with severe median neuropathy and the ulnar response from elbow stimulation is separate from the very slow median response.
From Rubin and Dimberg (2010), with permission.

Management

Management is by change in work activities and consideration for surgical exploration.

References

Bennett JB, Crouch CC. Compression syndrome of the recurrent motor branch of the median nerve. *J Hand Surg Am.* 1982;7:407–9.

Cartwright MS, Hobson-Webb LD, Boon AJ, Alter KE, Hunt CH, Flores VH, et al. Evidence-based guideline: neuromuscular ultrasound for the diagnosis of carpal tunnel syndrome. *Muscle Nerve.* 2012;46:287–93.

Cartwright MS, Walker FO. Neuromuscular ultrasound in common entrapment neuropathies. *Muscle Nerve.* 2013;48:696–704.

Chang MH, Wei SJ, Chiang HL, Wang HM, Hsieh PF, Huang SY. The cause of slowed forearm median conduction velocity in carpal tunnel syndrome: a Palmar stimulation study. *Clin Neurophysiol.* 2002;113:1072–6.

Dalton DM, Munigangaiah S, Subramaniam T, McCabe JP. Acute bilateral spontaneous forearm compartment syndrome. *Hand Surg.* 2014;19:99–102.

England JD, Sumner AJ. Neuralgic amyotrophy: an increasingly diverse entity. *Muscle Nerve.* 1987;10:60–8.

Jablecki CK, Andary MT, Floeter MK, Miller RG, Quartly CA, Vennix MJ, et al. Practice parameter: Electrodiagnostic studies in carpal tunnel syndrome. Report of the American Association of Electrodiagnostic Medicine, American Academy of Neurology, and the American Academy of Physical Medicine and Rehabilitation. *Neurology.* 2002;58:1589–92.

Keith MW, Masear V, Chung K, Maupin K, Andary M, Amadio PC, et al. Diagnosis of carpal tunnel syndrome. *J Am Acad Orthop Surg.* 2009;17:389–96.

Lesser EA, Venkatesh S, Preston DC, Logigian EL. Stimulation distal to the lesion in patients with carpal tunnel syndrome. *Muscle Nerve*. 1995;18:503–7.

Marshall S, Tardif G, Ashworth N. Local corticosteroid injection for carpal tunnel syndrome. *Cochrane Database Syst Rev*. 2007:CD001554.

Morris HH, Peters BH. Pronator syndrome: clinical and electrophysiological features in seven cases. *J Neurol Neurosurg Psychiatry*. 1976;39:461–4.

Oh SJ. *Clinical Electromyography: Nerve Conduction Studies*. 3rd ed. Philadelphia: Lippincott Williams & Wilkins; 2003.

O'Connor D, Page MJ, Marshall SC, Massy-Westropp N. Ergonomic positioning or equipment for treating carpal tunnel syndrome. *Cochrane Database Syst Rev*. 2012;1:CD009600.

Padua L, Di Pasquale A, Liotta G, Granata G, Pazzaglia C, Erra C, et al. Ultrasound as a useful tool in the diagnosis and management of traumatic nerve lesions. *Clin Neurophysiol*. 2013;124:1237–43.

Padua L, LoMonaco M, Gregori B, Valente EM, Padua R, Tonali P. Neurophysiological classification and sensitivity in 500 carpal tunnel syndrome hands. *Acta Neurol Scand*. 1997;96:211–17.

Page MJ, Massy-Westropp N, O'Connor D, Pitt V. Splinting for carpal tunnel syndrome. *Cochrane Database Syst Rev*. 2012a;7:CD010003.

Page MJ, O'Connor D, Pitt V, Massy-Westropp N. Exercise and mobilisation interventions for carpal tunnel syndrome. *Cochrane Database Syst Rev*. 2012b;6:CD009899.

Page MJ, O'Connor D, Pitt V, Massy-Westropp N. Therapeutic ultrasound for carpal tunnel syndrome. *Cochrane Database Syst Rev*. 2013;3:CD009601.

Pham M, Baumer T, Bendszus M. Peripheral nerves and plexus: imaging by MR-neurography and high-resolution ultrasound. *Curr Opin Neurol*. 2014;27:370–9.

Robinson LR, Micklesen PJ, Wang L. Strategies for analyzing nerve conduction data: superiority of a summary index over single tests. *Muscle Nerve*. 1998;21:1166–71.

Rubin DI, Dimberg EL. Martin-Gruber anastomosis and carpal tunnel syndrome: [corrected]

morphologic clues to identification. *Muscle Nerve*. 2010;42:457–8.

Sandin KJ, Asch SM, Jablecki CK, Kilmer DD, Nuckols TK. Clinical quality measures for electrodiagnosis in suspected carpal tunnel syndrome. *Muscle Nerve*. 2010;41:444–52.

Scholten RJ, Mink van der Molen A, Uitdehaag BM, Bouter LM, de Vet HC. Surgical treatment options for carpal tunnel syndrome. *Cochrane Database Syst Rev*. 2007:CD003905.

Seror P, Seror R. Severe and extreme idiopathic median nerve lesions at the wrist: new insights into electrodiagnostic patterns and review of the literature. *Muscle Nerve*. 2015;51:201–6.

Stevens JC. AAEM minimonograph #26: the electrodiagnosis of carpal tunnel syndrome. American Association of Electrodiagnostic Medicine. *Muscle Nerve*. 1997;20:1477–86.

Stevens JC, Smith BE, Weaver AL, Bosch EP, Deen HG, Jr., Wilkens JA. Symptoms of 100 patients with electromyographically verified carpal tunnel syndrome. *Muscle Nerve*. 1999;22:1448–56.

Sunagawa T, Nakashima Y, Shinomiya R, Kurumadani H, Adachi N, Ochi M. Correlation between "hourglass-like fascicular constriction" and idiopathic anterior interosseous nerve palsy. *Muscle Nerve*. 2017;55:508–12.

Suranyi L. Median nerve compression by Struthers ligament. *J Neurol Neurosurg Psychiatry*. 1983;46:1047–9.

Vasiliadis HS, Georgoulas P, Shrier I, Salanti G, Scholten RJ. Endoscopic release for carpal tunnel syndrome. *Cochrane Database Syst Rev*. 2014;1:CD008265.

Werner RA. Evaluation of work-related carpal tunnel syndrome. *J Occup Rehabil*. 2006;16:207–22.

Werner RA, Andary M. Electrodiagnostic evaluation of carpal tunnel syndrome. *Muscle Nerve*. 2011;44:597–607.

Witt JC, Hentz JG, Stevens JC. Carpal tunnel syndrome with normal nerve conduction studies. *Muscle Nerve*. 2004;29:515–22.

Yates SK, Yaworski R, Brown WF. Relative preservation of lumbrical versus thenar motor fibres in neurogenic disorders. *J Neurol Neurosurg Psychiatry*. 1981;44:768–74.

Ulnar Nerve Neuropathies

Introduction

Ulnar mononeuropathies are second in frequency to those of the median nerve, most commonly at the elbow, uncommon at the wrist, and very rare at proximal lesion sites (case reports). Nerve conduction studies, and recently ultrasound studies, are used to verify the lesion site, and ultrasound can provide information on underlying pathologic causes, especially if symptoms and electrodiagnostic findings are unusual. Much effort has been expended to designing nerve conduction testing protocols to improve sensitivity for detecting pathology at the elbow, but there is no "gold standard" test. Consequently, treatment, especially indications for surgical exploration, is not well sorted out.

Anatomy

The ulnar nerve is formed from both sensory and motor nerve fibers that enter and leave the spinal cord over the C8–T1 roots and sometimes the C7 root (Figure 9.1, Table 9.1). The nerve passes through the medial cord and lower trunk of the brachial plexus. In the arm, the nerve pierces a septum separating the flexor and extensor muscle groups, which includes an arcade (the arcade of Struthers) that is of variable thickness and can rarely compress the nerve. At the elbow, the nerve passes along a groove behind the medial epicondyle of the humerus, where it is vulnerable to external trauma and pressure. Another site of entrapment is between the two heads of the flexor carpi ulnaris muscle. A fibrous band crosses the two heads, and normal variations in muscle size and nerve trajectory can compress the nerve. This band is also called the humeroulnar arcade or Osborne's ligament. The nerve then traverses the cubital tunnel between the two heads of the flexor carpi ulnaris muscle, whose roof is the arcade. In the forearm, there are branches to the flexor carpi ulnaris and ulnar portion of the flexor digitorum profundus muscles, and sensory branches to the palm (palmar branch) and dorsum of the hand (dorsal cutaneous branch). When the nerve enters the hand, it passes between the hook of the hamate and the pisiform bones, through a 4-cm tunnel called Guyon's canal. The nerve divides into superficial and deep branches in the canal. The superficial sensory branch mediates sensation from the ulnar side of digit IV and all of digit V, and a deep motor branch innervates hypothenar and lumbrical muscles.

Pathology

Ulnar mononeuropathies are most often caused by focal nerve pressure (Table 9.2). External pressure includes habitual leaning on the elbow (medial epicondyle) or habitual/forced flexion or flexion/extension movements at the elbow (cubital tunnel). With elbow flexion, the flexor carpi ulnaris muscle contracts and the cubital tunnel tightens over the nerve and pressure increases in the tunnel. Direct trauma can be the consequence of elbow fractures, and bony overgrowth from remote fractures. The term "tardy ulnar palsy" denotes ulnar nerve injury following remote elbow trauma/fracture with a cubitus varus deformity of the elbow. Ganglion cysts occur at different sites within Guyon's canal. Vocational (holding a jackhammer) and avocational (bicycle riding) activities are associated with nerve injury at the wrist. There is an association of ulnar neuropathy with surgery, less likely from poor limb positioning during surgery and more likely from arm postures during convalescence (Stewart and Shantz, 2003). The degree of nerve damage is variable, and can include neurapraxic lesions or axonal damage. Ultrasound may be helpful to assess the nature and distribution of damage (Padua et al., 2013).

Elbow

The ulnar nerve is susceptible at several sites about the elbow, leading to the general term "ulnar neuropathy

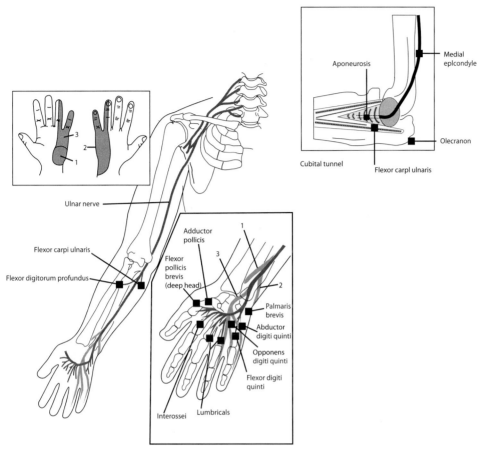

Figure 9.1 Ulnar nerve anatomy. Inset top left: cutaneous innervation (1 = palmar branch, 2 = dorsal cutaneous branch, 3 = superficial sensory branch). Inset top right: detail of cubital tunnel.
Modified from S Oh, MD, (2003), with permission.

at the elbow." There are a number of pathologic mechanisms, and the diagnostic challenges are accurate localization and determination of causation. However, it may not be possible to identify a cause, and idiopathic ulnar neuropathy at the elbow is a common conclusion.

Clinical Features

Assessment of clinical features to localize the lesion to the ulnar nerve at the elbow is important, as patients' reports of involvement may not be accurate. Symptoms of numbness are more common than weakness, and the areas most sensitive or painful at rest or to touch are frequently along the inner surface of the forearm. Testing the distribution of sensory loss among the three cutaneous portions of the ulnar nerve is valuable (digital, palmar, and dorsal branches) as involvement

of the palmar and dorsal branches places the lesion proximal to Guyon's canal, and more likely at the elbow. Muscle weakness and atrophy are less common as they occur with greater severity and longer duration of nerve damage. Localization to the ulnar nerve versus more proximal lesion sites (plexus and roots) is important as there are challenges in assessing for weakness in individual muscles: certain fascicles in the ulnar nerve tend to be more vulnerable at the elbow than others (see below); intrinsic hand muscles are more affected than forearm muscles; the first dorsal interosseous is more affected than hypothenar muscles; and flexor digital profundus muscle to digits IV and V more than flexor carpi ulnaris muscle (Stewart, 1987; Campbell et al., 1989).

It can be difficult to distinguish between lesion sites at the retroepicondylar groove, humeroulnar arcade, and the cubital tunnel. From cadaver studies,

Table 9.1 Predominant Root Innervation of Muscles Supplied by the Ulnar Nerve

Muscle	Root Innervation
Flexor carpi ulnaris	C8
Flexor digitorum profundus (digits IV–V)	C8–T1
Palmaris brevis	C8–T1
Abductor digiti quinti/minimi	C8–T1
Opponens digiti quinti/minimi	C8–T1
Flexor digiti quinti/minimi	C8–T1
Limbricals (digits III–IV)	C8–T1
Interossei (dorsal digits II–IV)	C8–T1
Interossei (volar digits II–IV)	C8–T1
Flexor pollicis brevis (deep head)	C8–T1
Adductor pollicis	C8–T1

the anatomy is variable: the humeroulnar arcade can be 3–20 mm distal to the medial epicondyle, and the intramuscular nerve course through the cubital tunnel can range from 18–70 mm in length (Campbell et al., 1991).

In the setting of surgery, symptoms suggestive of ulnar neuropathy are described after a variety of non-cardiac surgical procedures. A well-documented review indicates a true percentage of ulnar neuropathy at the elbow of about 0.5%, and among patients with hand numbness most proved to have a different lesion site (median neuropathies at the wrist, brachial plexopathy) and other causes (Warner et al., 1999). Most, but not all, symptoms spontaneously resolve over months. Males tend to be involved more than females, and there is an association with higher body weight. The time of symptom onset noted by the patient may not reconcile with hospital notes, and onset frequently occurs day after the operation. The cause is not clear, but postoperative and convalescent factors such as prolonged lying with pressure on the nerve at the elbow are suggested more often than pressure on the nerve from improper positioning during surgery (Barner et al., 2003; Stewart and Shantz, 2003).

Provocative clinical tests proposed to aid in the diagnosis include: Tinel's sign with various degrees of contact pressure and use of percussion objects (fingers, reflex hammer) applied to the epicondylar groove and clinical responses (patient report of paresthesias or twitch of first dorsal interosseous muscle); forced elbow flexion with pressure on the elbow for various intervals of time (1–5 min); and palpation of

the nerve for tenderness and thickening. Control tests include the contralateral asymmetric elbow or healthy subjects. A critical comparison of patients with electrodiagnostically confirmed ulnar neuropathy at the elbow showed sensitivities for provocative tests ranging from 0.28–0.62 and specificities from 0.40–0.87, and concluded that the diagnostic value is poor and not appropriate for clinical decision making (Beekman et al., 2009).

Diagnostic Evaluation

Electrodiagnostic Evaluation

A variety of nerve conduction techniques are available for diagnosing ulnar neuropathy at the elbow. While sensory symptoms predominate over motor symptoms, ulnar nerve sensory studies are less informative because attenuation of the normal SNAP amplitude at the elbow makes recording across the elbow responses unreliable, and localization is based on motor nerve studies demonstrating focal slowing across the elbow segment. There is no "gold standard" and an evidenced-based literature review supports the following guidelines (Campbell, 1999):

- Motor conduction velocity slowing >10 m/s across elbow segment (specific degree of slowing known) compared to forearm segment.
- Motor conduction velocity <50 m/s across elbow segment.
- CMAP area/amplitude reduction >20% across elbow segment compared to forearm segment.
- CMAP waveform shape change across elbow segment.

Traditional motor conduction studies record from the hypothenar eminence, but if inconclusive, recording from the first dorsal interosseous muscle may be more informative because fascicules innervating this muscle may be preferentially involved (Stewart, 1987). Comparisons of techniques are clouded by finding electrodiagnostic abnormalities in asymptomatic individuals, raising the question of normal nerve versus subclinical entrapment in control subjects.

Technical issues are a major component in interpreting test results (Campbell, 1999):

- Elbow joint position: Elbow flexed to 70–90 degrees and arm pronated, to make stretch of the nerve and conduction measurements uniform.
- Skin temperature: The ulnar nerve is superficial at the elbow, and low temperature can cause false

Table 9.2 Sites, Mechanisms, and Causes of Injury to the Ulnar Nerve

Site	Anatomy	Pathology	Causes
Axilla	Normal	Focal pressure	Crutch
			Sleep position
			Compartment Syndrome
		Trauma	Fracture
			Penetrating wound
			Hematoma
Arm	Normal		Sleep position
			Tourniquet
			Compartment Syndrome
		Trauma	Fracture
			Penetrating wound
			Fistula
Elbow	Normal	Idiopathic	
			Hyperflexion
			Elbow leaning
		Trauma	Fractures
			Old fracture
			Dislocation
	Anatomic variant	Focal pressure	Cubital tunnel
			Bone disease
Forearm	Normal	Focal pressure	Fistula
			Compartment Syndrome
		Trauma	Fracture
Wrist	Normal	Focal pressure	Handcuff
Hand	Normal	Focal pressure	Guyon canal
			Ganglion
			Cyst

slowing. In asymptomatic (normal) subjects, warming from an average of 31 to 34.5°C results in an increased conduction velocity across the elbow from a mean of 43 m/s to 48.5 m/s, but no significant change in conduction velocity amongst symptomatic subjects (Landau et al., 2005).

- Measurement errors: Despite controlled efforts, distance measurement errors around the elbow are greater than over similar straight-line distances in the forearm (Landau et al., 2002). The range of measurements can result in differences between forearm and across elbow conduction velocities up to 10 m/s in normal subjects.
- Optimum conduction distances: Conduction velocity across the elbow is traditionally measured over 10 cm, but shorter distances are more discriminating as the entrapment lesion is postulated to be ~1 cm in length, and mild slowing will be diluted by normal conduction velocities over flanking segments. Modeling indicates that conduction distances of 6–8 cm have good sensitivity and specificity, and sufficiently long to minimize measurement errors (Landau et al., 2003).
- Nerve position: The nerve may be displaced and not follow the predicted line across the elbow used for measurement, which can lead to a ±1 cm measurement error and subsequent ±7 m/s velocity error (Won et al., 2011).

Traditional motor nerve conduction studies can confirm the lesion site to the segment between the medial epicondyle or at the cubital tunnel. The close proximity of the two sites means that stimulation over short segments (1 cm increments) is more sensitive and accurate in detecting and localizing the lesion (Campbell et al., 1992). With short segment testing, the path of the ulnar nerve about the elbow is mapped using submaximal stimulating current and marked on the skin. Using the line between the medial epicondyle and the olecranon process as "0", marks at 1-cm intervals are made proximal and distal along the nerve path. Supramaximal CMAPs are elicited at each site, but with care that excessive current is not used that could result in activation of more distal nodes of Ranvier and hence negate detection of mild focal slowing. Waveform metrics at each stimulation site are CMAP distal latencies and unexpected prolongation reflects focal slowing, and changes in CMAP amplitude or area reflects elements of conduction block. However, despite care with surface recordings, precise localization may not be possible and intraoperative conduction studies may be required (Campbell et al., 1988).

Needle EMG has a lesser role, and cannot localize the lesion to the elbow, but can confirm denervation of ulnar innervated muscles and exclude more diffuse lesions. Not all ulnar innervated muscles are equally affected, and signs of denervation (positive waves and fibrillation potentials) were found in 84% in the first dorsal interosseous muscle, 52% in hypothenar eminence muscles, and only 16% in flexor carpi ulnaris or flexor digitorum profundus (Stewart, 1987). This pattern of greater denervation in hand muscles is attributed to greater vulnerability of specific fascicules in the nerve at the elbow.

Ultrasound Evaluation

Ultrasound can be used to aid in the diagnosis and determination of underlying pathology (Beekman et al., 2011). Two metrics are an increased nerve cross-sectional area and an increase in the ratio of the largest area at the elbow to the area of the nerve in the forearm or upper arm. Nerve echogenicity can also be assessed, with increases associated with pathology. Cross-sectional area and echogenicity can be measured at fixed locations or at its maximum. An evidence-based literature review shows that measurement of maximal cross-sectional area in normal nerves varies from 8.3–11.0 mm^2 and the ratio is 1.5, likely due to differences in techniques (Beekman et al., 2011). From the same study, for ulnar neuropathy at

the elbow based on a diagnosis by nerve conduction studies, ultrasound cross-sectional area had a sensitivity of 0.46–0.88 and specificity of 0.88–0.97, and measurement of the ratio a sensitivity of 1.00 and specificity of 0.97.

A comparison of the ability of the most sensitive electrodiagnostic technique (short-segment testing) to ultrasound to localize the site of the lesion shows that the site of maximal cross-sectional area and changes in echogenicity is frequently not in alignment with the site of focal nerve slowing (Simon et al., 2014). However, comparisons are confounded by variations in duration and severity of symptoms and the finding that asymptomatic elbows in both control subjects and asymptomatic contralateral can also have mild electrical and ultrasound abnormalities.

Pathology at the elbow can have a dynamic component, and ultrasound can assess both static structures and dynamic changes with elbow flexion (Beekman et al., 2011). Nerve movement can be assessed and the nerve can move from within the groove to the tip of the medial epicondyle (subluxation), or out of the groove (luxation), but these changes are also observed in normal individuals. Other rare factors that may cause ulnar nerve pathology and detected by ultrasound include snapping of the triceps muscle at the medial epicondyle, accessory anconeus muscle, ganglion cysts, osteophytes, and tumors (Beekman et al., 2011).

Management

It may not be possible to document a discrete nerve lesion site at the elbow by electrodiagnostic and ultrasound examinations, and ultrasound may not identify bony abnormalities, cysts, or other focal structural masses. When other causative factors such as postural pressure and nocturnal flexing at the elbow are excluded, a diagnosis of idiopathic ulnar neuropathy at the elbow is common.

Grading systems of severity have been proposed, and a combined system from the electrodiagnostic and surgical literature is a combination of symptoms, clinical signs, and electrodiagnostic signs (modified from Padua et al. (2001); Bartels et al. (2005)):

- Grade 1/negative (idiopathic):

  Clinical symptoms: intermittent numbness and paresthesias

  Clinical signs: may/may not have sensory loss; no muscle atrophy, slight weakness

Electrodiagnostic signs: normal SNAP and no motor slowing

- Grade 2/mild:

Clinical symptoms: constant numbness and paresthesias

Clinical signs: sensory loss; no muscle atrophy, slight weakness

Electrodiagnostic signs: normal SNAP, motor slowing

- Grade 3/moderate:

Clinical symptoms: constant numbness and paresthesias

Clinical signs: sensory loss; no muscle atrophy, mild weakness (≥4 MRC scale)

Electrodiagnostic signs: reduced SNAP, motor slowing

- Grade 4/marked:

Clinical symptoms: constant numbness and paresthesias

Clinical signs: sensory loss; moderate muscle atrophy, moderate weakness (<3 MRC scale)

Electrodiagnostic signs: absent SNAP, motor slowing

- Grade 5/severe:

Clinical symptoms: constant numbness and paresthesias

Clinical signs: sensory loss; marked muscle atrophy; claw hand; marked muscle weakness (<2 MRC scale)

Electrodiagnostic signs: absent SNAP, absent CMAP

Note: SNAP recorded from digit V; CMAP recorded from the abductor pollicis brevis muscle; motor slowing across elbow segment. Medical Research Counsel (MRC) grading scale.

Management outcomes are based on presumed etiology, management action (surgical/conservative), length of follow-up, and other factors. For lower grades of severity (grades 1–2, above), conservative management in the form of addressing common conditions that exert pressure on the nerve is appropriate. For more severe grades (grades 3–6, above), surgical intervention is reasonable to consider. There are two common surgical procedures: decompression of the cubital canal and ulnar nerve transposition. The former is the simpler of the two and has the least side effects. A randomized study of the two procedures showed both to be equally effective (Bartels et al., 2005).

Wrist

Four sites of focal entrapment at the wrist can be distinguished by patterns of motor and sensory branch involvement (Olney and Hanson, 1988). The palmar and dorsal branches are not involved as they leave the nerve proximal to the wrist. The term "Guyon's Canal Syndrome" is not specific and does not distinguish among the sites.

Guyon's Canal

Entrapment at or in Guyon's canal results in involvement of both sensory and motor branches, with paresthesias in the digits and weakness of all ulnar-innervated muscles in the hand (hypothenar, first dorsal interosseous and other interossei, opponens pollicis and portions of the flexor pollicis brevis and lumbrical muscles). Precipitating activities are associated with pressure at the wrist, particularly bicycle riding. Causative factors include ganglion cysts, lipomas, and synovial cysts.

Deep Motor Branch (Distal to Guyon's Canal)

Entrapment distal to the canal spares sensory nerves but involves motor branches with weakness of all ulnar-innervated hand muscles.

Deep Motor Branch (Sparing Hypothenar Muscles)

Entrapment more distal to the canal spares branches to hypothenar muscles but includes all other ulnar-innervated muscles, but no sensory loss. This is the most common site of entrapment and clinical pattern.

Superficial Terminal Branch (Sensory)

Entrapment very distal to the canal includes only sensory nerve to the digits.

Causes

Causes for lesions at all sites are similar and include ganglia, cysts, nerve tumors, and bony changes from arthritis and fractures. Imaging, including radiographs, CT, and ultrasound, can help determine causes.

Diagnostic Evaluation

Electrodiagnostic Evaluation

SNAP responses recorded from digit V that are reduced or absent supports axonal loss, and prolonged distal latency supporting demyelination. The dorsal ulnar sensory response should be normal. Motor nerve testing recording from hypothenar muscles can show reduced CMAP amplitude and prolonged distal latency. Since the first dorsal interosseous muscle is involved in most entrapments at the wrist, recording from this muscle can be informative (Olney and Hanson, 1988). A variety of other techniques have been described, including stimulating over short segments (McIntosh et al., 1998; Cowdery et al., 2002). Needle EMG can document denervation in hypothenar and first dorsal interosseous muscles. It is to be noted that many electrodiagnostic tests do not localize the lesion site to the wrist, and full consideration needs to be given to the more common lesion site at the elbow. Further, anomalous innervation of hand muscles can confound electrodiagnostic test interpretation.

Ultrasound

Ultrasound can be used to determine location, extent, and type of ulnar lesion in the hand (Tagliafico et al., 2012).

Management

Conservative approaches include modification of external physical factors. Surgical interventions are usually reserved for structural lesions.

References

Barner KC, Landau ME, Campbell WW. A review of perioperative nerve injury to the upper extremities. *J Clin Neuromuscul Dis.* 2003;4:117–23.

Bartels RH, Verhagen WI, van der Wilt GJ, Meulstee J, van Rossum LG, Grotenhuis JA. Prospective randomized controlled study comparing simple decompression versus anterior subcutaneous transposition for idiopathic neuropathy of the ulnar nerve at the elbow: Part 1. *Neurosurgery.* 2005;56:522–30.

Beekman R, Schreuder AH, Rozeman CA, Koehler PJ, Uitdehaag BM. The diagnostic value of provocative clinical tests in ulnar neuropathy at the elbow is marginal. *J Neurol Neurosurg Psychiatry.* 2009;80:1369–74.

Beekman R, Visser LH, Verhagen WI. Ultrasonography in ulnar neuropathy at the elbow: a critical review. *Muscle Nerve.* 2011;43:627–35.

Campbell WW. Guidelines in electrodiagnostic medicine. Practice parameter for electrodiagnostic studies in ulnar neuropathy at the elbow. *Muscle Nerve Suppl.* 1999;8:S171–205.

Campbell WW, Pridgeon RM, Riaz G, Astruc J, Leahy M, Crostic EG. Sparing of the flexor carpi ulnaris in ulnar neuropathy at the elbow. *Muscle Nerve.* 1989;12:965–7.

Campbell WW, Pridgeon RM, Riaz G, Astruc J, Sahni KS. Variations in anatomy of the ulnar nerve at the cubital tunnel: pitfalls in the diagnosis of ulnar neuropathy at the elbow. *Muscle Nerve.* 1991;14:733–8.

Campbell WW, Pridgeon RM, Sahni KS. Short segment incremental studies in the evaluation of ulnar neuropathy at the elbow. *Muscle Nerve.* 1992;15:1050–4.

Campbell WW, Sahni SK, Pridgeon RM, Riaz G, Leshner RT. Intraoperative electroneurography: management of ulnar neuropathy at the elbow. *Muscle Nerve.* 1988;11:75–81.

Cowdery SR, Preston DC, Herrmann DN, Logigian EL. Electrodiagnosis of ulnar neuropathy at the wrist: conduction block versus traditional tests. *Neurology.* 2002;59:420–7.

Landau ME, Barner KC, Campbell WW. Optimal screening distance for ulnar neuropathy at the elbow. *Muscle Nerve.* 2003;27:570–4.

Landau ME, Barner KC, Murray ED, Campbell WW. Cold elbow syndrome: spurious slowing of ulnar nerve conduction velocity. *Muscle Nerve.* 2005;32:815–17.

Landau ME, Diaz MI, Barner KC, Campbell WW. Changes in nerve conduction velocity across the elbow due to experimental error. *Muscle Nerve.* 2002;26:838–40.

McIntosh KA, Preston DC, Logigian EL. Short-segment incremental studies to localize ulnar nerve entrapment at the wrist. *Neurology.* 1998;50:303–306.

Oh SJ. *Clinical Electromyography: Nerve Conduction Studies.* 3rd edn. Philadelphia: Lippincott Williams & Wilkins; 2003.

Olney RK, Hanson M. AAEE case report #15: ulnar neuropathy at or distal to the wrist. *Muscle Nerve.* 1988;11:828–32.

Padua L, Aprile I, Mazza O, Padua R, Pietracci E, Caliandro P, et al. Neurophysiological classification of ulnar entrapment across the elbow. *Neurol Sci.* 2001;22:11–16.

Padua L, Di Pasquale A, Liotta G, Granata G, Pazzaglia C, Erra C, et al. Ultrasound as a useful tool in the diagnosis and management of traumatic nerve lesions. *Clin Neurophysiol*. 2013;124:1237–43.

Simon NG, Ralph JW, Poncelet AN, Engstrom JW, Chin C, Kliot M. A comparison of ultrasonographic and electrophysiologic "inching" in ulnar neuropathy at the elbow. *Clin Neurophysiol*. 2014.

Stewart JD. The variable clinical manifestations of ulnar neuropathies at the elbow. *J Neurol Neurosurg Psychiatry*. 1987;50:252–8.

Stewart JD, Shantz SH. Perioperative ulnar neuropathies: a medicolegal review. *Can J Neurol Sci*. 2003;30:15–19.

Tagliafico A, Cadoni A, Fisci E, Gennaro S, Molfetta L, Perez MM, et al. Nerves of the hand beyond the carpal tunnel. *Semin Musculoskelet Radiol*. 2012;16:129–36.

Warner MA, Warner DO, Matsumoto JY, Harper CM, Schroeder DR, Maxson PM. Ulnar neuropathy in surgical patients. *Anesthesiology*. 1999;90:54–9.

Won SJ, Yoon JS, Kim JY, Kim SJ, Jeong JS. Avoiding false-negative nerve conduction study in ulnar neuropathy at the elbow. *Muscle Nerve*. 2011;44:583–6.

Chapter 1

Radial Nerve Neuropathies

Chapter 10

Introduction

Radial nerve mononeuropathies are uncommon outside of obvious trauma. The radial nerve is implicated, but not clearly demonstrated to be involved, in painful conditions at the proximal forearm, and thus more likely represent musculoskeletal disorders.

Anatomy

The radial nerve is formed from both sensory and motor nerve fibers that enter and leave the spinal cord over C5–C8 roots and contribute to upper, middle, and lower trunks and merge to form the posterior cord. In the upper arm, motor branches innervate the three heads of the triceps muscles (Figure 10.1, Table 10.1). Sensory branches supply cutaneous innervation as the posterior cutaneous nerve of the arm and posterior cutaneous nerve of the forearm. The radial nerve then curves around the spinal groove in the humerus and passes through a fibrous arch. It gives motor branches to brachioradialis and anconeus muscles. Before reaching the elbow, it supplies the extensor carpi radialis longus and brevis muscles. The nerve passes into the forearm and divides into the posterior interosseous nerve (motor) and superficial radial nerve (sensory). The posterior interosseous nerve passes through an opening in the supinator muscle, the arcade of Frohse, where it gives of branches to the supinator muscle. Distally it branches to innervate the extensor digitorum communis, extensor ulnaris, extensor pollicis longus and brevis, abductor pollicis longus, extensor indicis, and extensor digiti minimi muscles. The superficial radial nerve branch supplies cutaneous innervation to the dorsolateral hand and portions of digits I–III.

Pathology

Proximal radial mononeuropathies are often caused by focal nerve pressure and represent neurapraxic

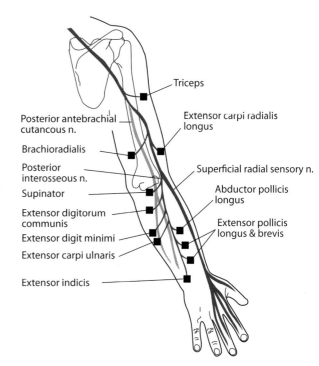

Figure 10.1 Radial nerve anatomy.
From S Oh, MD, (2003), with permission.

lesions. Rare causes are cysts and ganglia (Table 10.2). Humerus fractures cause axonal damage, and the degree of damage is variable, and ultrasound may be helpful to assess the nature and distribution of damage (Padua et al., 2013). Nerve damage attributed to the posterior interosseous syndrome is variable in degree, and is controversial. Chronic painful conditions about the elbow, also referred to as chronic tennis elbow or radial tunnel syndrome, are frequently ascribed to posterior interosseous nerve impingement, and thus are frequently treated by surgical release procedures. However, when no electrodiagnostic abnormalities are found and the underlying pathology is not known, these situations may not clearly represent

Table 10.1 Predominant Root Innervation of Muscles Supplied by the Radial Nerve

Muscle	Root Innervation
Triceps	C7–C8
Anconeus	C7–C8
Brachioradialis	C5–C6
Supinator (posterior interosseus nerve)	C6
Extensor carpi radialis longus/brevis	C6–C7
Extensor digitorum communis	C6–C8
Extensor carpi ulnaris (posterior interosseus nerve)	C7–C8
Abductor pollicis longus (posterior interosseus nerve)	C7–C8
Extensor indicis (posterior interosseus nerve)	C8–T1
Extensor pollicis longus/brevis (posterior interosseus nerve)	C7–C8

a radial mononeuropathy (Campbell and Landau, 2008). When there is axonal loss in the distribution of the posterior interosseous nerve and no obvious structural entrapment, the pathology may represent a microvasculitis affecting some fascicles, as postulated for Parsonage-Turner syndrome.

Another form of pathology, hourglass-like constrictions of nerve, has been described involving the radial nerve (as well as other nerves) that is encountered with ultrasound or at surgery (Nakamichi and Tachibana, 2007). Although the underlying pathologic factors affecting nerve function are not known, it may reflect another type of idiopathic neuropathy.

Axilla

Clinical Features

Sensory loss and weakness attributed to radial mononeuropathy at this site is uncommon as symptoms are usually combined with loss from the ulnar and median nerves as they are in close proximity. When only the radial nerve is involved, sensory loss includes the radial dorsum of the hand and forearm, and weakness includes muscles that extend the elbow, wrist, and all digits.

Diagnostic Evaluation

Electrodiagnostic studies cannot localize the lesion to the axilla, as proximal stimulation for nerve conduction studies cannot be readily performed. Needle EMG studies can document the degree of denervation, and determine if more than the radial nerve is involved. Imaging by x-ray, ultrasound, or MRI can help define structural issues and causes.

Management

Pressure palsies from abnormal use of crutches and from sleep postures generally resolve without intervention. Nerve damage from trauma is variable and can include axonal damage with variable degrees of recovery, and surgical consultation may be warranted.

Arm

Clinical Features

The radial nerve is susceptible to external pressure on the upper arm, especially along the medial side. In states of sleep or stupor (honeymoon palsy or Saturday night inebriation), pressure on the arm (arm draped over a chair, partner's head lying on the arm, sleeping lying over the arm) can cause varying degrees of weakness of the brachioradialis and wrist and finger extensor muscles and sensory loss in the distribution of the posterior cutaneous nerve of the forearm and the superficial radial nerve, but spares elbow extension (triceps muscles) (Trojaborg, 1970). Tourniquets used for blood pressure monitoring or to achieve a bloodless field can cause limb paralysis. While compression frequently affects median, ulnar, and radial nerves, the radial nerve is affected to the greatest degree (Landi et al., 1995).

Fractures of the humerus, and other forms of trauma, are obvious causes of nerve damage, and lesions are usually axonal. All radial innervated muscles and cutaneous distributions can be affected (Trojaborg, 1970).

Diagnostic Evaluation

Electrodiagnostic testing is indicated to assess for degree of axonal loss when suspected pathology is axonal or when recovery is slow. Electrodiagnostic testing with very proximal stimulation requires attention to technique with recording electrodes placed over the extensor pollicis longus–abductor pollicis longus muscle pair. Conduction block can be documented with stimulation proximal and distal to the spiral groove and at the elbow (Watson and

Table 10.2 Sites, Mechanisms, and Causes of Injury to the Radial Nerve

Site	Anatomy	Pathology	Causes
Axilla	Normal	Focal pressure	Crutch
			Sleep position
		Trauma	Fracture
			Dislocation
			Hematoma
Arm	Normal	Focal pressure	Sleep position
			Tourniquet
		Trauma	Fracture
			Dislocation
			Penetrating wounds
Forearm	Normal	Focal pressure	Fistula
			Arcade of Frohse
		Trauma	Fracture
			Dislocation
			Penetrating wound
Wrist	Normal	Focal pressure	Work-related

Brown, 1992). Electrodiagnostic studies can help with prognosis: the presence of a CMAP recorded from the extensor indicis muscle and full recruitment on needle EMG of the brachioradialis muscle portends to a good outcome (MRC grade >3); an absent evoked response and reduced recruitment is associated with a less favorable outcome (MRC grade 0–2); and those with poor evoked responses and recruitment tested three months from the injury have the worst outcome (Malikowski et al., 2007). Imaging studies can be helpful in determining cause and severity of nerve involvement.

Management

Causative factors are usually obvious. With compressive lesions, pathology usually represents neurapraxia with good recovery over eight weeks; however, with long-duration pressure such as in the setting of a coma, there may be axonal damage. With trauma, the pathology is usually axonal with recovery over many months consistent with nerve outgrowth, and recovery is variable. An evidence-based literature review supports a 70% spontaneous return of function. Surgical exploration may be helpful in the most severe cases (multiple injuries), and when there is no evidence for reinnervation after several months (Shao et al., 2005).

Elbow

Clinical Features

The radial nerve divides into superficial (superficial radial) and deep (posterior interosseous) branches at the elbow, and both branches are vulnerable to damage with radial bone fractures and elbow dislocations. The posterior interosseous nerve enters the extensor compartment of the forearm by passing through the arcade of Frohse, a fibrous band at the superior border of the supinator muscle. As the nerve travels distally it is said to pass for some distance through the "radial tunnel." It is hypothesized that the posterior interosseous nerve is vulnerable to focal pressure due to fibrous bands and adhesions in this area, and is said to account for idiopathic pain about the elbow, with or without finger extensor weakness. Surgical exploration frequently shows adhesions, and relief of symptoms after release has been used as verification of focal entrapment of the posterior interosseous nerve.

There are issues with the clinical features, anatomical findings, and surgically based conclusions. The clinical features include pain focal to the lateral elbow, exacerbated with extensor muscle activity, and some or no weakness of digital extension. Cadaver dissections reveal fibrous bands about the nerve at multiple sites in this region in a high percentage (>50%) and considerable variation in the course of the nerve, nerve branches, and vasculature (Konjengbam and Elangbam, 2004). The radial tunnel is an imprecisely defined structure (Campbell and Landau, 2008). In many clinical examples, no electrodiagnostic evidence is found for axonal nerve damage. The natural history of the posterior interosseous syndrome is not known, and symptoms of pain overlap with chronic/resistant tennis elbow syndrome (lateral epicondylitis). The entity of posterior interosseous nerve/radial tunnel syndrome can be divided into true entrapment with weakness of extension and electrodiagnostic findings of axonal loss, and disputed with only pain (Rosenbaum, 1999). Some cases with weakness and axonal loss may not reflect focal entrapment at this site, and are more likely examples of microvasculitis at more proximal sites along the nerve, as in the Parsonage-Turner or neuralgic amyotrophy syndrome (Rosenbaum, 1999; Bäumer, et al., 2016).

There are recent descriptions of hourglass-like constrictions of nerve that are not associated with focal compression, and represent another pathology.

Diagnostic Evaluation

Nerve conduction studies of the superficial radial nerve can confirm radial nerve involvement at or proximal to the elbow, and motor nerve conduction studies can confirm conduction block and axonal damage (Watson and Brown, 1992). When there is axonal loss, needle EMG can document whether the radial nerve is involved in isolation or whether there are other nerves such as a radiculopathy or plexopathy, and whether the lesion site is distal or proximal to the elbow by which muscles show denervation. The question of a complete or incomplete nerve transection can be answered from the EMG recruitment pattern or by imaging.

Nerve ultrasound can be helpful to document focal nerve changes, including hourglass-like constrictions (Nakamichi and Tachibana, 2007).

Management

Choosing among treatment options is difficult as an evidence-based literature review includes no controlled trials (Buchbinder et al., 2011). When there is no electrodiagnostic evidence for denervation, initial conservative treatment is appropriate. With persistent pain, imaging studies (ultrasound or MR neurography) may be helpful to define a structural

cause. If there is evidence for denervation, surgical exploration can be considered (Knutsen and Calfee, 2013). Surgery for conditions associated with hourglass-like constrictions may not lead to improvement (Nakamichi and Tachibana, 2007).

Wrist

The superficial radial nerve is vulnerable to external pressure over the radial aspect of the wrist, causing numbness over the dorsal radial hand, and has been called cheiralgia paresthetica. Causes include tight bands (watch, bracelet, rubber glove, plaster cast). Overly tight handcuffs can exert pressure on the superficial radial nerve, and also the ulnar and median nerves (Scott et al., 1989; Stone and Laureno, 1991).

Diagnostic Evaluation

The diagnosis is usually clinical, and electrodiagnostic studies can document involvement of the superficial radial nerve or additional nerves, and exclude a more proximal lesion site.

Management

Removal of tight bands is appropriate. Recovery from very tight bands can take months and may be incomplete (Stone and Laureno, 1991).

References

Bäumer P, Kele H, Xia A, Weiler M, Schwarz D, Bendszus, PM. Posterior interosseous neuropathy: Supinator syndrome vs fascicular radial neuropath. *Neurology*. 2016; 87:1884–91.

Buchbinder R, Johnston RV, Barnsley L, Assendelft WJ, Bell SN, Smidt N. Surgery for lateral elbow pain. *Cochrane Database Syst Rev*. 2011:CD003525.

Campbell WW, Landau ME. Controversial entrapment neuropathies. *Neurosurg Clin N Am*. 2008;19:597–608, vi–vii.

Knutsen EJ, Calfee RP. Uncommon upper extremity compression neuropathies. *Hand Clin*. 2013;29:443–53.

Konjengbam M, Elangbam J. Radial nerve in the radial tunnel: anatomic sites of entrapment neuropathy. *Clin Anat*. 2004;17:21–5.

Landi A, Saracino A, Pinelli M, Caserta G, Facchini MC. Tourniquet paralysis in microsurgery. *Ann Acad Med Singapore*. 1995;24:89–93.

Malikowski T, Micklesen PJ, Robinson LR. Prognostic values of electrodiagnostic studies in traumatic radial neuropathy. *Muscle Nerve*. 2007;36:364–7.

Nakamichi K, Tachibana S. Ultrasonographic findings in isolated neuritis of the posterior interosseous nerve: comparison with normal findings. *J Ultrasound Med*. 2007;26:683–7.

Oh SJ. *Clinical Electromyography: Nerve Conduction Studies*. 3rd edn. Philadelphia: Lippincott Williams & Wilkins, 2003.

Padua L, Di Pasquale A, Liotta G, Granata G, Pazzaglia C, Erra C, et al. Ultrasound as a useful tool in the diagnosis and management of traumatic nerve lesions. *Clin Neurophysiol*. 2013;124:1237–43.

Rosenbaum R. Disputed radial tunnel syndrome. *Muscle Nerve*. 1999;22:960–7.

Scott TF, Yager JG, Gross JA. Handcuff neuropathy revisited. *Muscle Nerve*. 1989;12:219–20.

Shao YC, Harwood P, Grotz MR, Limb D, Giannoudis PV. Radial nerve palsy associated with fractures of the shaft of the humerus: a systematic review. *J Bone Joint Surg Br*. 2005;87:1647–52.

Stone DA, Laureno R. Handcuff neuropathies. *Neurology*. 1991;41:145–7.

Trojaborg W. Rate of recovery in motor and sensory fibres of the radial nerve: clinical and electrophysiological aspects. *J Neurol Neurosurg Psychiatry*. 1970;33:625–38.

Watson BV, Brown WF. Quantitation of axon loss and conduction block in acute radial nerve palsies. *Muscle Nerve*. 1992;15:768–73.

Fibular/Peroneal Nerve Neuropathies

Introduction

The name "common peroneal nerve" was changed to "common fibular nerve" by the Terminologica Anatomica (International Anatomical Terminology). This was to prevent confusion with the perineal nerve. In this book, the nerve will be referred to as the fibular/peroneal nerve to cover all habits of appellation. The common fibular/peroneal nerve is the most frequent mononeuropathy in the leg.

Anatomy

The common fibular/peroneal nerve is formed from sensory and motor nerve fibers that enter and leave the spinal cord over L4–S3 nerve roots (Figure 11.1, Table 11.1). The nerve emerges from the lumbosacral plexus and joins with, but remains physically separate from, nerve fibers in the sacral plexus that form the tibial nerve. The two nerves are ensheathed by connective tissue to make up the sciatic nerve in the thigh, but distal to the popliteal fossa they separate into two nerves. Within the sciatic nerve, the common fibular/peroneal nerve is lateral to the tibial nerve. The branch of the sciatic nerve to the short head of the biceps femoris muscle comes from the common fibular/peroneal nerve. The next branch occurs in the popliteal fossa and is the sural communicating branch, which joins the medial sural nerve (from the tibial nerve) in the calf and contributes varying percentages of fibers to the sural nerve. The lateral cutaneous nerve of the calf innervates skin to the lateral aspect of the calf. The common fibular/peroneal nerve then wraps around the head of the fibula and is covered by minimal subcutaneous tissue for about 10 cm before it pierces the superficial head of the fibularis/peroneus longus muscle. At this site, there is a tendinous arch, the fibular tunnel, through which the nerve passes. The nerve then divides into the superficial and deep fibular/peroneal branches.

Motor fibers of the superficial branch innervate the fibularis/peroneus longus and fibularis/peroneus brevis muscles; sensory fibers innervate the skin of the anterolateral lower leg, and more distally innervates the skin of dorsal surface of the foot as the superficial fibular/peroneus nerve. Motor fibers of the deep fibular/peroneal nerve innervate the anterior tibialis, extensor hallucis longus, extensor digitorum longus, and fibularis/peroneus tertius muscles, and distally the extensor digitorum brevis muscle. Sensory fibers supply the medial and lateral surfaces of the first and second toes.

An accessory branch of the deep fibular/peroneal nerve occurs in about one-third of people. The accessory branch leaves the deep fibular/peroneal nerve at the fibular neck, descends along the lateral calf, passes under the lateral malleolus, and innervates all or part of the extensor digitorum brevis muscle. This anomalous innervation is important to be aware of when there is surgery at the lateral ankle. It most commonly comes to attention during electrodiagnostic studies when a CMAP of larger amplitude is recorded to stimulation at the fibular head compared to stimulation at the ankle. A full account can be made by stimulating at the lateral malleolus and the CMAP amplitude values from stimulation at the knee and at the malleolus should approximately equal the amplitude from stimulating at the ankle.

Pathology

The common fibular/peroneal nerve is damaged in the leg as part of sciatic nerve injuries as it occupies a lateral position and is more vulnerable (see Chapter 12). It is also most vulnerable at the fibular head due to its superficial location (Table 11.2). Causes may be obvious (trauma, fractures, dislocations) or subtle (crouching, sitting with crossed legs). The most common nerve pathology is pressure, mostly from external trauma, resulting in neurapraxic or

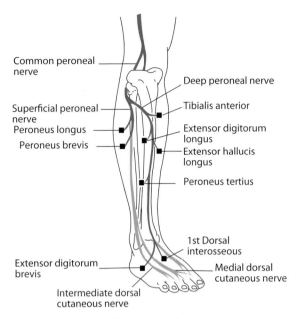

Figure 11.1 Common fibular/peroneal nerve anatomy. From S Oh,MD, (2003), with permission.

Table 11.1 Predominant Root Innervation of Muscles Supplied by the Common Fibular/Peroneal Nerve

Muscle	Root Innervation
Fibular/peroneal longus	L5–S1
Fibular/peroneal brevis	L5–S1
Anterior tibialis	L4–L5
Extensor hallucis longus	L5–S1
Extensor digitorum longus	L5–S1
Fibular/peroneal tertiius	L5–S1
Extensor digitorum brevis	L5–S1

neurotmesis lesions. The nature of the pressure varies, from mild to marked and from acute to chronic. The patient may not recognize the time course and degree of pressure, and examples are habitual leg crossing (mild but chronic) or a single episode of crouching (severe and acute). Focal compression attributed to a fibrous band at the fibular tunnel is controversial and difficult to verify as the cause because at surgery an observed band may not be exerting pressure. More severe trauma, including fractures and dislocations, frequently include axonal loss.

Foot drop can occur in the setting of a mononeuropathy multiplex due to diabetes, vasculitis, and more widespread neuropathies such as multifocal neuropathies with conduction block and hereditary neuropathy with liability to pressure palsies (discussed in chapters on these disorders).

Knee

Clinical Features

Clinical features are similar for causes in the popliteal fossa and fibular head, but variable in degree. A complete lesion causes paralysis of ankle dorsiflexion and eversion (foot drop) and toe extension, and sensory loss over the dorsum of the foot and rarely the lateral calf. Partial lesions cause variable patterns, and the

deep fibular/peroneal branch is more often involved than the superficial branch, and the explanation for this is that fascicles of the deep and superficial branches are separate, and those of the former are more anterior and susceptible to trauma. Sensory deficits are frequently less in magnitude or distribution than motor weakness (Sourkes and Stewart, 1991). Data from a formal assessment study indicates that neuropathies are four times more common in men than women, and causes are idiopathic (16%), related to surgery (22%), prolonged postures (23%), weight loss (15%), and trauma (10%) (Aprile et al., 2005).

Rapid or marked weight loss, from dieting or bariatric surgery (see Chapter 30), is associated with fibular/peroneal neuropathies at the fibular head, likely related to focal pressure from leg-crossing, prolonged sitting, and squatting (Cruz-Martinez et al., 2000). Weight loss ranges from 5–30 kg over a time range from two weeks to 12 months, and a rapid rate of loss may be a factor (Weyns et al., 2007). Spontaneous recovery is good in most patients.

The differential diagnosis of foot drop is broad, and lesion sites include L5 radiculopathy, lumbosacral trunk, sciatic nerve (lateral portion – fibular/peroneal nerve), and common fibular/peroneal nerve. Electrodiagnostic studies are helpful to localize the lesion site.

Diagnostic Evaluation

Electrodiagnostic Evaluation

Nerve conduction studies help determine lesion location, whether there is conduction block at the fibular head, and whether there is axonal loss (Wilbourn, 1986). Motor nerve conduction studies should be performed recording from the anterior tibialis muscle and not the extensor digitorum brevis muscle for the

Table 11.2 Sites, Mechanisms, and Causes of Injury to the Common Fibular/Peroneal Nerve

Site	Anatomy	Pathology	Causes
Hip	Normal	Trauma	Hip surgery
Knee	Normal	Focal pressure	Sleep
			Anesthesia
			Bed rest
			Cast
			Habitual leg crossing
			Squatting/kneeling
			Rapid weight loss
			Aneurysm
			Cyst, ganglion
			Tumor
		Trauma	Fracture
			Dislocation
			Blunt trauma
Ankle	Normal	Focal pressure	Compartment syndrome
			Ganglia
		Trauma	Fracture
			Dislocation
			Sprain

following reasons: the clinical condition is foot drop caused by weakness of the anterior tibialis muscle; the CMAP response maybe absent recording from the extensor digitorum brevis muscle; there may be an accessory deep fibular/peroneal nerve; and the degree of axonal loss may not be distributed equally to both muscles (Katirji and Wilbourn, 1988). Conduction block is evident when there is a loss of CMAP amplitude across the fibular head (stimulating in the popliteal fossa compared to stimulating below the fibular head). Axonal loss is evident when the CMAP amplitude is low to stimulation below the fibular head. Measurement of segmental conduction velocities adds little to determining lesion pathology, and conduction velocity across the fibular head is imprecise as it is difficult to accurately measure the distance along this nerve segment. For both sensory and motor conduction studies, distinguishing between axonal loss and conduction block may not be reliable if testing is performed within four days of an acute axonal lesion, because the distal CMAP amplitude may not show the effects of degeneration within this time period.

Sensory conduction studies of the superficial fibular/peroneal nerve, stimulating and recording distal to the knee, can indicate axonal loss with reduced SNAP amplitude. Sural SNAP is usually normal in the setting of severe common fibular/peroneal nerve lesions because most of the fibers are derived from the tibial nerve (Wilbourn, 1986).

Needle EMG can document axonal loss, but not reliably the degree nor the lesion site along the nerve, but denervation in the short head of the biceps femoris supports a proximal lesions site rather than at the fibular head. Denervation is usually found in one or more muscles innervated by the common fibular/peroneal nerve, but more frequently in those innervated by the deep fibular/peroneal nerve than the superficial fibular/peroneal nerve (Sourkes and Stewart, 1991). EMG of proximal muscles is important to verify that muscles innervated by other nerves (tibial nerve involvement in sciatic nerve lesions or gluteal nerves in lumbosacral plexus lesions) are not involved.

Ultrasound Evaluation

Ultrasound has been applied to common fibular/peroneal neuropathies at the knee as an aid to localization and determination of cause. Abnormalities in cross-sectional nerve area are found at the fibular head (Visser et al., 2013). When electrodiagnostic studies could not localize the lesion the addition of ultrasound identified a site in a substantial portion. In cases with electrodiagnostic evidence for conduction block at the fibular head, an increase in common fibular/peroneal cross-sectional nerve area was observed in about half of patients (Tsukamoto et al., 2014). Ultrasound can detect underlying anatomic causes, such as cysts.

Management

Clinical outcome data are biased to reports of surgical interventions. Large surgical series generally report favorable outcomes, but underlying causes are varied. Some situations clearly benefit from surgery, but similar large non-surgical (conservative) series are not available for comparison (Kim et al., 2004). A study of 25 patients with idiopathic common fibular/peroneal neuropathies at the fibular indicated that 78% had a good recovery (MRC grade ≥4) without surgery (Bsteh et al., 2013).

References

Aprile I, Caliandro P, Giannini F, Mondelli M, Tonali P, Foschini M, et al. Italian multicentre study of peroneal mononeuropathy at the fibular head: study design and preliminary results. *Acta Neurochir Suppl.* 2005;92:63–8.

Bsteh G, Wanschitz JV, Gruber H, Seppi K, Loscher WN. Prognosis and prognostic factors in non-traumatic acute-onset compressive mononeuropathies – radial and peroneal mononeuropathies. *Eur J Neurol.* 2013;20:981–5.

Cruz-Martinez A, Arpa J, Palau F. Peroneal neuropathy after weight loss. *J Peripher Nerv Syst.* 2000;5:101–5.

Katirji MB, Wilbourn AJ. Common peroneal mononeuropathy: a clinical and electrophysiologic study of 116 lesions. *Neurology.* 1988;38:1723–8.

Kim DH, Murovic JA, Tiel RL, Kline DG. Management and outcomes in 318 operative common peroneal nerve lesions at the Louisiana State University Health Sciences Center. *Neurosurgery.* 2004;54:1421–8; discussion 8–9.

Oh SJ. *Clinical Electromyography: Nerve Conduction Studies.* 3rd edn. Philadelphia: Lippincott Williams & Wilkins, 2003.

Sourkes M, Stewart JD. Common peroneal neuropathy: A study of selective motor and sensory involvement. *Neurology.* 1991;41:1029–33.

Tsukamoto H, Granata G, Coraci D, Paolasso I, Padua L. Ultrasound and neurophysiological correlation in common fibular nerve conduction block at fibular head. *Clin Neurophysiol.* 2014;125:1491–5.

Visser LH, Hens V, Soethout M, De Deugd-Maria V, Pijnenburg J, Brekelmans GJ. Diagnostic value of high-resolution sonography in common fibular neuropathy at the fibular head. *Muscle Nerve.* 2013;48:171–8.

Weyns FJ, Beckers F, Vanormelingen L, Vandersteen M, Niville E. Foot drop as a complication of weight loss after bariatric surgery: is it preventable? *Obes Surg.* 2007;17:1209–12.

Wilbourn AJ. AAEE case report #12: Common peroneal mononeuropathy at the fibular head. *Muscle Nerve.* 1986;9:825–36.

Sciatic Nerve Neuropathies

Introduction

The sciatic nerve is well protected, and mononeuropathies result mainly from trauma and a few other causes.

Anatomy

The sciatic nerve represents the common fibular/peroneal and tibial nerves in the segment proximal segment to the popliteal fossa (Figure 12.1, Table 12.1). Thus, it is composed of two separate trunks enclosed in a common sheath; the lateral trunk from L4–S2 roots (posterior division) becomes the common fibular/peroneal nerve, and the medial trunk from L4–S3 roots (anterior division) becomes the tibial nerve. The sciatic nerve begins at the inner wall of the pelvis and exits the pelvis through the sciatic foramen, which is formed by the bony greater sciatic notch and sacrospinus ligament. The nerve passes below the piriformis muscle, but portions of the nerve may pass through the muscle. In the thigh, branches from the medial trunk (tibial segment) innervate the hamstring muscles (semitendinosus, semimembranosus, long head biceps femoris, and adductor magnus), while a branch from the lateral trunk (common fibular/peroneal segment) innervates the short head of the biceps femoris. The nerve ends at the popliteal fossa.

Pathology

The term "sciatica" suggests involvement of the sciatic nerve, but is used indiscriminately for a range of symptoms, most commonly due to lumbar root disease (Ropper and Zafonte, 2015).

Axonal loss can occur from severe trauma to the pelvis. Stretching trauma can be associated with forced dislocation of the hip, stretching during hip arthroplasty surgery, and from focal pressure/ stretching from prolonged and unusual postures (lying with the leg across a firm object in the setting

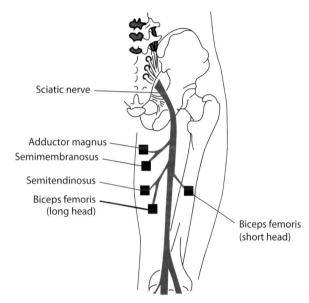

Figure 12.1 Sciatic nerve anatomy. From S Oh, MD, (2003), with permission.

Table 12.1 Predominant Root Innervation of Muscles Supplied by the Sciatic nerve

Muscle	Root Innervation
Semitendinosis	L4–L5–S1
Semimembranosis	L5–S1
Biceps femoris (long/short head)	L4–L5–S1
Adductor magnus	L4–L5–S1

of altered consciousness) (Table 12.2). Damage can occur from hardware fixation cement (heat from polymerization, direct nerve contact from spread). Neurapraxic damage also occurs in these settings.

The lateral division (common fibular/peroneal nerve) is affected more often than the medial division (tibial nerve), and thus can mimic common fibular/ peroneal nerve palsy. Anatomical and physiological

Table 12.2 Sites, Mechanisms, and Causes of Injury to the Sciatic Nerve

Site	Anatomy	Pathology	Causes
Pelvis	Normal	Focal pressure	Piriformis syndrome
		Trauma	Surgery
			Penetrating wound
			Fracture
Leg	Normal	Focal pressure	Tumor
		Trauma	Fracture
			Penetrating wound

explanations are based on differences between the lateral and medial divisions, and include: the lateral division is more superficial in the buttock and proximal thigh and more vulnerable; the lateral division is composed of a single fascicle along a part of its length and may have a single blood supply to this portion; and this division is more tightly tethered between the sciatic notch and neck of the fibula and has less slack during a stretch (Sunderland, 1953).

Sciatic entrapment neuropathy attributed to pressure from the piriformis muscle is controversial, but true neurogenic piriformis syndrome includes a combination of focal pressure and axonal damage (see below) (Stewart, 2003).

Hip

Clinical Features

Sciatic nerve damage in the setting of hip arthroplasty procedures occurs and is commonly mild (subclinical denervation), but may be severe (marked weakness, with greater involvement of common fibular/peroneal division) (Weber et al., 1976). Causes may be difficult to establish and are frequently inferred, and include stretching of the leg, retraction, and hardware fixation cement. Injury to the sciatic nerve can occur months to years after arthroplasty due migration of fixation hardware, and after revisions (Vastamaki et al., 2008).

A posterior thigh compartment syndrome (gluteal compartment syndrome), can result from prolonged pressure on the buttocks and posterior thigh related to unchanged sitting or lying position (floor, toilet seat) associated with stupor or coma (Henson et al., 2009).

The sciatic nerve can be damaged in the setting of endometriosis, due to endometrial tissue, fibrosis, and scar tissue (Torkelson et al., 1988).

Diagnostic Evaluation

Electrodiagnostic evaluation in severe neuropathies shows reduced or absent sural and motor responses in muscles innervated by the common fibular/peroneal motor responses and severe denervation with needle EMG; in mild (subclinical involvement) needle EMG shows the extent of denervation (Weber et al., 1976; Goldberg and Goldstein, 1998; Pekkarinen et al., 1999). Other nerves frequently damaged in addition to the sciatic nerve include the femoral and obturator nerves.

Management

Recovery is variable, from incomplete to complete, and improvement may continue for three years. Surgical intervention may be warranted when nerve damage is extreme (Yeremeyeva et al., 2009).

Pelvis-piriformis Syndrome

Clinical Features

Pressure on the sciatic nerve by the piriformis muscle is controversial because there are variations in definitions, vagueness of clinical features, uncertainty of the validity of test results considered to be diagnostic, and imaging findings that are not discriminating (Stewart, 2003). Criteria supportive of focal sciatic nerve damage (true neurogenic piriformis syndrome) include symptoms consistent with sciatic nerve dysfunction, electrodiagnostic evidence of axonal loss solely in the distribution of the sciatic nerve, and surgical confirmation of focal entrapment with symptomatic relief after decompression. Examples fulfilling the criteria represent rare case reports (Stewart, 2003). The concept of post-traumatic piriformis syndrome includes damage to several nerves (sciatic and gluteal), and does not strictly localized to the piriformis muscle (Benson and Schutzer, 1999).

The most controversial is a nonspecific piriformis syndrome, put forward to account for chronic buttock pain unassociated with objective sciatic nerve damage. Support for the piriformis muscle causing "functional" impairment of the sciatic nerve is largely based on symptoms of deep buttock pain, tenderness to deep palpation in the buttock–proximal thigh region.

The anatomic relationship of the piriformis muscle and sciatic nerve has been examined, and there is normal variation in whether the nerve, or a portion of the nerve, passes through, over, or under the piriformis muscle. Studies of cadavers and observations at surgery find an anomaly from the normal pattern of the nerve passing under the muscle in about 17% of subjects, and extrapolation suggests that a random individual has 23% chance of having a variation on one side (Smoll, 2010). MRI studies indicate that the S1 and S3 roots course above the muscle in most subjects, the S2 root traverses the muscle in 75% of subjects, and asymmetries of muscle size (up to 8 mm) occur in 19% of normal subjects (Russell et al., 2008).

Diagnostic Evaluation

Clinical Tests

Clinical diagnosis of nonspecific piriformis syndrome may be supported by pain with body and leg postures that are designed to intensify contact between the tendinous edge of the piriformis muscle and the sciatic nerve. Features of a true neurogenic piriformis syndrome are weakness of sciatic-innerved muscles.

Electrodiagnostic Evaluation

Electrodiagnostic tests purported to support sciatic nerve involvement that do not include axonal loss focus on prolonged H-wave latencies with the leg in provoking positions (Fishman and Zybert, 1992). Evaluation for a true neurogenic piriformis syndrome focuses on needle EMG abnormalities restricted to muscles innervated by the sciatic nerve.

Imaging Evaluation

If denervation in the distribution of the sciatic nerve is confirmed, imaging of the nerve from roots to the popliteal fossa is indicated as there are a number of etiologies, and entrapment of the nerve by the piriformis muscle is rare. If denervation is found in the distribution of the sciatic nerve the differential diagnosis includes benign and malignant nerve sheath tumors (Thomas et al., 1983; Petchprapa et al., 2010).

Management

Management of nonspecific piriformis syndrome is controversial. Support for the entity is reported symptomatic improvement with both surgical and nonsurgical treatment (Fishman et al., 2002; Fishman and Schaefer, 2003).

If denervation is found and imaging locates a causative lesion, surgery can be considered. If no denervation is found, conservative management is reasonable.

References

Benson ER, Schutzer SF. Posttraumatic piriformis syndrome: diagnosis and results of operative treatment. *J Bone Joint Surg Am.* 1999;81:941–9.

Fishman LM, Dombi GW, Michaelsen C, Ringel S, Rozbruch J, Rosner B, et al. Piriformis syndrome: diagnosis, treatment, and outcome – a 10-year study. *Arch Phys Med Rehabil.* 2002;83:295–301.

Fishman LM, Schaefer MP. The piriformis syndrome is underdiagnosed. *Muscle Nerve.* 2003;28:646–9.

Fishman LM, Zybert PA. Electrophysiologic evidence of piriformis syndrome. *Arch Phys Med Rehabil.* 1992;73:359–64.

Goldberg G, Goldstein H. AAEM case report 32: nerve injury associated with hip arthroplasty. *Muscle Nerve.* 1998;21:519–27.

Henson JT, Roberts CS, Giannoudis PV. Gluteal compartment syndrome. *Acta Orthop Belg.* 2009;75:147–52.

Oh SJ. *Clinical Electromyography: Nerve Conduction Studies.* 3rd edn. Philadelphia: Lippincott Williams & Wilkins, 2003.

Pekkarinen J, Alho A, Puusa A, Paavilainen T. Recovery of sciatic nerve injuries in association with total hip arthroplasty in 27 patients. *J Arthroplasty.* 1999;14:305–11.

Petchprapa CN, Rosenberg ZS, Sconfienza LM, Cavalcanti CF, Vieira RL, Zember JS. MR imaging of entrapment neuropathies of the lower extremity. Part 1. The pelvis and hip. *Radiographics.* 2010;30:983–1000.

Ropper AH, Zafonte RD. Sciatica. *N Engl J Med.* 2015;372:1240–8.

Russell JM, Kransdorf MJ, Bancroft LW, Peterson JJ, Berquist TH, Bridges MD. Magnetic resonance imaging of the sacral plexus and piriformis muscles. *Skeletal Radiol.* 2008;37:709–13.

Smoll NR. Variations of the piriformis and sciatic nerve with clinical consequence: a review. *Clin Anat.* 2010;23:8–17.

Stewart JD. The piriformis syndrome is overdiagnosed. *Muscle Nerve.* 2003;28:644–6.

Sunderland S. The relative susceptibility to injury of the medial and lateral popliteal divisions of the sciatic nerve. *Br J Surg.* 1953;41:300–302.

Thomas JE, Piepgras DG, Scheithauer B, Onofrio BM, Shives TC. Neurogenic tumors of the sciatic nerve. A clinicopathologic study of 35 cases. *Mayo Clin Proc.* 1983;58:640–7.

Torkelson SJ, Lee RA, Hildahl DB. Endometriosis of the sciatic nerve: a report of two cases and a review of the literature. *Obstet Gynecol*. 1988;71:473–7.

Vastamaki M, Ylinen P, Puusa A, Paavilainen T. Late hardware-induced sciatic nerve lesions after acetabular revision. *Clin Orthop Relat Res*. 2008;466:1193–7.

Weber ER, Daube JR, Coventry MB. Peripheral neuropathies associated with total hip arthroplasty. *J Bone Joint Surg Am*. 1976;58:66–9.

Yeremeyeva E, Kline DG, Kim DH. Iatrogenic sciatic nerve injuries at buttock and thigh levels: the Louisiana State University experience review. *Neurosurgery*. 2009;65:A63–6.

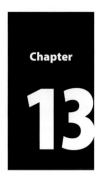

Femoral Nerve Neuropathies

Introduction

Femoral mononeuropathies are not common, and occur in the setting of pelvic surgery and major trauma. They also occur with retroperitoneal hemorrhage, and can be part of lumbosacral radiculoplexus neuropathies (see Chapter 7).

Anatomy

The femoral nerve includes sensory and motor fibers entering and leaving the spinal cord over L2–L4 roots (Table 13.1). The nerve is formed from the lumbar plexus (Figure 13.1), and emerges from the lateral border of the psoas muscle, and leaves the pelvis under the inguinal ligament. It branches in the proximal thigh to supply the quadriceps muscles (rectus femoris, vastus lateralis, vastus medialis, vastus intermedius) and the medial skin of the thigh. It continues down the medial leg to the foot as the saphenous nerve, a sensory nerve that supplies sensation along this band of skin (see Chapter 17)

Pathology

Pathology is frequently iatrogenic, associated with pelvic surgical procedures, and commonly due to stretching of the nerve from retractors (Table 13.2). Less common iatrogenic causes are inadvertent nerve laceration and heat from cement used in joint replacement. These represent axonotmesis or neurotmesis pathology, and, with the latter, nerve regrowth may lead to neuroma formation. Stretch injuries from hematomas likely represent neurapraxic lesions. Damage to the saphenous nerve occurs with harvesting of the saphenous vein for blood vessel grafts.

Muscles in the femoral nerve distribution are involved in diabetic and non-diabetic lumbosacral radiculoplexus neuropathies (see Chapter 28).

Table 13.1 Predominant Root Innervation of Muscles Supplied by the Femoral Nerve

Muscle	Root Innervation
Rectus femoris	L2–L4
Vastus lateralis	L2–L4
Vastus medialis	L2–L4
Vastus intermedius	L2–L4

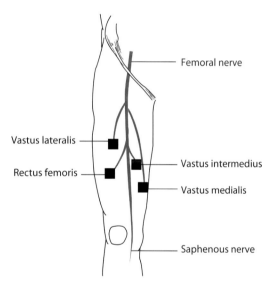

Figure 13.1 Femoral nerve anatomy.
From S Oh, MD, (2003), with permission.

Clinical Features

Femoral nerve lesions result in weakness of quadriceps muscles with difficulty extending the leg at the knee and frequent falls due to the leg giving way at the knee. Sensory loss includes the anterior-medial thigh and the medial aspect of the leg. With isolated saphenous nerve lesions, there is sensory loss along the medial aspect of the leg without weakness.

Table 13.2 Sites, Mechanisms, and Causes of Injury to the Femoral Nerve

Site	Anatomy	Pathology	Causes
Pelvis	Normal	Focal pressure	Hematoma
		Trauma	Surgery
			Pelvic trauma
Leg	Normal	Trauma	Surgery
			Penetrating wounds
			Lithotomy position

Diagnostic Evaluation

Motor nerve conduction studies of the femoral nerve are difficult to interpret as the muscles supplied are large, waveforms are of complex shape, and side-to-side amplitude comparisons are unreliable (Schubert and Keil, 1968). Nerve conduction studies cannot localize the lesion site, as it is not possible to stimulate proximal to the inguinal canal. Investigation relies on needle EMG studies to document denervation in the femoral nerve distribution. If the iliopsoas muscle shows signs of denervation, the lesion site is proximal to the inguinal canal. Sensory nerve conduction studies of the saphenous nerve can be performed to verify saphenous nerve involvement (see Chapter 17) (Wainapel et al., 1978). The medial femoral cutaneous nerve can be studied, and has been found to be abnormal more often than the femoral motor nerve (Oh et al., 2012).

Imagining Evaluation

For proximal lesion sites, when a hematoma is suspected, magnetic resonance imaging of the pelvis can be diagnostic (Weiss and Tolo, 2008).

Management

Management depends upon presumed cause. When a pelvic hematoma is verified, surgical evacuation can be considered. Surgical-based lesions are generally managed conservatively and many have complete functional recovery or significant improvement (Al-Ajmi et al., 2010).

References

Al-Ajmi A, Rousseff RT, Khuraibet AJ. Iatrogenic femoral neuropathy: two cases and literature update. *J Clin Neuromuscul Dis*. 2010;12:66–75.

Oh SJ. *Clinical Electromyography: Nerve Conduction Studies*. 3rd edn. Philadelphia: Lippincott Williams & Wilkins, 2003.

Oh SJ, Hatanaka Y, Ohira M, Kurokawa K, Claussen GC. Clinical utility of sensory nerve conduction of medial femoral cutaneous nerve. *Muscle Nerve*. 2012;45:195–9.

Schubert HA, Keil EW. Femoral nerve conduction velocity. *Am J Phys Med*. 1968;47:302–6.

Wainapel SF, Kim DJ, Ebel A. Conduction studies of the saphenous nerve in healthy subjects. *Arch Phys Med Rehabil*. 1978;59:316–19.

Weiss JM, Tolo V. Femoral nerve palsy following iliacus hematoma. *Orthopedics*. 2008;31:178.

Tibial Nerve Neuropathies

Introduction

The tibial nerve is protected and mononeuropathies are uncommon. Entrapment at the tarsal tunnel is controversial.

Anatomy

The tibial nerve is formed from sensory and motor nerve fibers that enter and leave the spinal cord over roots L5–S1–S2 (Figure 14.1, Table 14.1). The nerve emerges from the lumbosacral plexus and becomes part of the sciatic nerve where it joins with, but remains separate from, nerve fibers that form the common fibular/peroneal nerve. The two nerves travel together in the sciatic nerve to the distal thigh where the sciatic nerve bifurcates and the tibial nerve becomes separate. The tibial nerve leaves the popliteal fossa and travels deep to the two heads of the gastrocnemius muscle, and in the lower leg gives branches, in linear order, to each head of the gastrocnemius muscles, the soleus, posterior tibialis, flexor digitorum longus, and flexor hallucis longus muscles. At the ankle, it passes below the medial malleolus and through the tarsal tunnel, along with three tendons. The roof of the tarsal tunnel is a thin retinaculum. In or close to the tunnel the tibial nerve divides into the medial and lateral plantar nerves: the medial branch innervates the abductor hallucis, flexor digitorum brevis, and flexor hallucis brevis muscles; the lateral branch innervates the abductor digiti minimi, flexor digiti minimi, adductor halluces, and interossei muscles.

Sensory portions of the tibial nerve are the medial sural cutaneous nerve, which joins with the sural communicating nerve from the common fibular/peroneal nerve in the popliteal fossa to form the sural nerve (see Chapter 16). Distally, the calcaneal branch arises at the ankle and supplies sensation to the sole portion of the heel, while the medial and lateral plantar nerves branch in or around the tarsal tunnel and supply sensation to the sole of the foot, and distally form the interdigital nerves to innervate the toes

Pathology

In the popliteal fossa, Baker cysts can cause focal pressure on the nerve (Table 14.2). Nerve sheath tumors may occur anywhere along the nerve. Most lesions include axonal damage, and surgical exploration is common (Kim et al., 2003). Traumatic causes include fractures of long bones and intrinsic bones of the foot, and dislocations and sprains of the ankle.

Nerve damage localized to the tarsal tunnel can result from a variety causes. There is controversy as to whether focal pressure from the flexor retinaculum can account for foot pain unaccompanied by clinical signs of nerve damage. Controversy also exists for diagnostic tests to document this as a pathologic mechanism, and it is not clear whether or when surgical release is indicated (see below) (Campbell and Landau, 2008).

There is a related controversy as to whether nerves in a diabetic polyneuropathy are susceptible to double-crush pathology: metabolic stress from the diabetic neuropathy complicated by nerve compression at specific sites. This, in turn, has led to surgical release of the tibial nerve at the tarsal tunnel (and other nerves in the leg) as a treatment of diabetic polyneuropathy. An evidence-based literature review found no well-controlled studies, and the concept and procedure remain unsubstantiated (Chaudhry et al., 2006).

Knee

Clinical Features

Proximal tibial lesions at the knee cause weakness of all muscles supplied by the tibial nerve, with resultant calf muscle atrophy and weakness of ankle plantar flexion and inversion, and toe plantar flexion. In lesions of mild degree causing mild weakness, testing of toe flexion or having the patient repeatedly support the body on the toes of the affected side can be informative. Sensory loss is along the sole of the foot in the distribution of the sural nerve.

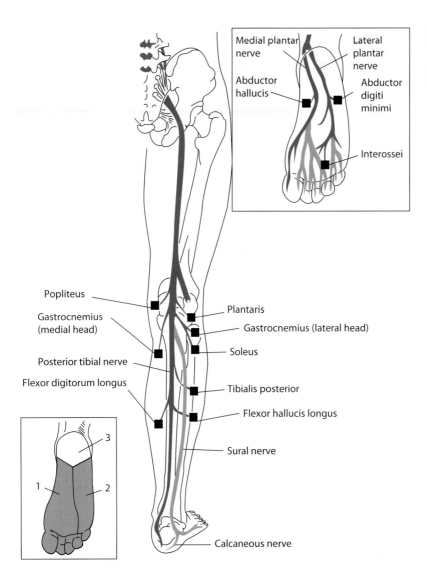

Figure 14.1 Tibial nerve anatomy. Insert lower left: cutaneous innervation (1 = medial plantar nerve, 2 = lateral plantar nerve, 3 = calcaneal branch). From S Oh, MD, (2003), with permission.

Diagnostic Evaluation

Electrodiagnostic Evaluation

Lesions distal to the popliteal fossa can be documented by recording absent or reduced CMAP responses to stimulation at the fossa, but the response to stimulation there is much lower in amplitude than the distal response in normal individuals, and should not be relied upon as sole evidence for such a lesion site (Barkhaus et al., 2011).

Distal tibial motor conduction studies, with comparison to the unaffected side, can document relative axonal loss. However, care must be taken to find the optimal position for the recording electrode on both sides for accurate comparisons (Bromberg and Spiegelberg, 1997). It may be difficult to activate the tibial nerve above the lesion site with stimulation at the popliteal fossa. F-wave and H-wave responses may be prolonged, but do not localize the lesion site.

Needle EMG can verify the distribution of tibial nerve denervation, but muscles innervated by the common fibular/peroneal nerve should also be studied.

Imaging Studies

MRI and ultrasound can be used to identify structural factors causing tibial neuropathies at the knee (Baker cyst) (Lopez-Ben, 2011).

Table 14.1 Predominant Root Innervation of Muscles Supplied by the Tibial Nerve

Muscle	Root Innervation
Gastrocnemius (medial/lateral)	S1–S2
Soleus	L5–S1–S2
Posterior tibialis	L5–S1
Flexor digitorum longus	S1–S2
Flexor halluces longus	S1–S2
Abductor hallucis	L5–S1
Flexor digitorum brevis	L5–S1
Flexor hallucis brevis	S1–S2
Abductor digiti minimi	S1–S2
Flexor digiti minimi	S1–S2
Adductor hallucis	S1–S2
Interossei	S1–S2

Table 14.2 Sites, Mechanisms, and Causes of Injury to the Tibial Nerve

Site	Anatomy	Pathology	Causes
Knee	Normal	Focal pressure	Cyst
			Tumor
		Trauma	Fracture
			Dislocation
			Penetrating wounds
			Injections
Leg	Normal	Focal pressure	Tumor
Ankle	Normal	Trauma	Sprain
	Tarsal tunnel	Focal pressure	Ill-fitting shoes
			Cyst
			Fibrous band
Foot	Normal	Focal pressure	Ganglia
		Trauma	Sprain
			Fracture

Management

Surgical exploration may be indicated when a causative factor is identified.

Ankle

Clinical Features

Nerve damage from trauma at the ankle is usually obvious, and there will be weakness of intrinsic foot muscles and sensory loss along the sole of the foot. There is controversy for idiopathic tarsal tunnel syndrome when there is no history of trauma (or minor trauma likely insufficient to cause nerve damage) and there are no clinical examination findings of nerve dysfunction. Foot and ankle pain may be mistaken for nerve damage.

Diagnostic Evaluation

Electrodiagnostic Evaluation

Nerve conduction studies are essential to support focal pathology at the tarsal tunnel. However, an evidence-based review revealed no adequately controlled studies to guide, which metrics are most sensitive and specific, and whether electrodiagnostic findings are helpful in management (Patel et al., 2005). In general, sensory nerve conduction studies of the medial and lateral plantar nerves can be performed orthodromically with the recording electrode proximal to the flexor retinaculum and stimulation of the great and little toe, respectively, but the responses are of very low amplitude and signals should be averaged to ensure a true nerve signal and achieve adequate resolution for marker placement (Oh et al., 1979). An absent response is supportive, but may also be found in asymptomatic (normal) limbs and in the unaffected limb of symptomatic individuals. The lateral plantar nerve more often than the medial nerve shows slowing of conduction. Use of near-nerve sensory recording techniques may be more sensitive, but technically challenging to perform (Oh et al., 1985). Motor responses may show prolonged distal latency to the abductor hallucis or abductor digiti minimi muscles, but sensory abnormalities may be more sensitive. A staging system has been proposed based on the severity of slowing of sensory and motor distal latencies (Mondelli et al., 2004).

The utility of needle EMG has not been studied. It is noted that abnormal spontaneous activity (positive waves and fibrillation potentials) and often neurogenic motor units (reduced recruitment and high amplitude) may be observed in tibial innervated foot muscles of asymptomatic subjects, and their presence alone cannot support an entrapment neuropathy (Falck and Alaranta, 1983).

Imaging Evaluation

Imaging has been used to help assess tarsal tunnel syndrome, and includes MRI and ultrasound imaging

(Lopez-Ben, 2011). Ultrasound has been used to demonstrate larger cross-sectional nerve diameters proximal to the tarsal tunnel in patients with diabetic neuropathy (Riazi et al., 2012).

Management

Management is dependent upon likely etiology. When there is no electrodiagnostic evidence for focal slowing, as in of suspected tarsal tunnel syndrome, conservative therapy is reasonable. With neurogenic tarsal tunnel syndrome, imaging can be used to guide management. In the setting of diabetes, nerve release surgery at the tarsal tunnel remains unproven (Chaudhry et al., 2006).

References

Barkhaus PE, Kincaid JC, Nandedkar SD. Tibial motor nerve conduction studies: an investigation into the mechanism for amplitude drop of the proximal evoked response. *Muscle Nerve.* 2011;44:776–82.

Bromberg MB, Spiegelberg T. The influence of active electrode placement on CMAP amplitude. *Electroencephalogr Clin Neurophysiol.* 1997;105:385–9.

Campbell WW, Landau ME. Controversial entrapment neuropathies. *Neurosurg Clin N Am.* 2008;19:597–608, vi–vii.

Chaudhry V, Stevens JC, Kincaid J, So YT. Practice Advisory: utility of surgical decompression for treatment of diabetic neuropathy: report of the Therapeutics and Technology Assessment Subcommittee of the American Academy of Neurology. *Neurology.* 2006;66:1805–8.

Falck B, Alaranta H. Fibrillation potentials, positive sharp waves and fasciculation in the intrinsic muscles of the foot in healthy subjects. *J Neurol Neurosurg Psychiatry.* 1983;46:681–3.

Kim DH, Ryu S, Tiel RL, Kline DG. Surgical management and results of 135 tibial nerve lesions at the Louisiana State University Health Sciences Center. *Neurosurgery.* 2003;53:1114–24; discussion 24–5.

Lopez-Ben R. Imaging of nerve entrapment in the foot and ankle. *Foot Ankle Clin.* 2011;16:213–24.

Mondelli M, Morana P, Padua L. An electrophysiological severity scale in tarsal tunnel syndrome. *Acta Neurol Scand.* 2004;109:284–9.

Oh SJ. *Clinical Electromyography: Nerve Conduction Studies.* 3rd edn. Philadelphia: Lippincott Williams & Wilkins, 2003.

Oh SJ, Kim HS, Ahmad BK. The near-nerve sensory nerve conduction in tarsal tunnel syndrome. *J Neurol Neurosurg Psychiatry.* 1985;48:999–1003.

Oh SJ, Sarala PK, Kuba T, Elmore RS. Tarsal tunnel syndrome: electrophysiological study. *Ann Neurol.* 1979;5:327–30.

Patel AT, Gaines K, Malamut R, Park TA, Toro DR, Holland N. Usefulness of electrodiagnostic techniques in the evaluation of suspected tarsal tunnel syndrome: an evidence-based review. *Muscle Nerve.* 2005;32:236–40.

Riazi S, Bril V, Perkins BA, Abbas S, Chan VW, Ngo M, et al. Can ultrasound of the tibial nerve detect diabetic peripheral neuropathy? A cross-sectional study. *Diabetes Care.* 2012;35:2575–9.

Lateral Femoral Cutaneous Nerve Neuropathies

Introduction

The lateral femoral cutaneous nerve is a sensory nerve. It is a common mononeuropathy, and is also referred to as meralgia paresthetica (Greek: "meros" – thigh; "algos" – pain).

Anatomy

The nerve inters the spinal cord via roots L2–L3 and leaves the lumbar plexus along the lateral edge of the psoas muscle (Figure 15.1). It passes under the lateral edge of the inguinal ligament, although it may pass over or have branches, which pass over and under the ligament. The nerve then divides into anterior and posterior branches that pass through the fascia lata and innervate the anterolateral skin of the thigh. There are variations in the area of innervated skin, and innervation may extend below the knee (Stewart, 2012).

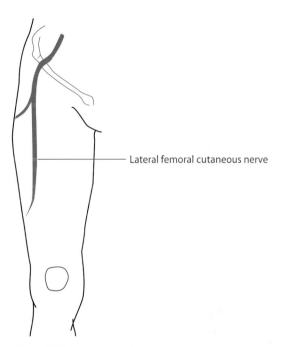

— Lateral femoral cutaneous nerve

Figure 15.1 Lateral femoral cutaneous nerve anatomy. Modified from S Oh, MD, (2003), with permission.

Pathology

Most clinical examples are without obvious cause (idiopathic). Obesity and diabetes are considered risk factors, and a population-based study supports both as associated factors, and thus a metabolic-based pathologic process may underlie some idiopathic cases (Parisi et al., 2011). Some likely represent focal pressure on the nerve reflecting neurapraxic damage with good recovery (Table 15.1) (Berini et al., 2014). Examples are tight and heavy tool belts that exert pressure on the nerve in the area of the inguinal ligament. Iatrogenic nerve damage from surgery on neighboring structures in the pelvis represents axonotmesis or neurotmesis, with delayed or incomplete recovery.

Clinical Features

Meralgia paresthetica may not be clearly recognized by the patient as a neuropathy, as the initial symptoms are frequently described as pain in the hip or in the muscle, and sometimes perceived as weakness. Consequently, another diagnosis is initially entertained (Seror and Seror, 2006). Further questioning reveals surface (cutaneous) pain or altered sensory perception to touch that may be exacerbated by standing and walking. The distribution of altered sensory perception may be smaller than expected from dermatomes (possibly reflecting damage to some and not all nerve fascicles), and may be very posterior (over the buttock) or distal (below the knee), but uncommonly is medial to the midline of the thigh. It may also be bilateral. There should not be objective weakness.

Diagnostic Evaluation

The diagnosis can be made by the history and examination findings.

Table 15.1 Sites, Mechanisms, and Causes of Injury to the Lateral Femoral Cutaneous Nerve

Site	Anatomy	Pathology	Causes
Pelvis	Normal	Focal pressure	Tumor
			Hematoma
		Trauma	Surgical injury
Inguinal ligament	Normal	Focal pressure	Tight clothes
		Trauma	Surgical injury
Thigh	Normal	Focal pressure	Tight clothes
		Trauma	Injections
			Surgical injury
			Wounds

Electrodiagnostic Evaluation

Sensory nerve conduction studies showing an absent lateral femoral cutaneous nerve evoked response are supportive, but there are difficulties in performing the test (Shin et al., 2006). The innervation area of the nerve is variable and there can be uncertainty that the recording electrode is appropriately positioned over nerve branches. Ultrasound can be used to identify proximal branches of the nerve (Boon et al., 2011). It is helpful to first elicit the response from the unaffected leg, and duplicate on the affected side the recording and stimulating electrode positions. However, in some normal subjects a response cannot be elicited on the unaffected side. Body habitus can be an added challenge, and a subdermal or more deeply placed monopolar electrode may record a response when a surface electrode cannot. Somatosensory evoked potential studies have been used in obese patients when routine sensory studies are not diagnostic (Seror, 2004).

Needle EMG is used to verify that the neuropathy is restricted to the sensory nerve and that there is no motor nerve (femoral nerve) involvement.

Management

Conservative care is appropriate for idiopathic cases with attention to lessening the use of tight items about the waist. Interventions may be non-surgical or surgical, but an evidence-based literature review showed no controlled trials to guide choice of interventions (Khalil et al., 2012). Non-surgical interventions include pulsed radiofrequency ablation (inducing focal nerve damage from focal heat) and nerve block. Surgical interventions include neurolysis and neurectomy, with controlled data to guide choices.

References

Berini SE, Spinner RJ, Jentoft ME, Engelstad JK, Staff NP, Suanprasert N, et al. Chronic meralgia paresthetica and neurectomy: a clinical pathologic study. *Neurology*. 2014;82:1551–5.

Boon AJ, Bailey PW, Smith J, Sorenson EJ, Harper CM, Hurdle MF. Utility of ultrasound-guided surface electrode placement in lateral femoral cutaneous nerve conduction studies. *Muscle Nerve*. 2011;44:525–30.

Khalil N, Nicotra A, Rakowicz W. Treatment for meralgia paraesthetica. *Cochrane Database Syst Rev*. 2012;12:CD004159.

Oh SJ. *Clinical Electromyography: Nerve Conduction Studies*. 3rd edn. Philadelphia: Lippincott Williams & Wilkins, 2003.

Parisi TJ, Mandrekar J, Dyck PJ, Klein CJ. Meralgia paresthetica: relation to obesity, advanced age, and diabetes mellitus. *Neurology*. 2011;77:1538–42.

Seror P. Somatosensory evoked potentials for the electrodiagnosis of meralgia paresthetica. *Muscle Nerve*. 2004;29:309–12.

Seror P, Seror R. Meralgia paresthetica: clinical and electrophysiological diagnosis in 120 cases. *Muscle Nerve*. 2006;33:650–4.

Shin YB, Park JH, Kwon DR, Park BK. Variability in conduction of the lateral femoral cutaneous nerve. *Muscle Nerve*. 2006;33:645–9.

Stewart JD. Meralgia paresthetica: Topography of the sensory deficit. *Muscle Nerve*. 2012;46:Abstract 64.

Sural Nerve Neuropathies

Introduction

The sural nerve is important as it is frequently assessed electrodiagnostically for evidence of a peripheral neuropathy and biopsied for assessment of underlying pathology for certain types of neuropathy. It is also harvested as a graft for injured nerves elsewhere in the body. Isolated neuropathies are rare.

Anatomy

The sural nerve is a sensory nerve formed in the popliteal fossa from the joining of branches of the tibial nerve (medial sural cutaneous nerve) and of the fibular/peroneal nerve (sural communication nerve) (Figure 16.1). The sural nerve descends in the posterior portion of the leg, between the two heads of the gastrocnemius muscle. Distally, it moves laterally and passes under the lateral malleoli. The nerve has several branches, including the lateral calcaneal nerve, which innervates the lateral portion of the heel, and, further distally, branches that innervate skin on the lateral side of the foot (from the heel to the little toe) and a dorsal branch to skin between toes IV–V.

Pathology

Nerve injuries result from pressure, trauma, or stretching (Table 16.1). Pressure injuries from ganglia and fibromas represent neurapraxia and usually recover after surgery if a structural cause is identified. Axonal injury from trauma includes penetrating wounds, as a consequence of surgery on close-by areas, or stretch injuries from strains, and recovery is variable (Flanigan and DiGiovanni, 2011; Yuebing and Lederman, 2014).

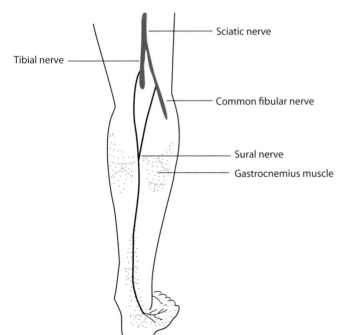

Figure 16.1 Sural nerve anatomy.
Modified from S Oh, MD, (2003), with permission.

Table 16.1 Sites, Mechanisms, and Causes of Injury to the Sural Nerve

Site	Anatomy	Pathology	Causes
Knee	Normal	Focal pressure	Cyst
Leg	Normal	Focal pressure	Casts
			Boots
		Trauma	Vein surgery
Ankle	Normal	Trauma	Fracture
			Dislocation
Foot	Normal	Trauma	Fracture

Clinical Features

Nerve damage is heralded by pain and numbness in the distribution of the nerve (Yuebing and Lederman, 2014).

Diagnostic Evaluation

There is anatomic variability in contributions to the sural nerve from the fibular/peroneal and tibial nerves, and a sensory nerve conduction study supports the majority of the SNAP response from stimulation of the tibial nerve (Kim et al., 2006). Routine sural nerve studies record antidromic conduction along the segment from the lateral portion of the foot to 13–14 cm up the leg. A modification records orthodromic responses with stimulation at the lateral portion of the foot and recording with surface electrodes between toes IV–V (Killian and Foreman, 2001). An ultrasound study of the pathway taken by the sural nerve indicates that a stimulation site 1 cm lateral to the midline of the calf at the level 14 cm from the lateral malleolus is optimal (Kim et al., 2014). Sural nerve damage is confirmed by showing a reduced or absent SNAP. Comparison with the asymptomatic side is helpful as a reduced or absent SNAP response may be part of a peripheral neuropathy.

Management

Removal of sources of focal pressure is appropriate when identified. Neuropathies with unclear cause can be localized and imaged for possible surgical exploration (Flanigan and DiGiovanni, 2011; Yuebing and Lederman, 2014).

References

Flanigan RM, DiGiovanni BF. Peripheral nerve entrapments of the lower leg, ankle, and foot. *Foot Ankle Clin*. 2011;16:255–74.

Killian JM, Foreman PJ. Clinical utility of dorsal sural nerve conduction studies. *Muscle Nerve*. 2001;24:817–20.

Kim CH, Jung HY, Kim MO, Lee CJ. The relative contributions of the medial sural and peroneal communicating nerves to the sural nerve. *Yonsei Med J*. 2006;47:415–22.

Kim KH, Yoo JY, You BC. Ultrasonographic evaluation of sural nerve for nerve conduction study. *Ann Rehabil Med*. 2014;38:46–51.

Oh SJ. *Clinical Electromyography: Nerve Conduction Studies*. 3rd edn. Philadelphia: Lippincott Williams & Wilkins, 2003.

Yuebing L, Lederman RJ. Sural mononeuropathy: a report of 36 cases. *Muscle Nerve*. 2014;49:443–5.

Saphenous Nerve Neuropathies

Introduction

The saphenous nerve can be inadvertently injured during surgical procedures.

Anatomy

The saphenous nerve is a sensory nerve and is a continuation of the femoral nerve (Figure 17.1). In the proximal thigh, it lies deep in Hunter's canal and becomes superficial as it pierces the fascia, about 10 cm above the knee. The infrapatellar branch supplies cutaneous sensation to the lateral part of the knee. The nerve continues down the medial aspect of the leg to the medial malleolus, and supplies sensation to the medial and lateral aspect of the leg, including the arch of the foot.

Pathology

Most causes are complications associated with surgical procedures. Damage can occur during femoral artery surgery in the thigh, and in the leg with saphenous varicose vein surgery and harvesting of the vein for vessel grafting (Table 17.1). Surgery at the knee can damage the infrapatellar branch. Most pathology represents axonal damage, and recovery is variable.

Clinical Features

Symptoms are mild and include sensory loss in the distribution of the infrapatellar branch or the saphenous nerve in the leg. Pain associated with infrapatellar branch damage may be vague, and described as knee pain (Trescot et al., 2013).

Diagnostic Evaluation

Sensory nerve conduction studies of the saphenous nerve can demonstrate an absent response (Wainapel et al., 1978). The infrapatellar nerve can also be studied, but due to anatomic variability, the response cannot always be recorded bilaterally in normal subjects

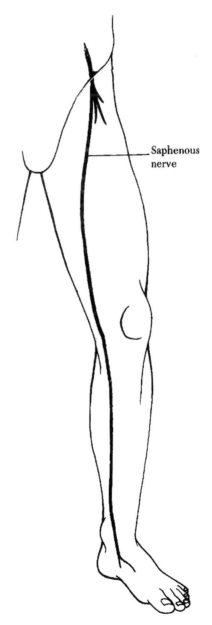

Saphenous nerve

Figure 17.1 Saphenous nerve anatomy.
From S Oh, MD, (2003), with permission.

Table 17.1 Sites, Mechanisms, and Causes of Injury to the Saphenous Nerve

Site	Anatomy	Pathology	Causes
Thigh	Normal	Trauma	Surgery
Knee	Normal	Trauma	Surgery
Leg	Normal	Trauma	Surgery

(Tsenter et al., 2012). To increase confidence in an absent response, verification of an intact response on the asymmetric side is appropriate.

Management

Conservative management is appropriate for surgically related saphenous nerve injuries. For infrapatellar neuropathies, diagnostic injections with local anesthetic may result in long-term pain relief (Trescot et al., 2013). If a compressive cause is considered ultrasound imaging may be helpful to identify a mass.

References

Oh SJ. *Clinical Electromyography: Nerve Conduction Studies*. 3rd edn. Philadelphia: Lippincott Williams & Wilkins, 2003.

Trescot AM, Brown MN, Karl HW. Infrapatellar saphenous neuralgia – diagnosis and treatment. *Pain Physician*. 2013;16:E315–24.

Tsenter J, Schwartz I, Katz-Leurer M, Meiner Z, Goldin D, Vatine JJ. A novel technique for conduction studies of the infrapatellar nerve. *Pm R*. 2012;4:682–5.

Wainapel SF, Kim DJ, Ebel A. Conduction studies of the saphenous nerve in healthy subjects. *Arch Phys Med Rehabil*. 1978;59:316–19.

Acute Immune Neuropathies

Acute immune-mediated neuropathies are characterized by a rapid time course (sudden onset to progression over four weeks) to maximal clinical impairment. They are important to diagnose as most forms are treatable. These neuropathies can be divided into those that reach their nadir within four weeks and those that have sudden onset. The acute progressive neuropathies usually have a polyneuropathy pattern, and are considered to be part of Guillain-Barré syndrome (GBS). The term GBS has evolved, and now includes a number of clinical patterns characterized by a monophasic time course, and caused by antibody-mediated primary demyelination or antibody-mediated pathology at the nodes of Ranvier (nodopathies). Both secondary and primary axonal loss occur, and vary from mild to severe. These are discussed in Chapters 19–21. The acute nonprogressive neuropathies are uncommon and usually involve individual nerves at focal sites. They include mononeuritis multiplex neuropathies, discussed in this section (Chapter 23), and immune-mediated plexopathies, which are discussed in Chapter 7. Nerve damage in these neuropathies is felt to be due to inflammation of microvasculature supplying the nerve, and nerve fiber damage is secondary to focal nerve ischemia.

Guillain-Barré Syndrome: General Features

Introduction

Landry described an acute ascending paralytic disorder with improvement without treatment in 1859. In 1916, Guillain, Barré, and Strohl added the clinical feature of areflexia and cerebral spinal fluid findings of increased protein but normal cell count (cytoalbuminologic dissociation), and the neuropathy has since then been known by the first two authors (Strohl was dropped, for unclear reasons). The term Guillain-Barré syndrome (GBS) initially described the clinical constellation of acute ascending weakness, absent reflexes, frequent weakness of facial muscles, altered bladder dysfunction, and laboratory findings of cytoalbuminologic disassociation in spinal fluid. The term "syndrome" has evolved, and GBS now refers to a number of related forms of acute polyneuropathy with interrelated and overlapping clinical features and pathologies.

Guillain-Barré Syndrome

GBS includes a variety of clinically recognized disorders characterized by progression of weakness, reaching a nadir over days to four weeks, with degrees of spontaneous resolution of impairments (Table 18.1). Acute inflammatory demyelinating polyradiculoneuropathy (AIDP) has traditionally been called GBS (see Chapter 19). Acute motor and sensory axonal neuropathy (AMSAN) is a fulminant form of AIDP (see Chapter 20). Acute axonal motor neuropathy (AMAN) is a motor-only neuropathy (see Chapter 21). It is to be noted that the distinction between AMSAN and AMAN is becoming blurred and they likely represent variations of a single entity. Fisher Syndrome (FS) includes the triad of ophthalmoplegia, ataxia, and areflexia, and occurs alone or combined with AIDP. Bickerstaff brainstem encephalitis (BEE) is similar to FS but includes altered consciousness (see Chapter 22). While the terms AIDP and GBS are used interchangeably in the literature, GBS in this book will

refer to the spectrum of neuropathies, while AIDP will be used for a specific type of GBS. There is overlap of symptoms among forms of GBS, with features of FS combined with AIDP, and distinction between AIDP and AMAN can be challenging: diagnostic criteria are evolving, and distinctions between them are based on electrophysiologic differences, which have support from immunology and experimental animal models (Uncini and Kuwabara, 2012). Despite diagnostic issues, treatment is similar for all forms of GBS.

General Clinical Features

All forms of GBS share features of rapid progression and a monophasic course. AIDP, AMSAN, and AMAN are characterized by symmetric weakness and varying amounts of sensory loss, while with AIDP variants, FS and BEE, weakness and dysfunction involves

Table 18.1 Variants of Acute Inflammatory Demyelinating Polyradiculoneuropathy (AIDP), Fisher Syndrome (FS), and Bickerstaff Brainstem Encephalopathy (BEE)

Type	Clinical Features
AIDP	
Prototypic AIDP	Weakness, sensory loss, areflexia in four limbs
Pharyngeal-cervical-brachal variant	Weakness of pharyngeal, cervical, brachal muscles
Pharyngeal weakness	Weakness of pharyngeal muscles
Paralytic weakness	Weakness of leg muscles
Sensory ataxia	Sensory loss, ataxic gait
AMSAN	Fulmanent weakness, sensory loss
AMAN	Weakness in four limbs
Fisher Syndrome	
Prototypic Fisher Syndrome	Ophthalmaloplegia, weakness, sensory loss, areflexia in four limbs
With AIDP	Ophthalmaloplegia, weakness
Prototypic Bickerstaff encephalopathy	Ophthalmaloplegia, ataxia, somulence

limited body regions. The severity of weakness varies amongst the types and within types of GBS. The natural (untreated) course is for recovery, but the degree varies based on underlying pathology and severity (amount of axonal damage). There may be associated demyelinating lesions in the central nervous system (Mao and Hu, 2014). While GBS is the most common cause of rapidly ascending paralytic disorders, consideration must also be given to a differential diagnosis (Wakerley and Yuki, 2015).

General Pathology

GBS is felt to represent an autoimmune disorder initiated by a systemic infection with production of antibodies that recognize epitomes on nerve gangliosides due to molecular mimicry with epitopes on the infectious agents. Infectious agents vary amongst the forms of GBS, with most data for *Campylobacter jejuni* associated with AMAN, but also cytomegalovirus, Epstein-Barr virus, *Mycoplasma pneumonia*, *Haemophilus influenza*, and influenza A virus, and case reports of other agents. There is recent support for an immunological response in nerves to the Zika virus. Specific antibodies to axonal and myelin gangliosides have been identified among different forms of GBS, but antibodies have not been found in all forms or in all patients (Table 18.2). There may be genetic differences within infectious agents and within patients that predispose to mimicry in the setting of relative common infection agents. An epidemiologic feature is differing geographic distributions amongst some forms of GBS, likely reflecting differences in distributions of infectious triggering agents, patient genetic susceptibilities, and also differences in disease definitions (Table 18.3).

The presence of antibodies leads to a cascade of immunologic events, with unique features among the different forms of GBS. The difference in antibodies and the distribution of antibody recognition sites along peripheral nerves may explain the diversity of clinical features. Consideration of differences in immunopathology is important in interpreting electrodiagnostic findings, and much of the understanding comes from animal models and analysis of serial nerve conduction studies (Uncini and Kuwabara, 2012). The pathology of AIDP is primary demyelination in a multifocal distribution along the nerve, which may include secondary axonal damage. AMAN and AMSAN have focal pathology at the node of Ranvier. This may lead to rapidly reversible

Table 18.2 Antibodies to Nerve Gangliosides Associated with Guillain-Barré Syndrome (GBS) Subtypes

Acute inflammatory demyelinating polyradiculopathy (AIDP)	No specific antibodies
Acute motor axonal neuropathy (AMAN)	GM1a, GM1b, GD1a, GalNAc-GD1a
Acute motor sensory axonal neuropathy (AMSN)	GM1, GD1a
Pharyngeal-cervical brachial variant	GTa, GQ1b, GD1a
Fisher Syndrome (FS)	GQ1b, GTa
Bickerstaff encephalitis	GQ1b, GTa

antibody-mediated alteration at the paranode regions or the nodal axon. Another factor at the node is primary axon loss without evidence for demyelination with subsequent Wallerian degeneration.

General Diagnostic Evaluation

The role of routine testing for ganglioside antibodies in the diagnosis of the various forms of GBS is poor as the frequency of specific antibodies is low and non-specific. The presence of anti-GQ1b antibodies is an exception as they are present in a high proportion of FS and BEE. On the practical side, testing for some antibodies may only be available in research laboratories, and methods of detection are evolving. Further, the time lag for the return of results also limits clinical utility (van den Berg et al., 2014).

Elevated cerebral spinal fluid protein with normal cell counts is a laboratory hallmark of most forms of GBS. However, there is a time course of elevation, and protein levels are frequently normal within the first week after symptom onset (Wong et al., 2015). The overall yield of elevated protein is ~50% for limb forms of GBS and lower for FS. The utility of a lumbar puncture in the diagnostic process is not clear; cytoalbuminologic dissociation within the first week is strongly supportive, but if spinal fluid is normal it is not clear that a second sample a week later provides greater diagnostic certainty than an electrodiagnostic evaluation (or a second nerve conduction study). Further, lumbar punctures are not without morbidity.

General Electrodiagnostic Features

Nerve conduction studies are most important for assessing underlying pathology and distinguishing among GBS forms. For all forms of GBS (except FS

Table 18.3 Geographic Distribution of Forms of Guillain-Barré Syndrome (GBS)

Country	AIDP	AMAN	AMSAN
North America	~90%	~4%	
Europe	~90%	~4%	
Israel	~63%	~22%	~15%
Pakistan	~46%	~31%	
Japan	~36%	~38%	~1–4%
Bangladesh	~22%	~56%	~11%
Mexico		~38%	

Source: Modified from Uncini and Kuwabara (2012).

and BEE) axonal loss, demyelination, and conduction block have a disproportionate effect on sensory nerves, frequently leading to no evoked responses for AIDP and AMSAN. When sensory responses are present, there is a pattern of sensory nerve responses that supports AIDP (see Chapter 19), and normal sensory responses distinguish between AMAN and AMSAN, but recent data indicate some degree of sensory nerve involvement in AMAN (Capasso et al., 2011). Diagnosing GBS and distinguishing between types is assessed by motor nerve conduction studies. Electrodiagnostic findings can evolve over 2–3 weeks (Albers et al., 1985), and two studies are more informative that a single one, and may result in a change in the type of GBS ultimately diagnosed (Uncini et al., 2010).

The main findings in AIDP are attributed to multifocal demyelination, and are slowed conduction greater than expected for the degree of axonal loss (measured by the CMAP amplitude). Metrics include: prolonged distal latency, prolonged F-wave latency, slowed conduction velocity, abnormal temporal dispersion (prolonged negative CMAP peak duration), and conduction block (CMAP area/amplitude loss to proximal stimulation compared to distal stimulation). Tables of electrodiagnostic criteria have been put forward (see Chapter 19).

The main findings in AMAN are severely reduced CMAP amplitude and normal SNAP amplitude. The findings in AMSAN are similar, but also with reduced or absent SNAP amplitude. However, some pathologic features change over the first weeks that affect electrodiagnostic interpretations: reversible conduction block can occur due to transient pathology at the node of Ranvier that blocks conduction but leaves myelin unaffected (non-demyelinating conduction block – nodopathy); pseudo conduction block due to focal axonal loss and nerve conduction testing soon thereafter (days) may result in a relative large distal CMAP and small proximal CMAP, that with retesting several weeks later may show reduction of the distal CMAP (and resolution of the apparent conduction block) due to the effects of Wallerian degeneration; apparent or reversible slowing (prolonged distal latencies and slow conduction velocities) due to temporary block of large-diameter nerve fibers (Uncini and Kuwabara, 2012) (see Chapters 20 and 21).

There may be no electrodiagnostic findings in FS or BEE. However, FS can be associated with AIDP, and will include electrodiagnostic findings for AIDP.

For all forms of GBS, needle EMG is informative for the presence of axonal loss but less so for the degree of loss. There will be some degree of secondary axonal loss in AIDP, marked in AMSAN and AMAN, and none in FS or BEE (Albers et al., 1985).

General Management

Recovery begins without treatment within weeks after reaching the nadir. Treatments with equal efficacy are IVIG and therapeutic plasma exchange (Guillain-Barré Syndrome Study Group, 1985; Hughes et al., 2014). Treatment can hasten the rate of improvement, but it is not clear if treatment within the first two weeks after onset is a factor in the ultimate level of improvement and recovery of function. The main pathologic factor affecting the rate and extent of weakness is the degree of axonal involvement, while older age is a general negative factor. Depending upon the degree of weakness at the nadir, outcomes vary, and 15% have near-normal function, 70% are left with some level of disability, and 15% have marked residual weakness (van den Berg, et al., 2014).

References

Alam TA, Chaudhry V, Cornblath DR. Electrophysiological studies in the Guillain-Barre syndrome: distinguishing subtypes by published criteria. *Muscle Nerve*. 1998;21:1275–9.

Albers JW, Donofrio PD, McGonagle TK. Sequential electrodiagnostic abnormalities in acute inflammatory demyelinating polyradiculoneuropathy. *Muscle Nerve*. 1985;8:528–39.

Aranyi Z, Kovacs T, Sipos I, Bereczki D. Miller Fisher syndrome: brief overview and update with a focus on electrophysiological findings. *Eur J Neurol.* 2012;19:15–20, e1–3.

Bromberg MB, Albers JW. Patterns of sensory nerve conduction abnormalities in demyelinating and axonal peripheral nerve disorders. *Muscle Nerve.* 1993;16:262–6.

Capasso M, Notturno F, Manzoli C, Uncini A. Involvement of sensory fibres in axonal subtypes of Guillain-Barre syndrome. *J Neurol Neurosurg Psychiatry.* 2011;82:664–70.

The Guillain-Barre syndrome Study Group. Plasmapheresis and acute Guillain-Barre syndrome. *Neurology.* 1985;35:1096–104.

Hughes RA, Swan AV, van Doorn PA. Intravenous immunoglobulin for Guillain-Barre syndrome. *Cochrane Database Syst Rev.* 2014:CD002063.

Kuwabara S, Yuki N. Axonal Guillain-Barre syndrome: concepts and controversies. *Lancet Neurol.* 2013;12:1180–8.

Mao Z, Hu X. Clinical characteristics and outcomes of patients with Guillain-Barre and acquired CNS demyelinating overlap syndrome: a cohort study based on a literature review. *Neurol Res.* 2014;36:1106–13.

Overell JR, Hsieh ST, Odaka M, Yuki N, Willison HJ. Treatment for Fisher syndrome, Bickerstaff's brainstem encephalitis and related disorders. *Cochrane Database Syst Rev.* 2007:CD004761.

Uncini A, Kuwabara S. Electrodiagnostic criteria for Guillain-Barre syndrome: a critical revision and the need for an update. *Clin Neurophysiol.* 2012;123:1487–95.

Uncini A, Manzoli C, Notturno F, Capasso M. Pitfalls in electrodiagnosis of Guillain-Barre syndrome subtypes. *J Neurol Neurosurg Psychiatry.* 2010;81:1157–63.

van den Berg B, Walgaard C, Drenthen J, Fokke C, Jacobs BC, van Doorn PA. Guillain-Barre syndrome: pathogenesis, diagnosis, treatment and prognosis. *Nat Rev Neurol.* 2014;10:469–82.

Wakerley BR, Uncini A, Yuki N. Guillain-Barre and Miller Fisher syndromes – new diagnostic classification. *Nat Rev Neurol.* 2014;10:537–44.

Wakerley BR, Yuki N. Mimics and chameleons in Guillain-Barre and Miller Fisher syndromes. *Pract Neurol.* 2015;15:90–9.

Wong AH, Umapathi T, Nishimoto Y, Wang YZ, Chan YC, Yuki N. Cytoalbuminologic dissociation in Asian patients with Guillain-Barre and Miller Fisher syndromes. *J Peripher Nerv Syst.* 2015;20:47–51.

Yuki N. Fisher syndrome and Bickerstaff brainstem encephalitis (Fisher-Bickerstaff syndrome). *J Neuroimmunol.* 2009;215:1–9.

Acute Inflammatory Demyelinating Polyradiculoneuropathy

Introduction

Acute inflammatory demyelinating polyradiculo-neuropathy (AIDP) is the prototypic form of Guillain Barré syndrome (GBS), and likely the form described by Guillain, Barré, and Strohl in 1916. Until other forms of GBS were described, the term GBS was equivalent to AIDP; in the current setting of a spectrum of disorders under GBS, AIDP should be considered a distinct form. AIDP is the most common form of GBS encountered in North America and Europe.

Pathology

An antibody-mediated attack on myelin with complement activation results in segmental or multifocal demyelination along the nerve, from roots to terminal branches. During the recovery phase, when axons are intact, there is proliferation of Schwann cells and subsequent remyelination. However, axons may also be damaged and recovery slowed and compromised. Changes may also occur at the node of Ranvier, which can lead to immune-mediated conduction block without structural damage. This differs from demyelination block in that block at the node can rapidly reverse (days) while remyelination takes more time (weeks). The relative severity of these processes varies amongst patients, and rapidly reversible conduction block is more characteristic of acute motor axonal neuropathy (AMAN) (see Chapter 21).

Clinical Features

Most patients reach their nadir of weakness within four weeks, and many within two weeks (van den Berg et al., 2014). Diffuse lower back pain may precede the onset of neurologic symptoms, presumed to be due to diffuse nerve root inflammation. Motor and sensory nerves are involved, although sensory variants occur (sensory ataxic variant) (Table 19.1). Motor and sensory symptoms are diffuse and symmetrically distributed in legs and arms, both distally and proximally, but

Table 19.1 Motor Nerve Conduction Criteria to Aid in the Diagnosis of AIDP Must Document ≥1 Finding in Each of ≥2 Nerves.

Conduction Velocity	<95% LLN if dCMAP amplitude >50% LLN
	<85% LLN if dCMAP amplitude <50% LLN
Distal Motor Latency	>110% ULN if dCMAP amplitude 100% LLN
	>120% ULN if dCMAP amplitude <100% LLN
pCMAP/dCAMP Amplitude Ratio	<0.7 any dCMAP amplitude
F-wave Latency	>120% any dCMAP amplitude

AIDP: acute inflammatory demyelinating polyradiculoneuropathy; dCMAP: distal compound muscle action potential; pCMAP: proximal compound muscle action potential; LLN: lower limit of normal; ULN: upper limit of normal.

Source: Modified from Albers et al. (1985).

with greater distal involvement in legs. Proximal limb involvement at onset separates this type of neuropathy from length-dependent polyneuropathies where distal arm segments are affected much later (years) than distal leg segments. Regional variations occur (pharyngeal-cervical-brachial, pharyngeal, leg variants – Table 19.1). Sensory abnormalities are numbness and tingling and altered proprioception, touch and vibration. Motor abnormalities are weakness in arms and legs. Tendon reflexes are absent globally, or at least absent in the legs and reduced in the arms. Occasionally patients may transiently exhibit pathologically brisk reflexes and extensor plantar responses. Gait is ataxic (proprioceptive loss) and patients may not be ambulatory due to sensory ataxia and weakness. The degree of severity (weakness) varies, and in the extreme patients may be quadriplegic with respiratory failure. Facial and bulbar weakness can occur, and can include elements of the FS. There is frequent autonomic nervous system involvement with irregular heart rhythms, blood pressure fluctuations, and bowel and bladder stasis. Pain,

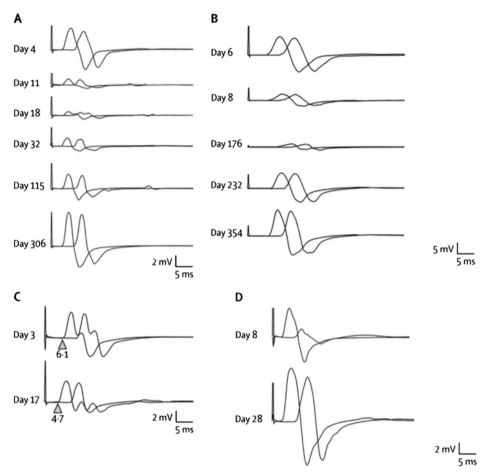

Figure 19.1 Serial nerve conduction studies showing evolution of changes associated with acute inflammatory demyelinating polyradiculoneuropathy (AIDP) and acute motor (and sensory) axonal neuropathies (AMSAN and AMAN). Panel A: AMAN with progressive decline in CMAP amplitude for distal and proximal stimulation without abnormal temporal dispersion or prolonged latencies (normal conduction velocities), followed by progressive increase in amplitude. Panel B: AIDP with progressive decline in CMAP amplitude, abnormal temporal dispersion and slowed conduction, followed by progressive normalization. Panel C: AMAN with reversible conduction block in distal segment with shortening of distal latency from 6.1 to 4.7 msec over 14 days. Panel D: AMAN with reversible conduction block of proximal segment with improvement in proximal CMAP over 20 days.
Modified from Kuwabara and Yuki (2013), with permission.

particularly back pain, is common, and likely reflects involvement of nerve roots.

Diagnostic Evaluation

The clinical pattern of rapid ascending distal and proximal weakness and sensory disturbance with absent or reduced reflexes is fairly distinct, but atypical forms may be more challenging to recognize. Cerebral spinal fluid with cytoalbuminologic dissociation is supportive, but protein levels may be normal in the first week.

Electrodiagnostic Evaluation

Motor nerve conduction studies are more informative than sensory studies. Electrodiagnostic criteria have been proposed, and refinements made based on applying criteria to nerve conduction data from sets of patients with the clinical diagnosis of AIDP, and making modifications to the criteria to include more patients in the test set. Amongst proposed criteria, diagnostic sensitivity reaches up to 75% as assessed in a set of patients with clinical AIDP (Alam et al., 1998). The criteria apply to prototypic AIDP, and fewer electrodiagnostic findings will be encountered amongst AIDP variants.

Electrodiagnostic features are length-dependent conduction changes greater than expected for the degree of axonal loss, and include: prolonged distal latency and F-wave latency, slowed conduction velocity, evidence for abnormal temporal dispersion, and conduction block. Sets of criteria to show primary demyeliation are proportional to distal CMAP amplitude (need to show greater slowing with reduced amplitude) and can be difficult to follow. A set of criteria with 75% sensitivity (Alam et al., 1998) and straightforward to follow is in Table 19.1 (Albers et al., 1985), and other sets are available (Hadden et al. 1998; Ho et al. 1995). Serial studies are important as pathologic changes can evolve over several weeks, and a sufficient spectrum of abnormal findings may not be apparent early on to make the diagnosis of AIDP (Albers et al., 1985) or some electrodiagnostic features may be transient and resolve and lead to a change in diagnosis from AIDP to AMAN (Figure 19.1) (see also Chapter 21) (Uncini et al., 2010).

Sensory nerve responses are frequently absent, but a pattern of normal sural SNAP and abnormal median nerve SNAP is encountered in one-third of patients with AIDP and is less common in length-dependent neuropathies (Bromberg and Albers, 1993). This is attributed to the recording of sural responses at a relatively more proximal site along the nerve compared to a more distal site along digital nerves.

Needle EMG shows evidence of distal axonal loss to varying degrees in the majority of patients (Albers et al., 1985).

Management

Treatment of AIDP by plasma exchange (~4 plasma apheresis treatments) has been shown in a placebo-controlled trial to be effective in hastening recovery when started within the first two weeks after onset (The Guillan Barré Study Group, 1985). Intravenous immunoglobulin (2 g/kg) has not been assessed in placebo-controlled trials, but is equally effective compared to plasma exchange (Hughes et al., 2014). Supportive care is important, and during the acute phase includes monitoring respiratory function, autonomic dysfunction, and pain control, and during rehabilitation, physical therapy, and evaluation for bracing (van den Berg et al., 2014).

References

Alam TA, Chaudhry V, Cornblath DR. Electrophysiological studies in the Guillain-Barre syndrome: distinguishing subtypes by published criteria. *Muscle Nerve*. 1998;21:1275–9.

Albers JW, Donofrio PD, McGonagle TK. Sequential electrodiagnostic abnormalities in acute inflammatory demyelinating polyradiculoneuropathy. *Muscle Nerve*. 1985;8:528–39.

Bromberg MB, Albers JW. Patterns of sensory nerve conduction abnormalities in demyelinating and axonal peripheral nerve disorders. *Muscle Nerve*. 1993;16:262–6.

The Guillain-Barre syndrome Study Group. Plasmapheresis and acute Guillain-Barre syndrome. *Neurology*. 1985;35:1096–104.

Hadden RD, Cornblath DR, Hughes RA, Zielasek J, Hartung HP, Toyka KV, et al. Electrophysiological classification of Guillain-Barre syndrome: clinical associations and outcome. Plasma Exchange/ Sandoglobulin Guillain-Barre Syndrome Trial Group. *Ann Neurol*. 1998;44:780–8.

Ho TW, Mishu B, Li CY, Gao CY, Cornblath DR, Griffin JW, et al. Guillain-Barre syndrome in northern China. Relationship to *Campylobacter jejuni* infection and anti-glycolipid antibodies. *Brain*. 1995;118 (Pt 3):597–605.

Hughes RA, Swan AV, van Doorn PA. Intravenous immunoglobulin for Guillain-Barre syndrome. *Cochrane Database Syst Rev*. 2014:CD002063.

Kuwabara S, Yuki N. Axonal Guillain-Barre syndrome: concepts and controversies. *Lancet Neurol*. 2013;12:1180–8.

Uncini A, Manzoli C, Notturno F, Capasso M. Pitfalls in electrodiagnosis of Guillain-Barre syndrome subtypes. *J Neurol Neurosurg Psychiatry*. 2010;81:1157–63.

van den Berg B, Walgaard C, Drenthen J, Fokke C, Jacobs BC, van Doorn PA. Guillain-Barre syndrome: pathogenesis, diagnosis, treatment and prognosis. *Nat Rev Neurol*. 2014;10:469–82.

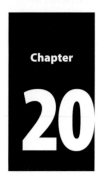

Acute Motor and Sensory Axonal Neuropathy

Introduction

Acute motor and sensory axonal neuropathy (AMSAN) is a very rare form of Guillain-Barré syndrome (GBS) characterized by a severe degree of weakness and sensory loss following a very rapid time course (over days) (Kuwabara and Yuki, 2013). Recovery is slow and incomplete due to marked axonal loss. The concept of AMSAN as a distinct clinical and pathologic entity is evolving because some features overlap with acute motor axonal neuropathy (AMAN) (see Chapter 21).

Clinical Features

The clinical pattern was initially called "axonal or fulminant GBS" because of rapid progression (<10 days) to quadriplegia and ventilatory failure associated with inexcitable nerves during nerve conduction testing. It is to be noted that all forms of AIDP have a degree of axonal loss, and AMSAN represents cases with extensive loss in the form of inexcitable nerves (see below).

Pathologic Features

AMSAN is characterized by extensive denervation with involvement of dorsal and ventral roots as well as more distal nerves. In the first cases described, nerve biopsy and postmortem examination showed extensive axonal loss and no evidence for demyelination, while in later cases there was evidence for primary demyelination and secondary axonal loss. Hence, inexcitable nerves can result from two fulminant pathologic processes (Feasby et al., 1993). There are also data in some patients supporting antibody-mediated pathology at the node of Ranvier as a possible third pathologic process (Uncini and Kuwabara, 2012).

Diagnostic Evaluation

Nerve conduction studies show early on very low amplitude or inexcitable sensory and motor nerve

Table 20.1 Electrodiagnostic Criteria for Acute Motor Axonal Neuropathy (AMAN)

No evidence for demyelination	
CMAP	<80% LLN
SNAP	<50% LLN

Source: Modified from Unicini and Kuwabara (Uncini and Kuwabara, 2012).

responses. Nerve conduction criteria have been proposed (Table 20.1). Electrodiagnostic findings in some patients include reversible conduction block in both motor and sensory nerves upon serial studies and serial studies are necessary to document reversible changes (Figure 19.1) (Uncini and Kuwabara, 2012). There is extensive denervation on needle EMG.

Management

There are minimal data on treatment with IVIG or plasma exchange, and many patients are quadriplegic and require respiratory support within days after onset of weakness. General patient care during prolonged ventilatory support is important, and mortality can be significant. With time (months) there is a degree of recovery, but given the degree of axonal involvement marked residual deficits are common.

References

Feasby TE, Hahn AF, Brown WF, Bolton CF, Gilbert JJ, Koopman WJ. Severe axonal degeneration in acute Guillain-Barre syndrome: evidence of two different mechanisms? *J Neurol Sci.* 1993;116:185–92.

Kuwabara S, Yuki N. Axonal Guillain-Barre syndrome: concepts and controversies. *Lancet Neurol.* 2013;12:1180–8.

Uncini A, Kuwabara S. Electrodiagnostic criteria for Guillain-Barre syndrome: a critical revision and the need for an update. *Clin Neurophysiol.* 2012;123:1487–95.

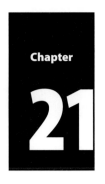

Acute Motor Axonal Neuropathy

Introduction

Acute motor axonal neuropathy (AMAN) is rare in North America and Europe and more common in Asia, Central America, and South America (Kuwabara and Yuki, 2013). Originally considered to involve only motor nerve fibers, subclinical involvement of sensory nerves can be demonstrated in some patients, and the distinction between AMAN and acute motor sensory axonal neuropathy (AMSAN) is less specific with overlap of features (see Chapter 20) (Uncini and Kuwabara, 2012).

Clinical Features

Progression of weakness is rapid (over weeks), frequently resulting in quadriplegia and respiratory failure, but without significant sensory symptoms. There is less cranial nerve involvement compared to acute inflammatory demyelinating polyradiculoneuropathy (AIDP). Tendon reflexes are preserved, and may be increased in a small percentage. Autonomic dysfunction is rare.

Pathologic Features

AMAN is characterized by antibody-mediated conduction block or axonal loss at the nodes of Ranvier (Uncini and Kuwabara, 2012). Underlying mechanisms, gleaned from experimental animal models, is complement deposition at the node with loss of sodium channels, resulting in conduction failure without damage to myelin, and this can explain relatively rapid improvements in strength in some patients. Axonal damage can also occur due to complement deposition and formation of membrane attack complex at the axolema at nodes of Ranvier, and this can explain slow improvements in strength in some patients. There is an association with *Campylobacter jejuni* infection and much of the data are from demonstrating molecular mimicry between epitopes on the bacterium and nerve.

Table 21.1 Electrodiagnostic Criteria for Acute Motor Axonal Neuropathy (AMAN)

No evidence for demyelination	
CMAP	<80% LLN
SNAP	<50% LLN

Source: Modified from Uncini and Kuwabara (Uncini and Kuwabara, 2012).

Diagnostic Evaluation

Motor nerve conduction criteria are similar to those for AMSAN (Table 21.1), but an element of reversible conduction block (reversible conduction failure) can be demonstrated with serial studies in some patients (Uncini and Kuwabara, 2012). The import of this is that, early on in the course, initial nerve conduction studies may show a pattern suggestive of primary demyelination, but a second study may show resolution of conduction block and a change in diagnosis from AIDP to AMAN in a proportion of patients (Figure 19.1). The presence of sensory nerve responses in AMAN distinguishes it from AMSAN, and SNAP amplitudes, if low, are above the lower limit of normal. However, patients with clinical AMAN can have subclinical electrodiagnostic involvement of sensory nerves demonstrated by increases in SNAP amplitude in serial nerve conduction studies (Capasso et al., 2011).

Management

There are no controlled trials, and treatment effects with IVIG or plasma exchange are inconsistent. However, it is appropriate to treat with IVIG or plasma exchange. Supportive care remains the most important element.

References

Capasso M, Notturno F, Manzoli C, Uncini A. Involvement of sensory fibres in axonal subtypes of Guillain-Barre syndrome. *J Neurol Neurosurg Psychiatry.* 2011;82:664–70.

Kuwabara S, Yuki N. Axonal Guillain-Barre syndrome: concepts and controversies. *Lancet Neurol.* 2013;12:1180–8.

Uncini A, Kuwabara S. Electrodiagnostic criteria for Guillain-Barre syndrome: a critical revision and the need for an update. *Clin Neurophysiol.* 2012;123:1487–95.

Chapter 22

Fisher Syndrome and Bickerstaff Encephalitis

Introduction

Fisher syndrome (FS) is frequently referred to as the Miller-Fisher syndrome, based on the erroneous assumption that the original description was by two individuals, but Charles Miller Fisher was a single individual. Guillain, after the initial report in 1916, recognized a spectrum of clinical presentations in 1938, including restricted involvement of cranial nerves, preceding Fisher's report in 1957 (Shahrizaila and Yuki, 2013). FS and Bickerstaff brainstem encephalitis (BEE) share clinical features, with the addition of altered consciousness in BEE. Features of FS may occur in conjunction with acute inflammatory demyelinating polyradiculoneuropathy (AIDP) and AIDP variants (Wakerley et al., 2014).

Pathologic Features

Initial efforts to localize the site of pathology focused on the central nervous system (cerebellum and brainstem) to account for ataxia and ophthalmoplegia (Shahrizaila and Yuki, 2013). In support are changes in brain MRI and electroencephalography (EEG), more with BEE than with FS. However, the discovery of anti-GQ1b and GT1b antibodies in a large percentage of patients with both disorders linked the two as a spectrum, and has been referred to as the "anti-GQ1b antibody syndrome." GQ1b is expressed at paranodes and neuromuscular junctions of cranial nerves III, IV, and VI to account for ophthalmoplegia, and cranial nerves IX and X to account for oropharyngeal involvement in variants. Anti-GQ1b antibodies label group Ia muscle spindle afferent fibers, and ataxia is thought to be due to loss of proprioception (Yuki, 2009).

The pathophysiology focuses on molecular mimicry linked most commonly with *Campylobacter jejuni* (also *Haemophilus influenzae*) infections in many patients with FS and BEE (Shahrizaila and Yuki, 2013). Within the anti-GQ1b antibody syndrome, the clinical presentation likely depends, in part, upon the infective bacterial strain and individual patient susceptibility. The expression of GQ1b at paranodes, combined with the association with the above infectious agents and the observation that some patients with FS have reversible conduction block demonstrated on serial nerve conduction studies, links FS and AMAN as nodopathies (see Chapter 21). Another aspect that may be a factor (speculative at this time) with BEE is reduced blood-brain barrier at the area postrema in the brain stem, allowing antibody access to the central nervous system.

Clinical Features

FS is a combination of ophthalmoplegia, ataxia, or areflexia, while BEE includes altered consciousness (drowsiness) and hypersomnolence (Odaka et al., 2003; Wakerley et al., 2014). BEE may also include upper motor neuron features (brisk tendon reflexes and extensor plantar responses). Patients with BEE may have marked weakness. Both progress over days to weeks, with a natural resolution. Both FS and BEE are rare amongst the full spectrum of GBS in North America and Europe (1–5%: BEE occurs less frequently than FS), but are more common in Asia (2025%) (Shahrizaila and Yuki, 2013). FS may remain restricted to the triad, or be combined over a time course of ~7 days with variants of AIDP (~15% with pharyngeal-cervical-brachial; see Chapter 19), or classic AIDP (~15%), or with altered consciousness to BEE (~15%) (Sekiguchi et al., 2016). There are reports of FS with acute motor axonal neuropathy (AMAN).

Diagnostic Evaluation

The triad features of FS, and the added feature of somnolence in BEE, are evident clinically. An antecedent illness is supportive (Shahrizaila and Yuki, 2013).

They may occur in combination with motor and sensory features of AIDP or variants.

Laboratory Evaluation

GQ1b and GT1a antibodies are found in 83–100% of patients (differences may represent laboratory and reporting techniques) in the first week (Yuki, 2009). Elevated CSF protein occurs more frequently during the second week. EEG abnormalities (diffuse slowing) are more common in BEE.

Electrodiagnostic Evaluation

Isolated FS and BEE have few electrodiagnostic abnormalities, which are mild in degree: motor nerve findings may include prolonged distal motor latency, slowed conduction velocity, reduced CMAP amplitude, and, most commonly, prolonged H-wave latency; sensory nerve findings are reduced SNAP amplitude (Aranyi et al., 2012).

Management

There are no randomized controlled treatment trials, but for isolated FS, comparisons between no treatment, treatment with IVIG, or plasma exchange, show no clinical differences in outcome, which is generally good (Overell et al., 2007). Treatment data are less clear for BEE, while outcome is generally good, treatment protocols have included no treatment, steroids, IVIG, and plasma exchange, either alone or in various combinations (Overell et al., 2007). A minority of patients with BEE require ventilator support and some have died, and thus it is reasonable to consider treating patients with IVIG (Yuki, 2009).

References

Aranyi Z, Kovacs T, Sipos I, Bereczki D. Miller Fisher syndrome: brief overview and update with a focus on electrophysiological findings. *Eur J Neurol*. 2012;19:15–20, e1–3.

Odaka M, Yuki N, Yamada M, Koga M, Takemi T, Hirata K, et al. Bickerstaff's brainstem encephalitis: clinical features of 62 cases and a subgroup associated with Guillain-Barre syndrome. *Brain*. 2003;126:2279–90.

Overell JR, Hsieh ST, Odaka M, Yuki N, Willison HJ. Treatment for Fisher syndrome, Bickerstaff's brainstem encephalitis and related disorders. *Cochrane Database Syst Rev*. 2007:CD004761.

Sekiguchi Y, Mori M, Misawa S, Sawai S, Yuki N, Beppu M, et al. How often and when Fisher syndrome is overlapped by Guillain-Barre syndrome or Bickerstaff brainstem encephalitis? *Eur J Neurol*. 2016;23:1058–63.

Shahrizaila N, Yuki N. Bickerstaff brainstem encephalitis and Fisher syndrome: anti-GQ1b antibody syndrome. *J Neurol Neurosurg Psychiatry*. 2013;84:576–83.

Wakerley BR, Uncini A, Yuki N. Guillain-Barre and Miller Fisher syndromes – new diagnostic classification. *Nat Rev Neurol*. 2014;10:537–44.

Yuki N. Fisher syndrome and Bickerstaff brainstem encephalitis (Fisher-Bickerstaff syndrome). *J Neuroimmunol*. 2009;215:1–9.

Vasculitic Neuropathy

Introduction

Vasculitic neuropathy refers to neuropathies where the underlying pathology is inflammation of blood vessels that supply nerves (microvasculitis), and the resultant ischemia leads to focal nerve damage. Nerve involvement is usually a single nerve (mononeuropathy), but there can be progression to involve other nerves (mononeuritis multiplex). There are a number of classification schemes based on the presence or absence of an underlying systemic autoimmune disease, or based on the size of vessels involved (Table 23.1) (Jennette et al., 2013; Gwathmey et al., 2014). Vasculitis of peripheral nerves can occur with or without systemic autoimmune disease. The frequency of a vasculitic neuropathy in the setting of a system autoimmune disease is not clear and depends upon criteria used, but is high when there is active vasculitis of large vessels; uncommonly the vasculitis it can be restricted to small vessels in peripheral nerves. However, in the clinical setting of an unusual mononeuropathy or several mononeuropathies (mononeuropathy multiplex) it is important to consider a vasculitic cause as it may be treatable, or at least progression can be impeded.

Proximal neuropathies (cervical and lumbosacral radiculoplexus neuropathy, with or without diabetes) are also considered to be vasculitic neuropathies (microvasculitis) (Collins et al., 2010), and are considered in Chapters 7 and 28.

Pathology

The pathologic finding in involved nerves or neighboring muscles is necrosis of blood vessel walls resulting in occlusion and focal ischemia of small vessels. There is inflammation of the vessel wall and necrosis of the tunica median intima, hemosiderin-laden macrophages, complement deposition, and the presence of fibrinogen (Collins et al., 2010). This causes nerve fiber loss, and evidence for subsequent nerve fiber regeneration.

Table 23.1 Classification of Vasculidities Based on Size of Blood Vessels Involved (Left) and Frequently Associated Systemic Diseases (Right)

Vessel Size	Systemic Diseases
Large vessel	Takayasu
	Giant cell
Medium vessel	Polyartritis nodosa
Small vessel	ANCA-associated
	Wegeners
	Churg-Strauss
Variable vessel	Behçet
Systemic diseases	Lupis erythematosis
	Rheumatoid arthritis
	Sarcoid
	Hepatitis C
	Cancer-related

Clinical Features

The key clinical feature is pain, sensory loss, and weakness in the distribution of a single nerve (mononeuritis) or multiple nerves (mononeuritis multiplex). The most common nerve involved in the legs is the common fibular/peroneal nerve, and in the arms the ulnar nerve, but proximal nerves affecting hip and shoulder strength are also involved (Collins et al., 2003). Pain is deep, with or without cutaneous pain, and weakness is in the distribution of the nerve. Only a portion of a nerve's sensory and motor territory may be involved. There can be progression over days to involve other nerves. However, if smaller nerves are involved, progression may be slower and the patient may not seek medical attention until there is confluence of mononeuropathies into an asymmetric or symmetric distal polyneuropathy, or the neuropathy can progress as a distal symmetric polyneuropathy (Collins et al., 2003; Lacomis and Zivkovic, 2007). In this situation, it may be difficulty to determine a stepwise progression, and a vasculitic neuropathy may not be considered.

Diagnostic Evaluation

Laboratory Evaluation

A consensus recommendation for laboratory investigation for suspected vasculitic neuropathy has been put forward (Table 23.2), but abnormalities are supportive and not definitive (Collins et al., 2010). Erythrocyte sedimentation rate is the most commonly abnormal test, and other tests are not elevated in a consistent pattern (Collins et al., 2003).

Nerve Biopsy

The definitive test is a nerve biopsy, seeking evidence for inflammatory cells in vessel walls and some combination of fibrinoid necrosis, disrupted endothelium, altered internal elastic lamina, thrombosis, and vascular or perivascular hemorrhage (see Chapter 2) (Collins et al., 2010). Findings are sought almost always in a sensory nerve as excision of the nerve and the resultant further loss of sensory perception can be tolerated by the patient. It is important that the nerve be clinically involved, as verified by an absent or low-amplitude SNAP response on nerve conduction studies (Lacomis and Zivkovic, 2007). The most commonly biopsied nerve is the sural nerve, but the superficial fibular/superficial peroneal or superficial radial nerves are appropriate if affected. Vasculitic lesions can involve limited segments of the nerve (skipped lesions), and may be missed when only a small number of histologic sections are assessed, and microscopic sections along a length of nerve may need to be viewed. Inclusion of a neighboring muscle can improve the chance of finding pathology by ~20% (Agadi et al., 2012).

Electrodiagnostic Evaluation

Nerve conduction studies classically show an asymmetric and non-length-dependent pattern (mononeuritis multiplex), but other patterns are described, such as symmetric or asymmetric polyneuropathy, and mononeuropathy (Lacomis and Zivkovic, 2007). Involvement is supported by absent sensory and motor responses. When the pathology is less severe, asymmetric responses are supportive, but there should be a >50% side-to-side difference in response amplitude to be clinically significant (Bromberg and Jaros, 1998). Since nerve infarcts can occur abruptly, nerve conduction studies performed

Table 23.2 Basic Laboratory Tests in the Setting of Peripheral Nerve Vasculitis

Complete blood count
Erythrocyte sedimentation rate
C-reactive protein
Rheumatoid factor
Antinuclear antibodies
Myeloperoxidase
Anti-neurrophil cytoplasmic antibodies
Vascular endothelial growth factor
Serum protein electrophoresis
Cryoglobulins
Hepatitis B & C antigens

within days after the event may show apparent focal conduction block across the site; however, block is transient as it resolves when retested days to a week later due to the fact that it takes days for the distal segment to degenerate and stop conducting impulses (Chaudhry and Cornblath, 1992). Needle EMG will show evidence for axonal loss (positive waves and fibrillation potentials), but may take several weeks from the event. Needle EMG can help define denervation in proximal muscles whose innervating nerve cannot be easily stimulated during nerve conduction studies.

Management

Pharmacologic treatment of a vasculitic neuropathy is imperative, and should be aggressive. This is particularly so in cases with both large and small vessel disease as there is a significant mortality associated with the underlying systemic autoimmune disease, and the neuropathy can progress with significant morbidity (Collins et al., 2003). Treatment can be divided into induction and maintenance phases, and consensus guidelines are available (Collins et al., 2010). The duration of each phase is governed by patient response. Induction is commonly with corticosteroids, 1 gm/kg for several months followed by a very slow taper. Cyclophosphamide pulse therapy or rituximab may be needed in severe cases. Methotrexate can be added to steroids in milder cases. Maintenance therapy includes lower doses of corticosteroids, methotrexate, azathioprine, and mycophenolate. In cases with hepatitis C-related cyroglobulins, antiviral drugs are added.

Treatment of microvasculitides involving only peripheral nerves includes similar doses of corticosteroids for induction, and for maintenance a more rapid taper with lower doses of corticosteroids, plus the addition of methotrexate, azathioprine, and mycophenolate as needed.

The response to treatment is slow, with initial reduction in pain, but it may take one to three years for improvements in strength due to the slow pace of axonal regrowth. Patients must be monitored for relapses, and treated accordingly. The long-term prognosis includes mortality from a variety of causes, and only ~10% are symptom-free while the majority have some degree of disability (Collins et al., 2003).

References

Agadi JB, Raghav G, Mahadevan A, Shankar SK. Usefulness of superficial peroneal nerve/peroneus brevis muscle biopsy in the diagnosis of vasculitic neuropathy. *J Clin Neurosci.* 2012;19:1392–6.

Bromberg MB, Jaros L. Symmetry of normal motor and sensory nerve conduction measurements. *Muscle Nerve.* 1998;21:498–503.

Chaudhry V, Cornblath DR. Wallerian degeneration in human nerves: serial electrophysiological studies. *Muscle Nerve.* 1992;15:687–93.

Collins MP, Dyck PJ, Gronseth GS, Guillevin L, Hadden RD, Heuss D, et al. Peripheral Nerve Society Guideline on the classification, diagnosis, investigation, and immunosuppressive therapy of non-systemic vasculitic neuropathy: executive summary. *J Peripher Nerv Syst.* 2010;15:176–84.

Collins MP, Periquet MI, Mendell JR, Sahenk Z, Nagaraja HN, Kissel JT. Nonsystemic vasculitic neuropathy: insights from a clinical cohort. *Neurology.* 2003;61:623–30.

Gwathmey KG, Burns TM, Collins MP, Dyck PJ. Vasculitic neuropathies. *Lancet Neurol.* 2014;13:67–82.

Jennette JC, Falk RJ, Bacon PA, Basu N, Cid MC, Ferrario F, et al. 2012 revised International Chapel Hill Consensus Conference Nomenclature of Vasculitides. *Arthritis Rheum.* 2013;65:1–11.

Lacomis D, Zivkovic SA. Approach to vasculitic neuropathies. *J Clin Neuromuscul Dis.* 2007;9:265–76.

Chronic Immune Neuropathies

Immune neuropathies can be divided by time course of progression into acute and chronic time courses, and the former are discussed in Chapters 18–22. The time course of chronic immune neuropathies is progression over >8 weeks. The chronic immune neuropathies can be divided into two general patterns, one with diffusely distributed nerve involvement (chronic inflammatory demyelinating polyradiculoneuropathy – CIDP and variants), and the other a mono- or multiplex nerve pattern with focal conduction block (multifocal motor neuropathy – MMN and multifocal acquired demyelinating and sensory neuropathy – MADSAM or Lewis-Sumner syndrome – LSS) (Table 24.1). Within the CIDP division are variants associated with systemic disorders. The underlying pathology is felt to be immune-mediated, affecting myelin or nodes of Ranvier. There are patterns of nerve conduction abnormalities that help distinguish them from primary axonal neuropathies. These neuropathies are rare, but potentially treatable with immunomodulating therapies.

Chronic Inflammatory Demyelinating Polyradiculoneuropathy

Introduction

Chronic inflammatory demyelinating polyradiculo-neuropathy (CIDP) is the prototypic chronic immune-mediated polyneuropathy, and the most common form. There are variations with sensory or motor predominance, ataxia, distal distribution, and rare forms that are restricted to one limb (Table 24.1).

Pathology

The primary pathology is multifocal demyelination. Pathology data are mostly from distal leg sensory nerve biopsies, but postmortem studies indicate pathology distributed along the entire length of nerves (see Chapter 2). However, there may be a predilection at proximal and distal sites. There is evidence for repeated Schwann cell proliferation and remyelination leading to onion bulb formations, and secondary axonal loss. Proximal nerves may be enlarged on imaging studies.

Supportive data for immune mechanisms come from clinical responses to immunomodulating treatment regimens and plasmapheresis. The underlying pathologic mechanisms are complex and involve combinations of cell-mediated and humoral interactions, and vary amongst types of CIDP (Mathey et al., 2015). Features include breakdown of the blood-nerve barrier allowing accumulations of T-cells and macrophages and inflammatory proteins. T-cells are activated and are involved in destruction of myelin and axons. Antibodies are involved, but specific types are uncommonly identified. Recent data focuses on antibody involvement specific to non-compact myelin and the axon at nodes of Ranvier, causing functional conduction block that can be readily reversed with treatment, more rapidly than expected for remyelination after demyelination (nodopathy).

Clinical Features

Symptoms of weakness and sensory loss affect both distal and proximal limb segments of legs and arms

Table 24.1 Patterns and Variants of Chronic Immune-Mediated Neuropathies

Neuropathy	Patterns and Variants
CIDP	Prototypic, distal and proximal, motor > sensory, symmetric
	Sensory-predominant
	Motor-predominant
	Focal limb distribution
	Associated with monoclonal gammopathy
	Associated with myelin-associated glycoprotein antibodies (anti-MAG)
	Polyneuropathy, organomegaly, endocrinology, monoclonal gammopathy, skin changes (POMES)
	Chronic ataxic neuropathy, ophthalmoplegia, IgM paraprotein, cold aggultinins, disialosyl antibodies (CANOMAD)
DADS	Distal, sensory > motor, symmetric
MMN	Mononeuritis multiplex, motor, focal conduction block
MADSAM or LSS	Mononeuritis multiplex, motor and sensory, focal conduction block

Chronic inflammatory demyelinating polyradiculopathy (CIDP); distal predominant axonal demyelinating sensory neuropathy (DADS); multifocal motor neuropathy with conduction block (MMN); multifocal acquired demyelinating sensory and motor neuropathy (MADSAM) or Lewis-Sumner Syndrome (LSS).

early in the course, although weakness and sensory loss is greatest distally in the legs and arms. Symptoms and signs are usually symmetric in distribution. Patients have difficulty with ambulation due to weakness of leg muscles and proprioceptive loss. Bulbar dysfunction and respiratory compromise are uncommon, and mild if present. Tendon reflexes are absent or reduced (Dyck et al., 1975). This pattern differs from the stocking-glove loss in primary axonal polyneuropathies, where only ankle reflexes

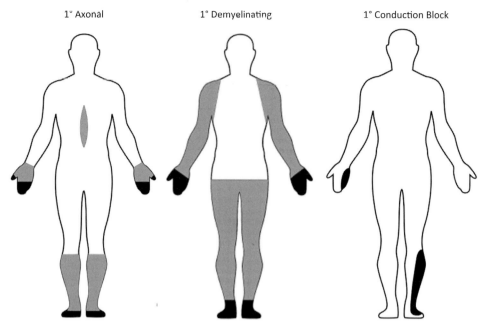

1° Axonal   1° Demyelinating   1° Conduction Block

Figure 24.1 Figurines of the distribution of nerve involvement, contrasting primary axonal (length-dependent), with primary demyelinating (distal > proximal), and focal conduction block away from sites of entrapment (mononeuritis or mononeuritis multiplex) (modified from Bromberg and Brownell, 2012).

are reduced or lost (Figure 24.1). The time course is progressive, and may include a step-wise or rarely relapsing and remitting pattern, and progression is over a relatively few months compared to slowly progressive stocking-glove polyneuropathies over years. Approximately 5% of CIDP presents acutely (within weeks) and are given an initial diagnosis of acute inflammatory demyelinating polyradiculoneuropathy (AIDP), but symptoms relapse and require additional treatments beyond eight weeks (Ruts et al., 2010).

Diagnostic Evaluation

Nerve conduction studies are the most important test to support primary demyelination. Cerebrospinal fluid may have an increased protein due to breakdown of the blood-nerve barrier but normal cell count. Optional nerve biopsy can directly show segmental demyelination (Van den Bergh et al., 2010).

Electrodiagnostic Evaluation

Electrodiagnosis is mainly based on motor nerve conduction studies demonstrating features of primary demyelination in the form of conduction slower than expected for the degree of axonal loss. These include prolonged distal and F-wave latencies,

slowed conduction velocities, abnormal temporal dispersion, and conduction block. At least 16 sets of electrodiagnostic criteria have been proposed, and sensitivity and specificity are 60–90% (Bromberg, 2011). Fulfillment of criteria is based on documenting a number of demyelinative features in a number of nerves, and the required numbers vary amongst criteria. The heterogeneous nature of underlying pathology amongst patients results in diagnoses of definite, probable, possible CIDP, designations perhaps more important for research or clinical trials than in the clinic. A comparison of 14 sets of criteria (Breiner and Brannagan, 2014) favored the European Federation of Neurological Societies/Peripheral Nerve Society (EFNS/PNS) criteria as having a reasonable balance between sensitivity (73%) and specificity (91%) (Hughes et al., 2006) (Table 24.2). Sets of criteria vary in complexity and can be cumbersome to use, and one approach is to consider nerve conduction values based on guideline limits of slowing greater than in primary axonal neuropathies as a trigger for considering CIDP (Table 4.3 and see Chapter 4), after which one of the formal criteria can be consulted (Bromberg, 2011).

Sensory nerves are involved, and ~50% of CIDP patients have absent responses. When responses are present, patterns of sensory involvement can be

Table 24.2 European Federation of Neurological Societies/Peripheral Nerve Society (EFNS/PNS) for Chronic Inflammatory Demyelinating Polyradiculoneuropathy (CIDP)

Either conditions I, II, or III:

I: For definite CIDP at least one of the following:

Prolonged distal latency in two or more nerves: >150% of ULN

Reduced conduction velocity in two or more nerves: <70% of LLN

Prolonged F-wave in two nerves (10–15 trials):
>120% of ULN if CMAP amplitude >80% of LLN
>150% of ULN if CMAP amplitude <80% of LLN

or

Absent F-wave in two nerves:
>120% of ULN if CMAP amplitude <80% of LLN

plus

at least one other demyelinating feature

Partial conduction block in two nerves:

Proximal:distal duration ratio <0.5 if CMAP amplitude >20% of LLN

or

Partial conduction block in one nerve plus at least one other feature

Abnormal temporal dispersion in two nerves:

Proximal:distal duration >130%

or

Distal CMAP duration >9 ms in one nerve plus

and

At least one other demyelinating feature in one or more nerves

II: For probable CIDP:

Partial conduction block in two nerves:

Proximal:distal duration ratio <0.7 with if CMAP amplitude >20% of LLN (excluding posterior tibial nerve)

or

Partial conduction block in one nerve plus at least one other feature

III: For Possible CIDP:

As in I, but in only one nerve

Compound muscle action potential (CMAP); lower limit of normal (LLN); upper limit of normal (ULN).

Source: Modified from Hughes et al. (2006; EFNS/PNS, 2010).

supportive of a primary demyelinating neuropathy. One pattern is greater involvement of the median nerve (digital nerves) compared to the sural or superficial radial nerves (Bromberg, 2011). The pattern of abnormal median/normal sural or radial nerve conduction metrics is felt to be due to greater pathologic involvement of distal nerve segments recorded from digital median nerves compared to more proximal recording sites for sural or radial nerves. This pattern is observed in about >25% of CIDP patients,

and is less common in length-dependent axonal polyneuropathies.

Needle EMG frequently shows evidence for axonal loss attributed to secondary pathology and is encountered more commonly in distal muscles.

Ultrasound

While motor nerve conduction studies have a primary role in documenting nerve abnormalities, ultrasound has been used, especially to assess proximal nerve segments that are difficult to study electrodiagnostically (Jang et al., 2014). Nerve cross-sectional area is increased in about half of nerves, and is higher in nerve segments with slowed conduction (Di Pasquale et al., 2015).

Magnetic Resonance Imaging

Magnetic resonance imaging (MRI) frequently shows enlargement of nerve roots and in the plexuses (Beydoun et al., 2012), and may be helpful in cases of atypical CIDP to show nerve root enlargement in affected limbs (Lozeron et al., 2016).

Laboratory Studies

Spinal fluid analysis is supportive with increased protein and normal cell counts, but is elevated only in ~25% of patients. Cytoalbuminologic dissociation does not exclude other causes of neuropathy, such as diabetic neuropathy.

A clinically unsuspected monoclonal gammopathies is found in 10–30% of patients with CIDP, commonly IgM or IgG and rarely IgA subtypes (Bromberg et al., 1992). There are no clinical or electrodiagnostic differences between those with and without a gammopathy. However, there are rare demyelinating neuropathies associated with plasma cell dyscrasias, including POEMS syndrome (polyneuropathy, organomegaly, endocrinopathy, monoclonal gammopaty, and skin changes), multiple myeloma, plasmacytomas, Waldenström macroglobulinema, malignant lymphoma, and amyloidosis (EFNS/PNS, 2010). If a paraprotein is found, an evaluation for a subclinical plasma cell dyscrasia by quantitative testing of immunoglobulins in serum and urine and a skeletal x-ray survey is warranted. If no dyscrasia is found, the paraprotein can be considered a monoclonal gammopathy of uncertain significance (MGUS); however yearly surveillance by quantitative immunoglobulins is importance as there is a 1%-per-year conversion to a dyscrasias (EFNS/PNS, 2010).

A portion of patients with an IgM gammopathy also have antibodies to myelin-associated glycoprotein (anti-MAG) (EFNS/PNS, 2010). With this combination, there is frequently a unique clinical pattern of slowly progressive sensory ataxia and an electrodiagnostic pattern of symmetric distal-predominant demyelination (distal acquired demyelinating symmetric – DADS), which is discussed in Chapter 25.

Nerve biopsy is helpful when electrodiagnostic studies are equivocal, showing onion bulb formations and alternations of myelin profiles on teased fiber preparations (Dyck et al., 1975).

Management

A number of first-line treatment modalities are available that include corticosteroids, immunoglobulins, and plasmapheresis, but with no consensus for order, dosing, or taper schedules. Selection considerations are cost, side effects, and convenience. A treatment trial of immunosuppression is warranted when there is supportive evidence for CIDP. However, it is recommended that clear measureable treatment endpoints be established as ~25% of patients achieve remission but continue to be treated, and a sizable portion of patients "feel" a need for continued treatment (Cornblath et al., 2013; Querol et al., 2013). Principles of treatment strategies and use of endpoint measures are considered in Chapter 48.

Corticosteroids

Corticosteroids have been shown to be effective, largely based on empiric evidence and small open-label trials (Hughes and Mehndiratta, 2015). Oral prednisone (or prednisolone) has traditionally been given as initial doses of 60 mg daily or 120 mg every other day, followed by a taper based on patient response, but with no consensus on taper schedules (see also Chapter 48) (Bromberg and Carter, 2004). The onset time of improvement is within weeks. An advantage of oral corticosteroids is their very low cost and ease of delivery. Corticosteroids are associated with significant side effects and there have been attempts at different formulations and protocols to reduce them. Oral methylprednisolone (500 mg) weekly or four days per month has been used for varying lengths of time, followed by a slow taper (Muley et al., 2008), but with no consensus for these variables. Intravenous methylprednisolone (1000 mg monthly) has also been

given (Eftimov et al., 2012; Boru et al., 2014) to reduce side effects from more frequent dosing.

Immunoglobulin

Immunoglobulin is pooled and processed gammaglobulin fraction from over 10,000 donors. Randomized and placebo-controlled trials of immunoglobulin administered intravenously (IVIG) show an improvement in function and strength within two to six weeks (Eftimov et al., 2013). Some patients respond rapidly, suggesting functional conduction block at the node of Ranvier, while most improve slowly attributed to remyelination and require periodic infusions. Maximal improvement with treatment occurs at about six months (Hughes et al., 2008). There are no objective data on initial or subsequent dosing or tapering, but traditional dosing carried over from other diseases is an initial dose of 2 gm/kg in divided infusions over several days, followed by maintenance doses of 1 gm/kg in a single infusion over one day (see also Chapter 48). Maintenance doses are traditionally scheduled at three- to four-week intervals until maximal response is achieved. Taper schedules may maintain the 1 gm/kg dose and increase the interval, or keep the interval at four weeks (immunoglobulin half-life) and decrease the dose (Rajabally, 2015). Due to high cost, dosing by ideal body weight over total weight is a consideration, and a large trial indicates that a maximum of 160 gm for the 2 gm/kg and 80 gm for 1 gm/kg are effective (Hughes et al., 2008; Anderson and Olson, 2015). Intravenous infusions are administered by a nurse in a medical setting (infusion center), but can be administered in a patient's home with a nurse supplied by a home infusion company. The cost of IVIG is high.

Immunoglobulin can be infused into subcutaneous tissue as this route may be more convenient for the patient as it does not require a venipuncture and side effects may be less. Subcutaneous infusions are more convenient for the patient as they are infused by the patient at home and take place at night. There is no difference in half-life based on route of administration. From a small number of cases, smaller doses infused more frequently are well tolerated and effective (Rajabally, 2014).

Plasmapheresis

Plasmapheresis or therapeutic plasma exchange is a process where whole blood is removed from the patient, cells are separated and infused back into the patient, and a fraction of plasma is discarded. The rationale is that the discarded plasma contains immune factors, including antibodies and proteins, which results in a reduction in the inflammatory process. Plasmapheresis is performed as a series, usually four to six exchanges on an every-other-day schedule. An evidence-based review indicates a prompt response (within days), but of short duration (lasting 7–14 days), presumably because production of pathogenic antibodies and proteins is not reduced (Mehndiratta and Hughes, 2012). Peripheral access for two catheters is required (one for withdrawal and the other for infusion), which can be difficult to maintain in many patients, and central venous access is usually required. Most patients are hospitalized for the infusion series, and the overall cost is high. Plasmapheresis is usually reserved for reversing marked weakness, and is used in conjunction with immunosuppression medications.

Treatment Outcome

The clinical response to corticosteroids, intravenous immune globulin, and plasmapheresis is generally good and ~80% of patients have improvement in strength and function, although in many trials response is assessed over a relatively short time period (~12 weeks), whereas CIDP is a chronic disease. Plasmapheresis is generally considered a temporary treatment modality, as the immune system is not modified, while corticosteroids and immunoglobulins have a modulating effect on immune function. Long-duration follow-ups show general equivalence between corticosteroids and intravenous immune globulin (Rajabally, 2015).

Other Treatment Options

About 20% of CIDP patients do not respond to corticosteroids, IVIG, or plasmapheresis. It is to be noted that some patients may respond to corticosteroids and not IVIG, and vice versa. While an evidence-based review found no support for other immunomodulating drugs due to a lack of placebo controls (Mahdi-Rogers et al., 2013), there are reports of responses to azathioprine, methotrexate, cyclophosphamide, cyclosporine A, mycophenolate mofetil, interferon beta-Ia, entanercept, alemtuzumab, rituximab, and allogeneic blood stem cell transplantation. From a series of patients not responding to steroids or IVIG, 37% responded to one of the following drugs either alone or switched from one to another if no response: azathioprine, methotrexate, cyclophosphamide, cyclosporine A, mycophenolate mofetil, interferon beta-Ia, rituximab (Cocito et al., 2011). Accordingly, if the diagnosis of CIDP is secure, different immunomodulating agents can be considered.

References

European Federation of Neurological Societies/Peripheral Nerve Society Guideline on management of paraproteinemic demyelinating neuropathies. Report of a Joint Task Force of the European Federation of Neurological Societies and the Peripheral Nerve Society – first revision. *J Peripher Nerv Syst.* 2010;15(3):185–95.

Anderson CR, Olson JA. Correlation of weight-based i.v. immune globulin doses with changes in serum immunoglobulin G levels. *Am J Health Syst Pharm.* 2015;72(4):285–9.

Beydoun SR, Muir J, Apelian RG, Go JL, Lin FP. Clinical and imaging findings in three patients with advanced inflammatory demyelinating polyradiculoneuropathy associated with nerve root hypertrophy. *J Clin Neuromuscul Dis.* 2012;13(3):105–12.

Boru UT, Erdogan H, Alp R, Tasdemir M, Yildirim S, Bilgic A, et al. Treatment of chronic inflammatory demyelinating polyneuropathy with high dose intravenous methylprednisolone monthly for five years: 10-Year follow up. *Clin Neurol Neurosurg.* 2014;118:89–93.

Breiner A, Brannagan TH, III. Comparison of sensitivity and specificity among 15 criteria for chronic inflammatory demyelinating polyneuropathy. *Muscle Nerve.* 2014;50(1):40–6.

Bromberg MB. Review of the evolution of electrodiagnostic criteria for chronic inflammatory demyelinating polyradicoloneuropathy. *Muscle Nerve.* 2011;43(6):780–94.

Bromberg MB, Brownell AA. Role of electroidagnosis in the evaluation of peripheral neuropathies. *Intestbook of Peripheral Neuropathy*, Donofrio PD (ed). New York: Demosmedical; 2012.

Bromberg MB, Carter O. Corticosteroid use in the treatment of neuromuscular disorders: empirical and evidence-based data. *Muscle Nerve.* 2004;30(1):20–37.

Bromberg MB, Feldman EL, Albers JW. Chronic inflammatory demyelinating polyradiculoneuropathy: comparison of patients with and without an associated monoclonal gammopathy. *Neurology.* 1992;42(6):1157–63.

Cocito D, Grimaldi S, Paolasso I, Falcone Y, Antonini G, Benedetti L, et al. Immunosuppressive treatment in refractory chronic inflammatory demyelinating polyradiculoneuropathy. A nationwide retrospective analysis. *Eur J Neurol.* 2011;18(12):1417–21.

Cornblath DR, Gorson KC, Hughes RA, Merkies IS. Observations on chronic inflammatory demyelinating polyneuropathy: A plea for a rigorous approach to diagnosis and treatment. *J Neurol Sci.* 2013;330(1–2):2–3.

Di Pasquale A, Morino S, Loreti S, Bucci E, Vanacore N, Antonini G. Peripheral nerve ultrasound changes in CIDP and correlations with nerve conduction velocity. *Neurology.* 2015;84(8):803–809.

Dyck PJ, Lais AC, Ohta M, Bastron JA, Okazaki H, Groover RV. Chronic inflammatory polyradiculoneuropathy. *Mayo Clin Proc.* 1975;50(11):621–37.

Eftimov F, Vermeulen M, van Doorn PA, Brusse E, van Schaik IN. Long-term remission of CIDP after pulsed dexamethasone or short-term prednisolone treatment. *Neurology.* 2012;78(14):1079–84.

Eftimov F, Winer JB, Vermeulen M, de Haan R, van Schaik IN. Intravenous immunoglobulin for chronic inflammatory demyelinating polyradiculoneuropathy. *Cochrane Database Syst Rev.* 2013;12:CD001797.

Hughes RA, Bouche P, Cornblath DR, Evers E, Hadden RD, Hahn A, et al. European Federation of Neurological Societies/Peripheral Nerve Society guideline on management of chronic inflammatory demyelinating polyradiculoneuropathy: report of a joint task force of the European Federation of Neurological Societies and the Peripheral Nerve Society. *Eur J Neurol.* 2006;13(4):326–32.

Hughes RA, Donofrio P, Bril V, Dalakas MC, Deng C, Hanna K, et al. Intravenous immune globulin (10% caprylate-chromatography purified) for the treatment of chronic inflammatory demyelinating polyradiculoneuropathy (ICE study): a randomised placebo-controlled trial. *Lancet Neurol.* 2008;7(2):136–44.

Hughes RA, Mehndiratta MM. Corticosteroids for chronic inflammatory demyelinating polyradiculoneuropathy. *Cochrane Database Syst Rev.* 2015;1:CD002062.

Jang JH, Cho CS, Yang KS, Seok HY, Kim BJ. Pattern analysis of nerve enlargement using ultrasonography in chronic inflammatory demyelinating polyneuropathy. *Clin Neurophysiol.* 2014;125(9):1893–9.

Lozeron P, Lacour MC, Vandendries C, Theaudin M, Cauquil C, Denier C, et al. Contribution of plexus MRI in the diagnosis of atypical chronic inflammatory demyelinating polyneuropathies. *J Neurol Sci.* 2016;360:170–5.

Mahdi-Rogers M, van Doorn PA, Hughes RA. Immunomodulatory treatment other than corticosteroids, immunoglobulin and plasma exchange for chronic inflammatory demyelinating polyradiculoneuropathy. *Cochrane Database Syst Rev.* 2013;6:CD003280.

Mathey EK, Park SB, Hughes RA, Pollard JD, Armati PJ, Barnett MH, et al. Chronic inflammatory demyelinating polyradiculoneuropathy: from pathology to phenotype. *J Neurol Neurosurg Psychiatry.* 2015.

Mehndiratta MM, Hughes RA. Plasma exchange for chronic inflammatory demyelinating polyradiculoneuropathy. *Cochrane Database Syst Rev.* 2012;9:CD003906.

Muley SA, Kelkar P, Parry GJ. Treatment of chronic inflammatory demyelinating polyneuropathy with pulsed oral steroids. *Arch Neurol.* 2008;65(11):1460–4.

Querol L, Rojas-Garcia R, Casasnovas C, Sedano MJ, Munoz-Blanco JL, Alberti MA, et al. Long-term outcome in chronic inflammatory demyelinating polyneuropathy patients treated with intravenous immunoglobulin: a retrospective study. *Muscle Nerve.* 2013;48(6):870–6.

Rajabally YA. Subcutaneous immunoglobulin therapy for inflammatory neuropathy: current evidence base and future prospects. *J Neurol Neurosurg Psychiatry.* 2014;85(6):631–7.

Rajabally YA. Long-term Immunoglobulin therapy for chronic inflammatory demyelinating polyradiculoneuropathy. *Muscle Nerve.* 2015;51(5):657–61.

Ruts L, Drenthen J, Jacobs BC, van Doorn PA. Distinguishing acute-onset CIDP from fluctuating Guillain-Barre syndrome: a prospective study. *Neurology.* 2010;74(21):1680–6.

Van den Bergh PY, Hadden RD, Bouche P, Cornblath DR, Hahn A, Illa I, et al. European Federation of Neurological Societies/Peripheral Nerve Society guideline on management of chronic inflammatory demyelinating polyradiculoneuropathy: report of a joint task force of the European Federation of Neurological Societies and the Peripheral Nerve Society – first revision. *Eur J Neurol.* 2010;17(3):356–63.

Chronic Inflammatory Demyelinating Polyradiculoneuropathy: Variants and Syndromes

Introduction

Among chronic inflammatory demyelinating polyradiculoneuropathies, classic chronic inflammatory demyelinating polyradiculoneuropathy (CIDP) is the most common form (~50%), but variants are recognized and include a distal-predominant variant, pure sensory variant (~35%), pure motor variant (~10%), and focal limb variant (rare). They are considered variants of CIDP because of moderately rapid progression (more rapid than distal-predominant polyneuropathies), electrodiagnostic findings of primary demyelination in motor nerves, sensory nerve biopsy supporting demyelination, monoclonal proteins in ~20%, and high response rate (~90%) to corticosteroids or IVIG (Viala et al., 2010; Nobile-Orazio, 2014). CIDP can also part of a syndrome involving other organ systems (see below).

CIDP Variants

Distal Acquired Demyelinating Symmetric Neuropathy

Distal acquired demyelinating symmetric neuropathy (DADS) is characterized by symptoms and signs in a distal-predominant, sensory > motor (or sensory only), and legs > arms distribution (Katz et al., 2000). Those with only sensory symptoms and signs may overlap with the sensory CIDP variant (see below). The majority of DADS patients are male and progression leading to the diagnosis is slower than for those with a diagnosis of CIDP. Many patients have an IgM paraprotein (which is uncommon in CIDP), and a large percentage have antibodies to myelin-associated glycoprotein (anti-MAG) (EFNS/PNS, 2010). Pathologically, there is a widening of myelin lamellae on nerve biopsy felt due to the anti-MAG antibody. The clinical issue is distinguishing DADS patients from those with length-dependent axonal polyneuropathy.

Electrodiagnostic features are prolonged distal motor latencies, low or absent SNAPs, and no abnormal temporal dispersion in motor nerves. The response to immunomodulating treatments for patients with DADS patients without an IgM protein is similar to CIDP, while the response is less for those with an IgM protein.

Sensory Variant

In sensory variant CIDP, sensory symptoms predominate despite motor nerve conduction abnormalities of primary demyelination (Ayrignac et al., 2013). Symptoms are paresthesias, pain, proprioceptive ataxia, reduced reflexes or areflexia, and progression to include arm involvement. Somatosensory evoked potentials were uniformly abnormal. Response to immunotherapy is good.

Motor Variant

Motor variant CIDP is rare with symptoms of weakness, and it is unclear if they represent multifocal motor neuropathy (Nobile-Orazio, 2014).

Focal Limb Variant

There are rare reports of chronic and progressive unilateral or asymmetric arm weakness and sensory loss, associated with motor nerve conduction abnormalities consistent with primary demyelination, and with response to immune-modulating treatment (Thomas et al., 1996).

CIDP as Part of a Syndrome

Chronic neuropathies with primary demyelinating features can be part of a syndrome with involvement of other organ systems. The pathology is felt to involve the immune system as the syndromes frequently include a monoclonal gammopathy and respond to immunomodulating therapy.

POEMS Syndrome

POMES syndrome consists of polyneuropathy, organomegaly, endocrinopathy, monoclonal gammopathy, and skin changes and is considered a paraneoplastic syndrome (Dispenzieri, 2014). Other names encountered for this syndrome are osteosclerotic myeloma, Takatsuki syndrome, and Crow-Fukase syndrome. Not all features are required for the diagnosis, and it can be challenging to make it. Two required mandatory major criteria are: CIDP-like neuropathy and a monoclonal gammopathy (the majority of patients also have lambda light chains). One major criterion is also required: sclerotic bone lesions or elevated vessel endothelial growth factor (VEGF). Finally, one or more minor criteria are also required: organomegaly, extravascular volume overload, endocrinopathy, skin changes, papilledema, thrombocytosis, or erythrocytosis.

Castleman disease is a lymphoproliferative disorder (angiofollicular lymph node hyperplasia), without a monoclonal gammopathy, and is part of POEMS syndrome in ~20%.

Management is based on the spectrum of associated features, and treatment focuses on agents that address the monoclonal gammopathy.

CANOMAD

CANOMAD is the collection of chronic (sensory) ataxic neuropathy, ophthalmoplegia, IgM paraprotein, cold agglutinins, and disialosyl antibodies (Willison et al., 2001). The clinical features are male predominance, slow progression of disabling ataxia frequently affecting legs (preventing ambulation) and arms, paresthesias affecting limbs and trigeminal nerve distributions, relative preservation of strength, and weakness of eye movements.

Electrodiagnostic findings are prominent sensory nerve abnormalities, and either primary demyelination or axonal motor nerve abnormalities. IgM anti-ganglioside antibodies against disialosyl gangliosides are present, as is an IgM monoclonal protein. It is interesting that antibody specificity includes GQ1b,

which is also encountered in Fisher Syndrome. The presence of cold agglutinins occurs in ~50%. Case reports of successful treatment include IVIG, rituximab, and plasmapheresis.

References

Ayrignac X, Viala K, Koutlidis RM, Taieb G, Stojkovic T, Musset L, et al. Sensory chronic inflammatory demyelinating polyneuropathy: an under-recognized entity? *Muscle Nerve.* 2013;48(5):727–32.

Dispenzieri A. POEMS syndrome: 2014 update on diagnosis, risk-stratification, and management. *Am J Hematol.* 2014;89(2):214–23.

European Federation of Neurological Societies/Peripheral Nerve Society Guideline on management of paraproteinemic demyelinating neuropathies. Report of a Joint Task Force of the European Federation of Neurological Societies and the Peripheral Nerve Society – first revision. *J Peripher Nerv Syst.* 2010;15(3):185–95.

Katz JS, Saperstein DS, Gronseth G, Amato AA, Barohn RJ. Distal acquired demyelinating symmetric neuropathy. *Neurology.* 2000;54(3):615–20.

Magy L, Kabore R, Mathis S, Lebeau P, Ghorab K, Caudie C, et al. Heterogeneity of Polyneuropathy Associated with Anti-MAG Antibodies. *J Immunol Res.* 2015;450391.

Nobile-Orazio E. Chronic inflammatory demyelinating polyradiculoneuropathy and variants: where we are and where we should go. *J Peripher Nerv Syst.* 2014;19(1):2–13.

Thomas PK, Claus D, Jaspert A, Workman JM, King RH, Larner AJ, et al. Focal upper limb demyelinating neuropathy. *Brain.* 1996;119 (Pt 3):765–74.

Viala K, Maisonobe T, Stojkovic T, Koutlidis R, Ayrignac X, Musset L, et al. A current view of the diagnosis, clinical variants, response to treatment and prognosis of chronic inflammatory demyelinating polyradiculoneuropathy. *J Peripher Nerv Syst.* 2010;15(1):50–6.

Willison HJ, O'Leary CP, Veitch J, Blumhardt LD, Busby M, Donaghy M, et al. The clinical and laboratory features of chronic sensory ataxic neuropathy with anti-disialosyl IgM antibodies. *Brain.* 2001;124(Pt 10):1968–77.

Chronic Immune Motor and Sensory Neuropathies with Conduction Block

Introduction

Prototypic chronic inflammatory demyelinating polyradiculoneuropathy (CIDP) involves demyelination distributed along the lengths of nerve (multifocal demyelination), possibly with greater involvement distally and proximally (Kuwabara et al., 2015). This distribution can cause conduction block of individual nerve fibers anywhere along the nerve. In contrast, there are neuropathies characterized by conduction block of a large number of motor or sensory fibers at focal regions away from common entrapment sites, and thus individual nerves are affected in a mononeuritis multiplex pattern (multifocal conduction block). These two patterns differ in pathology, with demyelination causing conduction block in the former, and changes at the node of Ranvier in the latter. The distinction between the two patterns is based on electrodiagnostic studies.

Within neuropathies with focal conduction block are two patterns recognized clinically; one affecting only motor nerve fibers (multifocal motor neuropathy – MMN), and the other affecting both motor and sensory nerves (multifocal acquired demyelinating sensory and motor neuropathy – MADSAM, which is also referred to as the Lewis-Sumner syndrome – LSS). However, the distinction between the two patterns is becoming blurred.

Multifocal Motor Neuropathy with Conduction Block

MMN with conduction block is very rare, but frequently considered when amyotrophic lateral sclerosis (ALS) is part of the differential diagnosis due to apparent overlap of clinical features; although, with careful consideration, the clinical features of MMN differ from those observed in ALS.

Pathology

Focal conduction block in this setting implies normal nerve fiber conduction in segments distal and proximal

to the block, and that the block is not at entrapment sites. Data support dysfunction at the node of Ranvier, with or without elements of segmental demyelination (usually relatively minor). There can be axonal loss of mild degree developing over time (Leger et al., 2015). The underlying mechanism of block may be combinations of membrane hyperpolarization or depolarization, abnormal temporal dispersion (supporting a demyelinating component), or block related to the discharge rate of nerve activity. These mechanisms at the node of Ranvier are similar to those described for several acute neuropathies (acute motor axonal neuropathy–AMAN and motor and sensory neuropathies–AMSAN) (see Chapter 21). Functional block may be due to specific antibodies acting at the node, and MMN is associated with elevated GM1 ganglioside antibodies in ~50% of patients, but clinical and electrodiagnostic features do not differ between those with and without GM1 antibodies.

Clinical Features

MMN involves conduction block in individual nerves, and is very slowly progressive with greater numbers of named nerves involved leading to a mononeuritis multiplex pattern. Nerves in the arms are more often involved than those in the legs, and weakness in the radial nerve distribution with digital and wrist extension weakness is common. Weakness is out of proportion to muscle atrophy, and fasciculations may be observed in weak muscles. While considered a motor neuropathy, vague sensory symptoms may be reported and abnormalities are encountered during nerve conduction studies (see below). Tendon reflexes are normal or reduced in involved muscles (Leger et al., 2015).

Diagnostic Evaluation

Conduction block documented by nerve conduction studies is the key feature. Block is more readily demonstrated in distal nerve segments for technical reasons, but block may occur in proximal segments where it is difficult to document. Ganglioside titers are helpful when positive.

Electrodiagnostic Evaluation

Focal conduction block is estimated by a reduction of the CMAP area or amplitude (area is the preferred metric) across the site, but must be distinguished from reduced CMAP area due to abnormal temporal dispersion from slowed conduction velocities due to demyelination (see Chapter 4) (EFNS/PNS, 2010). Focal conduction block is demonstrated more often in nerves innervating weak muscles, but also occurs in nerves innervating strong muscles (Van Asseldonk et al., 2003). There are technical issues with nerve conduction studies that can lead to over-diagnosis of conduction block (Bromberg and Franssen, 2015). One is ensuring supramaximal nerve stimulation without overstimulation that would active neighboring nerves. Supramaximal stimulation is difficult with deep-lying proximal nerve segments as the current output of the stimulator is limited. Thus, block is most commonly documented in distal nerve segments. Care must be taken in analyzing CMAP metrics to ensure that the loss in area or amplitude across the site is not related to abnormal temporal dispersion. With these cautions in mind, there are levels of certainty for the presence of conduction block based on consensus and modeling (Table 26.1) (Olney et al., 2003). Demonstrating conduction block is difficult when the number of blocked fibers is small, and definite block is based on >50% of fibers being blocked.

Conduction block should leave distal axons intact but motor axonal loss occurs late in the course, and MMN is progressive despite treatment (Van Asseldonk et al., 2006).

MMN is considered a motor neuropathy, but patients may experience paresthesias, and sensory nerve conduction studies can show evidence for reduced SNAP amplitude over time (Lambrecq et al., 2009; Capasso et al., 2011). Axonal sensory loss corresponds with motor axonal loss.

Imaging Evaluation

Given the challenges in documenting focal conduction block, ultrasound has been used to identify sites of nerve enlargement as a proxy for conduction block, particularly at proximal locations not amenable to nerve conduction testing. While nerve cross-sectional area is greater among patients with MMN compared to control subjects, there are no consistent correlations between electrodiagnostic and ultrasound abnormalities (Kerasnoudis et al., 2014; Pitarokoili et al., 2015).

Laboratory Evaluation

High titers of antibodies to GM1 gangliosides are detected in ~50% (Leger et al., 2015).

Management

IVIG has been shown to improve strength and function (van Schaik et al., 2005). MMN is a chronic disease and continuous treatment is commonly required (EFNS/PNS, 2010). Most importantly, despite long-term treatment, effectiveness of IVIG frequently diminishes over time, despite increasing doses. This deteriorating effectiveness is felt to be reflected in part as progressive axonal loss over time (Van Asseldonk et al., 2006). Other forms of immunomodulation treatment have not been found to be effective, although treatment trials involve few patients (Umapathi et al., 2015). There are reports of patients receiving no benefit or experiencing worsening of weakness taking corticosteroids (EFNS/PNS, 2010).

There are descriptions of patients with a similar pattern of multiple motor nerve involvement but who have no demonstrable conduction block but who also respond to IVIG (Delmont et al., 2006).

Table 26.1 Criteria for Focal Conduction Block, Based on Expert Opinion

	CMAP Segment Amplitude Reduction	CMAP Segment Area Reduction	CMAP Negative Peak Duration Segment Increase
Definite CB	⇓ >50%	⇓ >40%	⇑ <30%
Probable CB	⇓ >40%	⇓ >30%	⇑ <30%
Possible CB	⇓ >50%	⇓ >40%	⇑ 31–60%

Source: Adapted from Olney et al. (2003).

Multifocal Acquired Demyelinating Sensory and Motor Neuropathy

Multifocal acquired demyelinating sensory and motor neuropathy (MADSAM) or Lewis-Sumner syndrome (LSS) is characterized by multiple sites of focal conduction block involving both motor and sensory fibers (Lewis et al., 1982; Saperstein et al., 1999). It is not clear if MADSAM/LSS represents a variant of CIDP or one end of a spectrum of conduction block neuropathies with MMN on the other end.

Clinical Features

Similar to MMN, progression in MADSAM/LSS is chronic, and follows a stepwise pattern of weakness and sensory loss in the distribution of individual nerves (mononeuritis multiplex), and affecting arms more than legs (Saperstein et al., 1999). Neuropathic pain can be marked. Tendon reflexes are reduced or absent in affected muscles. Cranial neuropathies (VII, IX, X, XII) are observed (Verschueren et al., 2005).

Diagnostic Evaluation

Electrodiagnostic Evaluation

Attention to nerve conduction details also applies to MADSAM/LSS. Motor nerve conduction studies show focal conduction block away from common sites of entrapment, and also evidence for primary demyelination (Saperstein et al., 1999). Further, sensory nerve action potentials were commonly absent or reduced.

Laboratory Evaluation

The majority of patients have elevated cerebral spinal fluid protein but few or none have elevated GM1 gangliosides (Saperstein et al., 1999).

Management

Some patients respond to treatment with corticosteroids (Lewis et al., 1982), although there are reports of worsening while on steroids (Attarian et al., 2011). Small patient series report a response to IVIG (Attarian et al., 2011). Long-term prognosis is dependent upon continued treatment, and there may be progression of symptoms despite treatment. Long-term subcutaneous immunoglobulin has been effective (Bayas et al., 2013).

References

European Federation of Neurological Societies/Peripheral Nerve Society guideline on management of multifocal motor neuropathy. Report of a joint task force of the European Federation of Neurological Societies and the Peripheral Nerve Society – first revision. *J Peripher Nerv Syst.* 2010;15(4):295–301.

Kuwabara S, Isose S, Mori M, Mitsuma S, Sawai S, Beppu M, et al. Different electrophysiological profiles and treatment response in "typical" and "atypical" chronic inflammatory demyelinating polyneuropathy. *J Neurol Neurosurg Psychiatry.* 2015;86(10):1054–9.

Leger JM, Guimaraes-Costa R, Iancu Ferfoglia R. The pathogenesis of multifocal motor neuropathy and an update on current management options. *Ther Adv Neurol Disord.* 2015;8(3):109–22.

Van Asseldonk JT, Van den Berg LH, Van den Berg-Vos RM, Wieneke GH, Wokke JH, Franssen H. Demyelination and axonal loss in multifocal motor neuropathy: distribution and relation to weakness. *Brain.* 2003;126(Pt 1):186–98.

Bromberg MB, Franssen H. Practical rules for electrodiagnosis in suspected multifocal motor neuropathy. *J Clin Neuromuscul Dis.* 2015;16(3):141–52.

Olney RK, Lewis RA, Putnam TD, Campellone JV, Jr. Consensus criteria for the diagnosis of multifocal motor neuropathy. *Muscle Nerve.* 2003;27(1):117–21.

Van Asseldonk JT, Van den Berg LH, Kalmijn S, Van den Berg-Vos RM, Polman CH, Wokke JH, et al. Axon loss is an important determinant of weakness in multifocal motor neuropathy. *J Neurol Neurosurg Psychiatry.* 2006;77(6):743–7.

Lambrecq V, Krim E, Rouanet-Larriviere M, Lagueny A. Sensory loss in multifocal motor neuropathy: a clinical and electrophysiological study. *Muscle Nerve.* 2009;39(2):131–6.

Capasso M, Notturno F, Manzoli C, Uncini A. Involvement of sensory fibres in axonal subtypes of Guillain-Barre syndrome. *J Neurol Neurosurg Psychiatry.* 2011;82(6):664–70.

Kerasnoudis A, Pitarokoili K, Behrendt V, Gold R, Yoon MS. Multifocal motor neuropathy: correlation of nerve ultrasound, electrophysiological, and clinical findings. *J Peripher Nerv Syst.* 2014;19(2):165–74.

Pitarokoili K, Gold R, Yoon MS. Nerve ultrasound in a case of multifocal motor neuropathy without conduction block. *Muscle Nerve.* 2015;52(2):294–6.

van Schaik IN, van den Berg LH, de Haan R, Vermeulen M. Intravenous immunoglobulin for multifocal motor neuropathy. *Cochrane Database Syst Rev.* 2005(2):CD004429.

Umapathi T, Hughes RA, Nobile-Orazio E, Leger JM. Immunosuppressant and immunomodulatory treatments for multifocal motor neuropathy. *Cochrane Database Syst Rev.* 2015;3:CD003217.

Delmont E, Azulay JP, Giorgi R, Attarian S, Verschueren A, Uzcnot D, et al. Multifocal motor neuropathy with and without conduction block: a single entity? *Neurology.* 2006;67(4):592–6.

Lewis RA, Sumner AJ, Brown MJ, Asbury AK. Multifocal demyelinating neuropathy with persistent conduction block. *Neurology.* 1982;32(9):958–64.

Saperstein DS, Amato AA, Wolfe GI, Katz JS, Nations SP, Jackson CE, et al. Multifocal acquired demyelinating sensory and motor neuropathy: the Lewis-Sumner syndrome. *Muscle Nerve.* 1999;22(5):560–6.

Verschueren A, Azulay JP, Attarian S, Boucraut J, Pellissier JF, Pouget J. Lewis-Sumner syndrome and multifocal motor neuropathy. *Muscle Nerve.* 2005;31(1):88–94.

Attarian S, Verschueren A, Franques J, Salort-Campana E, Jouve E, Pouget J. Response to treatment in patients with Lewis-Sumner syndrome. *Muscle Nerve.* 2011;44(2):179–84.

Bayas A, Gold R, Naumann M. Long-term treatment of Lewis-Sumner syndrome with subcutaneous immunoglobulin infusions. *J Neurol Sci.* 2013;324(1–2):53–6.

Length-Dependent Polyneuropathies

Length-dependent polyneuropathies are by far the most common type of polyneuropathy, and are caused by or attributed to a large number of causes. The basic distinction when evaluating polyneuropathies is between primary axonal and primary demyelinating neuropathies. While all neuropathies affect longer nerves initially, length-dependent, primary axonal polyneuropathies progress in a stocking-glove distribution over a long period of time, usually over years. In contrast, primary demyelinating neuropathies affect both long- and short-length nerves in both legs and arms early on, usually over months. This distinction is important as primary demyelinating neuropathies are

considered to be immune-mediated, and hence may be treatable. In general, length-dependent neuropathies are not treatable, but those due to neurotoxic drugs or toxins, vitamin deficiencies, or medical conditions may exhibit reduction of progression or some remission when causes are managed. It is important to be aware that in 25% or more of length-dependent neuropathies, a cause cannot be identified and remain idiopathic.

Epidemiologically, the most common type of length-dependent neuropathy is attributed to diabetes. Hereditary neuropathies are also of this type, but are considered in Chapter 42.

Chapter

27

Length-Dependent Polyneuropathies: General Features

Introduction

Length-dependent polyneuropathies primarily affect the longest nerves first and represent a prototypic form of a primary axonal neuropathy. They are also referred to as "stocking-glove" distribution neuropathies because as the pathologic process progresses, shorter nerves are affected, and the length of nerve from the spine to the knee is equal to the length from the neck to the fingers. Since the underlying pathology is thought primarily to affect the cell body or axon, longer nerves are metabolically more vulnerable. Another name is "toxic-metabolic" neuropathies, although the underlying metabolic-pathologic factors are rarely identified or understood. Further, some length-dependent neuropathies also include involvement of myelin, and two examples are the most common form of diabetic neuropathy, which has mildly reduced conduction velocities in addition to distal axonal loss, and type 1 hereditary neuropathies, which have markedly slow conduction velocities but weakness and sensory loss are due to length-dependent axonal loss. There are variations in the length-dependent pattern, and some toxic neuropathies due to medications, such as cancer chemotherapeutic drugs, cause an early effect on distal segments of nerve in both arms and legs.

The clinical symptoms and signs and electrodiagnostic features of a prototypic axonal polyneuropathy generally apply to most such neuropathies, but variations occur, and the prototypic neuropathy is a construct.

Pathology

It is assumed that the longest nerve fibers are affected earliest due to metabolic vulnerability linked to fiber length, and that over time shorter fibers are affected. It is also assumed that both large- and smaller-diameter fibers are affected, but possibly to differing degrees. The underlying pathophysiology varies amongst causes, accounting for differences in rates of progression and variations in patterns of involvement (Cashman and Hoke, 2015).

Clinical Features

Length-dependent neuropathies generally follow a chronic time course, months to years, and early findings are emphasized because they relate to the time when patients seek diagnosis. Sensory symptoms and signs occur earlier and predominate over motor because there is no collateral reinnervation of sensory fibers to blunt the effects of nerve loss as there is with collateral reinnervation of motor nerves. Positive sensory symptoms (burning pain, paresthesias) are more noticeable than negative symptoms (numbness, impaired balance), while motor symptoms are likely missed although there may be an increase in muscle cramps. Clinical signs follow symptoms with a distal to proximal gradient of altered light touch, perception of the tuning fork vibration, and joint position sense. Achilles tendon reflexes may be reduced or absent. For motor signs, the foot may appear to be thinner than expected, and distal toe extension and flexion may be mildly weak.

Electrodiagnostic Evaluation

Symptoms and signs may be mild early on, and nerve conduction studies are useful to confirm peripheral nerve involvement, but may not be abnormal early in the course. Testing a distal sensory nerve is the most sensitive for axonal loss. The sural nerve is reasonable and practical to study, while more distal nerves, such as the plantar sensory nerves, may be more sensitive but may be abnormal in asymptomatic people. The sural SNAP amplitude is dependent upon the number of nerve fibers, and amplitude falls in a linear manner and is below the lower limits of normal when ~80% of fibers at the recording site have been lost (Perkins and Bril, 2014). The CMAP may remain above the lower limit of normal until the sural SNAP falls below the lower limit. With early assessment and mild symptoms and signs sensory and motor nerve conduction metrics may remain with laboratory limits, but may be closer to the limits of normal than expected.

A key issue in interpreting nerve conduction data is determining whether mildly prolonged distal latencies and slowed conduction velocities represent loss of the largest and most rapidly conducting nerve fibers (primary axonal neuropathy) or secondary to myelin involvement (primary demyelinating neuropathy), and interpretation errors are common (Allen and Lewis, 2015). The general principles of distinguishing between the two types of neuropathy are discussed in Chapter 4. Complicating interpretation is a neuropathy with mixed pathology, such as with diabetic neuropathy, and is discussed in Chapter 28.

References

Allen JA, Lewis RA. CIDP diagnostic pitfalls and perception of treatment benefit. *Neurology*. 2015;85:498–504.

Cashman CR, Hoke A. Mechanisms of distal axonal degeneration in peripheral neuropathies. *Neurosci Lett*. 2015;596:33–50.

Perkins B, Bril V. Electrophysiologic testing in diabetic neuropathy. *Handb Clin Neurol*. 2014;126:235–48.

Diabetic Neuropathies

Introduction

Diabetes mellitus, types 1 and 2 both, is associated with a variety of neuropathies (Table 28.1). Classification can be by time course (chronic: sensorimotor, distal small-fiber, autonomic; or acute: severe distal sensory, insulin neuritis, cranial nerve) or by distribution patterns (length-dependent: symmetric sensorimotor or small-fiber, cachexia, hypoglycemic; or asymmetric: radiculoplexopathy, mononeuropathy, cranial nerve). The range of autonomic nerve involvement is difficult to document, as multiple organ systems can be affected (cardiovascular, gastrointestinal, genitourinary, central nervous system) and symptoms may not come to light during evaluation for a neuropathy, or be managed by other medical disciplines. For type 1 diabetes, elevated glucose is the most likely factor, but, for type 2 diabetes, the setting for the most common of the diabetic neuropathies, the pathophysiologic role of elevated glucose is not known and likely is one element in a multifactorial pathologic process. This chapter focuses on symptomatic length-dependent large-fiber and small-fiber polyneuropathies as they are most common, and proximal neuropathies (radiculoplexopathy) are considered in Chapter 7. The lifetime incidence of symptomatic polyneuropathy is ~45% for type 1 and ~60% for type 2. Overall, neuropathies associated with diabetes have the highest prevalence worldwide.

Diabetic Symmetric Polyneuropathy

Diabetic symmetric polyneuropathy (DSPN) is the most common neuropathy associated with diabetes types 1 or 2. It generally becomes clinically evident over years after the diagnosis of diabetes, but subclinical evidence for a neuropathy may be detected by electrodiagnostic tests (de Souza et al., 2015) and screening tests, such as fasting glucose or hemaglobin A1c (discussed in Chapter 5). DSPN follows a length-dependent pattern, but progression is slow and it may

Table 28.1 Types of Neuropathy Associated with Diabetes Mellitus

Distal symmetric sensorimotor
Distal small-fiber
Acute severe distal sensory
Autonomic
Neuropathic cachexia
Hypoglycemic
Treatment-induced (insulin neuritis)
Polyradiculopathy
Radiculoplexopathy
Mononeuropathy (entrapment of median, ulnar)
Cranial neuropathies

take years for the stocking distribution to unroll up the legs to a glove distribution in the arms.

Pathology

Despite the marked prevalence of DSPN, a full understanding of causes has been elusive. For patients with type 1 diabetes, hyperglycemia is a major factor, and pathologic features can resolve with pancreatic transplantation (Kennedy et al., 1990). For patients with type 2 diabetes, a combination of factors associated with the metabolic syndrome is implicated in the underlying pathology of nerve damage (three of the following, even if treated: elevated glucose, elevated lipids, cholesterol, blood pressure, and truncal obesity) (Smith and Singleton, 2013). Microscopically, there is evidence for both axonal degeneration and demyelination, and there may be altered function at nodes of Ranvier. Sural nerve biopsies show axonal loss of large and small fibers with alterations to myelin and evidence for nerve fiber regeneration, but the pattern is not specific for diabetes. Ultrastructural studies support hypoxia or ischemia to the nerve as likely pathologic factors.

Clinical Features

Sensory loss is the initial symptom and is perceived as decreased feeling or tingling in the toes and feet. A percentage of patients experience distal pain, which can be burning or a feeling of tightness about the foot. An uncomfortable increased sensitivity to pressure (standing) at the soles of the feet may accompany pain. Progressive loss of touch and proprioception can lead to gait or standing instability, and, while troubling to the patient, is not commonly severe. There is also loss of motor fibers, but significant distal leg weakness is uncommon early on. Progression is very slow, but follows a length-dependent pattern, and sensory loss and muscle atrophy and weakness in the hands can occur at late stages. Autonomic nerves are involved to varying degrees, with changes to skin about the foot (decreased sweating, coolness, dry and cracked skin) and impotence in men.

Clinical testing reveals loss of light touch, vibration perception, and pin perception in the feet, with a gradation to normal sensory perception proximally up the shin. Joint-position perception at the great toe is frequently impaired. The Achilles tendon reflex is frequently absent. Loss of motor nerve fibers can be appreciated by the presence of thinness of the feet and weakness of toe extension and flexion.

Diagnostic Evaluation

The diagnosis is largely clinical, based on the above clinical features when concurrent diabetes is known (types 1 or 2). However, symptoms may be present when diabetes type 2 is undiagnosed, and it is important to assess for elements of the metabolic syndrome (England et al., 2009) (see Chapter 5).

Electrodiagnostic Evaluation

Electrodiagnostic testing is useful to confirm DSPN in the setting of early diabetes type 2, and particularly when evaluating an idiopathic neuropathy in the setting of prediabetes (metabolic syndrome). Early on, nerve conduction changes are small in magnitude and technical factors such as adequate limb temperature for accurate SNAP responses and recording electrode position for CMAP responses is important to detect abnormalities (see Chapter 4). Nerve conduction changes are first noted in longest sensory nerves (sural nerve), and the first changes between normal subjects and presymptomatic diabetic subjects are a mild reduction in SNAP amplitude

and mild slowing of conduction velocity, but detection may be difficult as values frequently remain within laboratory limits (de Souza et al., 2015). Similar small changes (within laboratory limits) may occur in the fibular/peroneal motor responses. With the clinical progression of presymptomatic diabetes to symptomatic neuropathy and clinical diabetes, nerve conduction findings are more marked with reduced response amplitudes and conduction velocity slowing in a length-dependent manner. Slowing of conduction velocities are more apparent when measured over longer distances, and F-wave latencies are prolonged in tibial and fibular/peroneal nerves in presymptomatic diabetic subjects (Pan et al., 2014). The greater loss of SNAP amplitude than CMAP amplitude is attributed to the effects of collateral reinnervation in the later. Needle EMG study in intrinsic foot muscles will show evidence for varying degrees of chronic, mild denervation.

Conduction slowing in diabetic neuropathy must be interpreted with some caution, and should not be attributed to a primary demyelinating neuropathy (chronic demyelinating polyradiculoneuropathy – CIDP) as distal latency, conduction velocity, and F-wave latency may overlap with those encountered in CIDP, but the severity of slowing and number of nerves with slowing do not meet CIDP criteria (Figure 28.1). An approach when evaluating a neuropathy in the setting of diabetes to distinguish a primary demyelination neuropathy versus DSPN is to rely on guideline motor nerve values for primary demyelination neuropathy. Specifically, for primary demyelinating neuropathy the distal latency and F-wave distal latency should be >125% of the laboratory upper limit of normal, and conduction velocity <75% of the lower limit (see Chapters 4 and 24). DSPN values rarely are in the demyelinating range (Figure 28.1). Diabetic neuropathy and CIDP can occur in the same patient, and clinical and diagnostic features have been set forward to separate the two (see below).

Laboratory Evaluation

The diagnosis of type 1 diabetes is usually established before a neuropathy is clinically evident. When the laboratory diagnosis of type 2 diabetes has not been made, evidence for glucose dysregulation should be assessed by a two-hour glucose tolerance test (GTT) because hemoglobin A1c and fasting glucose testing is less sensitive (Singleton et al., 2001). A lipid profile is helpful for evidence of the metabolic syndrome. Other

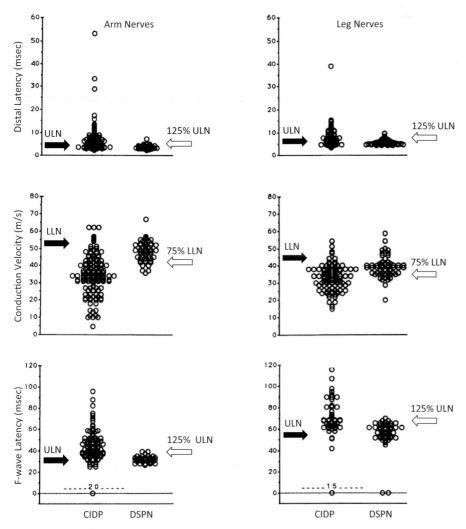

Figure 28.1 Distribution of motor nerve conduction metrics for distal latency, conduction velocity, and F-wave latency from patients comparing patients with chronic demyelinating polyradiculoneuropathy (CIDP) and diabetic symmetric polyneuropathy (DSPN). Solid arrows represent upper and lower limits of normal (solid arrows); and open arrows represent 125% or 75% of upper and lower limits, respectively, which indicate greater slowing than expected for the degree of axonal loss.
Modified from Bromberg (1991).

informative laboratory tests include vitamin B12 and serum immunofixation (England et al., 2009).

Management

There is no disease-altering medication for neuropathy from type 1 or 2 diabetes. In the setting of type 1 diabetes, tight glucose control reduces the risk of developing a neuropathy by modest percentages, but may be challenging for the patient to manage, as hypoglycemic episodes are to be avoided (DCCT, 1993). With type 2 diabetes, the risk of developing a neuropathy is also reduced with tight glucose control, and, additionally, there is a reduction of microvascular complications and reduced risk of amputations (Callaghan et al., 2012). In the setting of prediabetes, efforts to reduce metabolic syndrome factors may be helpful in forestalling the onset of neuropathy. Change from a sedentary to an active life style and regular exercise can be effective in reducing pain (Singleton et al., 2015). Pain can be controlled with a number of medications effective for neuropathic pain (see Chapter 48). Foot care is important and is discussed in Chapter 47.

Diabetes Neuropathy and Chronic Inflammatory Demyelinating Polyradiculoneuropathy

The issue of the prevalence of diabetes and CIDP is difficult to study because diabetes is common, is associated with a neuropathy that develops over time in a high percentage of patients, and the diagnosis of CIDP relies in part on nerve conduction studies whose values overlap between DSPN and CIDP (Figure 28.1). Issues in interpreting reports for or against an association include small numbers of patients and retrospective nature of the reports. A large study based on insurance claims data, with acknowledgement that the diagnosis of CIDP could not be confirmed, showed a nine-fold increase in the prevalence of CIDP amongst patients with a concurrent diagnosis of diabetes compared to non-diabetics (Bril et al., 2016).

With the association of CIDP and diabetes, CIDP can coexist with DSPN. The likelihood is that DSPN precedes the onset of CIDP, and the challenge is identifying the development of CIDP and distinguishing it from DSPN. An algorithm has been developed based on documenting numbers of clinical features (proximal weakness progressing over less than months, involvement of lower and upper limbs) and electrodiagnostic features (prolonged distal latency >150% of the upper limit, prolonged F-wave latency >130% of the upper limit, slowed conduction velocity <70% of the lower limit, evidence for practical conduction block, prolonged negative peak >9 msec) demonstrated in several nerves (Lotan et al., 2015).

Diabetic Painful Neuropathy

This type of neuropathy may occur in isolation without numbness or as a component of DSPN.

Clinical Features

It is characterized by distal and symmetric symptoms of prickling, deep aching, sharp electric shock-like pains, and burning, frequently of greater severity late in the day, which can disturb sleep. Pain may be increased with walking. Distal hyperesthesia is common. Signs may be minimal and restricted to altered perception of sharp stimuli. Progression of nerve damage may lead to less pain and more numbness.

Pathology

Damage is felt to be largely restricted to unmyelinated and thinly myelinated fibers, but there may be associated large-fiber involvement in the setting of DSPN.

Diagnostic Evaluation

Electrodiagnostic findings when symptoms are pain without numbness may be normal, or distal sensory responses mildly reduced (Singleton et al., 2001). Skin biopsy may show reduced density of intraepidermal nerve fibers (Sommer, 2008). The differential diagnosis of painful small-fiber neuropathies is considered in Chapter 38.

Laboratory Evaluation

In the setting of known diabetes, a symmetric distal pattern of pain is supportive of the diagnosis. Without known diabetes, the pattern raises the question of impaired glucose tolerance, and a two-hour glucose tolerance test (GTT) is a more sensitive test for glucose metabolism abnormalities than hemoglobin A1c or fasting glucose tests (Singleton et al., 2001).

Management

Exercise may help with symptoms (Singleton et al., 2015). Management of neuropathic pain is considered in Chapter 48

Acute Painful Neuropathy Associated with Insulin Treatment

A rare form of neuropathy occurs within weeks after starting insulin therapy, and includes patients with either type 1 or 2 diabetes (Gibbons and Freeman, 2010). The pain is severe and is associated with autonomic involvement, both clinically and by autonomic testing. Other names applied to neuropathies with similar clinical features include "insulin neuritis" and "diabetic neuropathic cachexia," but there is no evidence for nerve inflammation and the patient may not be in a cachexic state.

Routine nerve conduction studies are not reported. The pain subsides over 12+ months. The pathology is not clear, but involves both small myelinated and unmyelinated autonomic fibers.

References

Bril V, Blanchette CM, Noone JM, Runken MC, Gelinas D, Russell JW. The dilemma of diabetes in chronic inflammatory demyelinating polyneuropathy. *J Diabetes Complications*. 2016;30:1401–7.

Bromberg MB. Comparison of electrodiagnostic criteria for primary demyelination in chronic polyneuropathy. *Muscle Nerve* 1991;14(10):968–76.

Callaghan BC, Little AA, Feldman EL, Hughes RA. Enhanced glucose control for preventing and treating diabetic neuropathy. *Cochrane Database Syst Rev*. 2012:CD007543.

de Souza RJ, de Souza A, Nagvekar MD. Nerve conduction studies in diabetics presymptomatic and symptomatic for diabetic polyneuropathy. *J Diabetes Complications*. 2015;29:811–17.

The Diabetes Control and Complications Trial Research Group. The effect of intensive treatment of diabetes on the development and progression of long-term complications in insulin-dependent diabetes mellitus. *N Engl J Med*. 1993;329:977–86.

England JD, Gronseth GS, Franklin G, Carter GT, Kinsella LJ, Cohen JA, et al. Practice Parameter: evaluation of distal symmetric polyneuropathy: role of laboratory and genetic testing (an evidence-based review). Report of the American Academy of Neurology, American Association of Neuromuscular and Electrodiagnostic Medicine, and American Academy of Physical Medicine and Rehabilitation. *Neurology*. 2009;72:185–92.

Gibbons CH, Freeman R. Treatment-induced diabetic neuropathy: a reversible painful autonomic neuropathy. *Ann Neurol*. 2010;67:534–41.

Kennedy WR, Navarro X, Goetz FC, Sutherland DE, Najarian JS. Effects of pancreatic transplantation on diabetic neuropathy. *N Engl J Med*. 1990;322:1031–7.

Lotan I, Hellman MA, Steiner I. Diagnostic criteria of chronic inflammatory demyelinating polyneuropathy in diabetes mellitus. *Acta Neurol Scand*. 2015;132:278–83.

Pan H, Jian F, Lin J, Chen N, Zhang C, Zhang Z, et al. F-wave latencies in patients with diabetes mellitus. *Muscle Nerve*. 2014;49:804–8.

Singleton JR, Smith AG, Bromberg MB. Increased prevalence of impaired glucose tolerance in patients with painful sensory neuropathy. *Diabetes Care*. 2001;24:1448–53.

Singleton JR, Smith AG, Marcus RL. Exercise as Therapy for Diabetic and Prediabetic Neuropathy. *Curr Diab Rep*. 2015;15:120.

Smith AG, Singleton JR. Obesity and hyperlipidemia are risk factors for early diabetic neuropathy. *J Diabetes Complications*. 2013;27:436–42.

Sommer C. Skin biopsy as a diagnostic tool. *Curr Opin Neurol*. 2008;21:563–8.

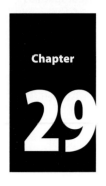

Acquired Amyloid Neuropathy

Introduction

Neuropathies due to the deposition of amyloid can be divided into rare acquired forms and more common hereditary forms (familial amyloid polyneuropathy – FAP), which are discussed in Chapter 44 (Shin and Robinson-Papp, 2012). Acquired amyloid neuropathies result from the production of amyloid due to plasma cell dyscrasias or B-cell lymphoproliferative disorders. Amyloid produced by these aberrant cells is deposited in multiple organs, and in a percentage deposition occurs in peripheral nerves.

Pathologic Features

Deposited amyloid can be composed of different forms, and the AL form is the most common found in peripheral nerves (Matsuda et al., 2011). AL amyloidosis has also been called light-chain or primary amyloidosis as it is usually lambda or kappa light chains that are misfolded and accumulate either in a restricted distribution (median nerve at the wrist) or a systemic distribution.

Clinical Features

Involvement of peripheral nerves occurs in one-third of patients with amyloidosis, most commonly with sensory disturbances and with pain (Matsuda et al., 2011). The pattern is length-dependent, and patients may or may not have median mononeuropathy at the wrist.

Diagnostic Evaluation

The diagnosis of AL amyloidosis is based on initial systemic features due to involvement of other organs, which include fatigue, weight loss, proteinuria, congestive heart failure, and hepatomegaly. The evaluation leads to detection of a plasma cell dyscrasias or B-cell lymphoproliferative disorder, and confirmed by finding elevated lambda or kappa light changes in the urine or a lambda to kappa ratio of 3:1. AL amyloidosis may coexist with IgG (less commonly IgA or IgM) monoclonal gammopathies of uncertain clinical significance (MGUS) (Rajabally, 2011). Confirmation is by demonstrating amyloid by Congo red staining from tissue.

Electrodiagnostic Evaluation

Nerve conduction studies show a distal-predominant neuropathy of mild degree (Matsuda et al., 2011). There may be a higher incidence of median mononeuropathy at the wrist.

Management

Treatment for the underlying plasma cell disorder is difficult and leads to high mortality. Treatment is based on protocols for multiple myeloma, melphalan, and dexamethasone, but stem cell treatment and bortezomib and thalidomide has improved survival (Kumar et al., 2011).

References

Kumar SK, Gertz MA, Lacy MQ, Dingli D, Hayman SR, Buadi FK, et al. Recent improvements in survival in primary systemic amyloidosis and the importance of an early mortality risk score. *Mayo Clin Proc.* 2011;86:12–18.

Matsuda M, Gono T, Morita H, Katoh N, Kodaira M, Ikeda S. Peripheral nerve involvement in primary systemic AL amyloidosis: a clinical and electrophysiological study. *European journal of neurology.* 2011;18:604–10.

Rajabally YA. Neuropathy and paraproteins: review of a complex association. *European journal of neurology.* 2011;18:1291–8.

Shin SC, Robinson-Papp J. Amyloid neuropathies. *Mt Sinai J Med.* 2012;79:733–48.

Chapter 30

Neuropathy Associated with Bariatric Surgery

Introduction

Bariatric surgery is defined as surgical procedures to restrict food intake, and can lead to peripheral nerve disorders in ~15% of patients (Thaisetthawatkul et al., 2004). The most common indication for surgery is severe obesity (Body Mass Index >40 or >30 in the setting of heart disease or diabetes), and there are several surgical procedures available (Koffman et al., 2006). Most neuropathies are related to vitamin deficiencies, and patients can have preexisting low levels or deficiencies prior to surgery or polyneuropathies related to preexisting diabetes (Thaisetthawatkul et al., 2004). Thiamine deficiency can lead to Wernicke encephalopathy in the setting of prolonged vomiting in the postoperative period.

Pathology

Few affected nerves have been biopsied, and the pathology may vary amongst the types of neuropathies (Thaisetthawatkul et al., 2004). Sensory-dominant neuropathies are characterized by active axonal loss in distal sensory nerve biopsies. There are varying amounts of inflammatory cells but no evidence for a vasculitis. Mononeuropathies have not been biopsied, and causes likely vary amongst the different nerves and sites. Biopsies from patients with radicoloplexopathies support a microvasculitis, as observed in diabetic and non-diabetic radicoloplexopathies.

There are few clear-risk general medical factors, other than the presence of diabetes. Clinical factors associated with the postoperative period include rapid weight loss, postoperative vomiting and diarrhea, and not attending postoperative nutritional clinics for adequate supplementation (Thaisetthawatkul et al., 2004). Unassociated factors are preoperative BMI and total amount of weight lost.

Clinical Features

Three types of neuropathies are encountered (Thaisetthawatkul et al., 2004). The most common form is a sensory distal-predominant polyneuropathy, usually with insidious onset and slow progression, but which occasionally may be subacute or acute in presentation. Mononeuropathies are the next most common type, most frequently the median nerve at the wrist, but also involving other nerves at other sites, and are encountered with greater frequency in patients with preexisting diabetes. Radicoloplexopathies are the least common and may involve either cervical or lumbosacral roots in an asymmetric pattern.

Diagnostic Evaluation

Laboratory Evaluation

Preoperative and postoperative vitamin levels are not remarkable, and not different from patients with similar degrees of obesity undergoing cholecystectomy (Thaisetthawatkul et al., 2004). However, elevated hemoglobin A1c and triglyceride levels are associated as a risk factor (Thaisetthawatkul et al., 2010).

Electrodiagnostic Evaluation

Nerve conduction study of sensory-dominant polyneuropathy shows large-fiber loss with no evidence for demyelination. Some patients have normal studies, supporting small-fiber loss. Needle EMG findings of radicoloplexopathies show denervation.

Management

Postoperative management with vitamin supplementation can reduce the rate of sensory-dominant neuropathies by ~50% (Thaisetthawatkul et al., 2010). General guidelines are available (Rudnicki, 2010).

References

Koffman BM, Greenfield LJ, Ali LL, Pirzada NA. Neurologic complications after surgery for obesity. *Muscle Nerve*. 2006;33:166–76.

Rudnicki SA. Prevention and treatment of peripheral neuropathy after bariatric surgery. *Curr Treat Options Neurol*. 2010;12:29–36.

Thaisetthawatkul P, Collazo-Clavell ML, Sarr MG, Norell JE, Dyck PJ. A controlled study of peripheral neuropathy after bariatric surgery. *Neurology*. 2004;63:1462–70.

Thaisetthawatkul P, Collazo-Clavell ML, Sarr MG, Norell JE, Dyck PJ. Good nutritional control may prevent polyneuropathy after bariatric surgery. *Muscle Nerve*. 2010;42:709–14.

Neuropathy Associated with Critical Illness

Introduction

In the setting of intensive care for multiorgan failure and sepsis, a large percentage of patients develop weakness. Although the mechanisms are not understood, based on the underlying medical comorbidities being treated, the weakness has been named "systemic inflammatory response syndrome" (SIRS) (Bolton, 2005). In most patients, there is evidence for both a polyneuropathy and myopathy contributing to weakness (Khan et al., 2006), and this chapter focuses on the former. The incidence of neuropathy is high, affecting >50% of patients who are being treated in the intensive care setting for 1–3 weeks.

Pathology

The pathophysiology is complex and varies amongst patient based on comorbidities (which organs are failing), precipitating events (burns, trauma), and other factors (types of infections) (Bolton, 2005). Sepsis, and the systemic inflammatory response, includes cellular and humoral factors that affect capillary integrity with impaired delivery of essential factors (glucose, oxygen). The specific pathologic processes relating to damage to axons and myelin are not clear.

Clinical Features

Weakness is global but may have a distal predominance (Lacomis, 2013). Weakness is frequently recognized when medical conditions are responding to treatment and patients fail attempts to be weaned off of the ventilator. There may be a distal sensory loss, but in the setting of very ill patients it is difficult to elicit subtleties of sensory and motor symptoms and signs as many patients have an encephalopathy and are on a ventilator.

Diagnostic Evaluation

General laboratory testing is abnormal across a wide spectrum of tests due to features of sepsis and organ failure, but no specific laboratory abnormality is associated with the development of critical illness neuropathy.

Electrodiagnostic Evaluation

It can be difficult to record low-amplitude sensory responses in the intensive care unit due to electrical interference from life support equipment. Further complicating recording both low sensory and motor responses is limb edema associated with sepsis. Another issue is distinguishing among other factors that could reduce motor response amplitudes, such as extreme disuse muscle atrophy due to several weeks of bed rest and critical illness myopathy. Changes in sensory responses can occur within three to four days of being critically ill, and there is further loss with longer disease duration (Khan et al., 2006). Information from serial testing suggests a progression of nerve conduction abnormalities in a distal to proximal distribution.

Critical illness neuropathy and myopathy frequently co-exist, and two nerve conduction findings can favor myopathy over neuropathy or the presence of a myopathic component. One is a preserved distal leg sensory response in the setting of a low motor response, indicating a relatively mild neuropathy. The second is a CMAP whose waveform is broad and has a prolonged negative peak duration, frequently twice as long as in normal motor potentials, a finding indicating direct muscle involvement (Goodman et al., 2009). Another discriminating electrodiagnostic test is to assess CMAP amplitude by comparing the response to nerve stimulation with the response to direct muscle stimulation, and a low response to nerve stimulation and a larger response to muscle stimulation supports a greater neuropathic component (Lacomis, 2013).

Management

Management is based on treating the underlying causes of sepsis and organ failure, which is difficult, and mortality is ~50%. Low-amplitude CMAP portends poor survival (Khan et al., 2006). If the patient survives, the neuropathy gradually improves, but the extent of improvement depends upon the degree of nerve (axonal) damage, and some patients remain markedly and permanently weak (Lacomis, 2013). Critical illness neuropathy has a worse prognosis for recovery than critical illness myopathy or a combination of both.

References

Bolton CF. Neuromuscular manifestations of critical illness. *Muscle Nerve.* 2005;32:140–63.

Goodman BP, Harper CM, Boon AJ. Prolonged compound muscle action potential duration in critical illness myopathy. *Muscle Nerve.* 2009;40:1040–2.

Khan J, Harrison TB, Rich MM, Moss M. Early development of critical illness myopathy and neuropathy in patients with severe sepsis. *Neurology.* 2006;67:1421–5.

Lacomis D. Electrophysiology of neuromuscular disorders in critical illness. *Muscle Nerve.* 2013;47:452–63.

Neuropathy Associated with Environmental Toxins

Introduction

A number of polyneuropathies are associated with toxins, which include neurotoxic substances ingested and inadvertent exposure to those in the environment. The incidence of exposure to and development of a neuropathy from environmental toxins is rare.

Alcohol (Ethanol)

The contribution of alcohol to a neuropathy is difficult to assess, and likely requires very high amounts of alcohol consumed over long periods of time. The toxic properties of ethanol on peripheral nerves have been difficult to sort out from concurrent nutritional deficiencies (malnutrition and thiamine deficiency) in humans (Mellion et al., 2011). However, there appears to be a primary painful sensory neuropathy associated with large and chronic amounts of ethanol consumption (>100 gms per day for >10 years) in patients who have no nutritional deficiencies (Koike et al., 2001).

Pathology

Sural nerve biopsy indicates loss of small myelinated and unmyelinated fibers (Koike et al., 2001).

Clinical Features

Burning pain affects distal portions of the lower extremities, and the pain can be disabling. Weakness of distal muscles can occur in extreme cases (Koike et al., 2001).

Diagnostic Evaluation

Sensory and motor responses in distal nerves in the legs are reduced and conduction velocities are moderately slowed (Koike et al., 2001).

Lead

Lead toxicity affects broad areas of the nervous system, and symptoms and signs vary by age of the individual and rate and degree of exposure (Thomson and Parry, 2006). A mild polyneuropathy from chronic low-level lead exposure in industrial settings has been studied, and mild changes in conduction velocity of distal leg nerves are recorded. Nerve damage from higher levels of lead exposure over a subacute time course is very rare (case reports).

Pathology

There is no predictable relationship between lead serum and urine levels and the degree of neuropathy. Few nerves have been examined with modern pathologic techniques, and the mechanism remains unclear.

Clinical Features

Classic findings of acute or subacute exposure are a motor neuropathy with early weakness of finger extension (third digit, later involvements of other digits) and wrist extension, and less commonly weakness of ankle dorsiflexion. The pattern is asymmetric, and with time there is muscle atrophy (Thomson and Parry, 2006). With chronic exposure, there can be mild distal sensory loss (Wu et al., 1995).

Diagnostic Evaluation

There are few studies documenting electrodiagnostic findings (Oh, 1975; Thomson and Parry, 2006). With mild weakness, motor responses are reduced but conduction velocities are normal, or slowed in proportion to axonal loss. With progression and greater degrees of weakness, motor responses decline but with no change in conduction velocity. Limited data on sensory responses indicate reduced or absent responses (Oh, 1975). Needle EMG supported distal denervation.

Management

Removal from exposure is essential. If lead levels are high, treatment with chelating agents can be considered, but there are little data for the threshold to treat. Recovery may be slow and incomplete (Oh, 1975).

Arsenic

Arsenic has a long history of intentional abuse leading to death (suicide or homicide), but acute exposure short of death can cause a peripheral neuropathy. Chronic environmental exposure can also lead to a peripheral neuropathy (Vahidnia et al., 2007).

Pathology

The pathology of peripheral nerve toxicity is not known (Vahidnia et al., 2007), but appears to be toxic to axons with initial segmental demyelination (Donofrio et al., 1987).

Clinical Features

Acute high doses are associated with abdominal pain, vomiting and diarrhea, and light-headedness and delirium. Symptoms of a polyneuropathy may be delayed by several weeks, and cause a rapid onset of painful dysesthesias with marked distal sensory loss, which can affect gait (Donofrio et al., 1987).

Diagnostic Evaluation

In the setting of acute onset, an early electrodiagnostic study may have a pattern consistent with an acute primary demyelinating neuropathy (AIDP), but subsequent studies several weeks later support a primary axonal neuropathy (Donofrio et al., 1987).

Management

There is a progressive recovery, but may be incomplete due to extensive axonal loss.

References

Donofrio PD, Wilbourn AJ, Albers JW, Rogers L, Salanga V, Greenberg HS. Acute arsenic intoxication presenting as Guillain-Barre-like syndrome. *Muscle Nerve.* 1987;10:114–20.

Koike H, Mori K, Misu K, Hattori N, Ito H, Hirayama M, et al. Painful alcoholic polyneuropathy with predominant small-fiber loss and normal thiamine status. *Neurology.* 2001;56:1727–32.

Mellion M, Gilchrist JM, de la Monte S. Alcohol-related peripheral neuropathy: nutritional, toxic, or both? *Muscle Nerve.* 2011;43:309–16.

Oh SJ. Lead neuropathy: case report. *Arch Phys Med Rehabil.* 1975;56:312–17.

Thomson RM, Parry GJ. Neuropathies associated with excessive exposure to lead. *Muscle Nerve.* 2006;33:732–41.

Vahidnia A, van der Voet GB, de Wolff FA. Arsenic neurotoxicity – a review. *Hum Exp Toxicol.* 2007;26:823–32.

Wu PB, Kingery WS, Date ES. An EMG case report of lead neuropathy 19 years after a shotgun injury. *Muscle Nerve.* 1995;18:326–9.

33

Chapter

Neuropathy Associated with Drugs

Introduction

A number of drugs can cause a peripheral neuropathy. Some affect nerves with high predictability and in a dose-dependent manner, such as chemotherapeutic drugs. Several commonly prescribed drugs infrequently cause a neuropathy, but should be considered when other causes have been excluded. The neuropathies are due to focal disturbances of nerve metabolism that affects cell body or axonal function, and hence the clinical pattern is a primary axonal length-dependent neuropathy. Drugs that alter dorsal root ganglia cells cause sensory neuropathies that affect nerves in the arms and legs at onset, but have greatest pathologic effect in the longest nerves. Drugs that affect axonal function cause a sensory and motor neuropathy, with the greatest involvement of the longest nerves in the legs. For some drugs, the neuropathy progresses for several months after stopping the drug (coasting phenomena). Amelioration of symptoms after stopping a drug is better for those that affect axonal function, and poor for those that affect and cause the death of nerve cell bodies (Windebank and Grisold, 2008).

Cancer Chemotherapeutic Drugs

Most chemotherapeutic drugs affect sensory nerves, and the onset of the neuropathy is dependent upon the accumulated dose. Neurotoxicity frequently limits the dose with respect to treatment of the underlying cancer. Comorbidities are a factor for a more severe neuropathy and include alcohol consumption, diabetes, and inherited neuropathies (which may not be known to the patient) (Chaudhry et al., 2003). Patients frequently received more than one neurotoxic chemotherapeutic drug.

Platinum-Containing Drugs

These include cisplatin, carboplatin, and oxaliplatin.

Pathology

This group of drugs binds to DNA, and if the amount of DNA damage exceeds the ability to repair, cell death ensures. Dorsal root ganglia cells are particularly vulnerable, and large-diameter nerve fibers are involved (Windebank and Grisold, 2008).

Clinical Features

There is a threshold for a neuropathy, with doses of ~250–350 mg/m^2 for cisplatin and 500–650 mg/m^2 for oxaliplatin. Symptoms are numbness and paresthesias in distal extremities, and ankle reflexes are frequently absent. Sensory loss can lead to dystaxia. Lhermitte's phenomena may be noted with neck flexion: while Lhermitte's phenomena is traditionally encountered in the setting of cervical cord pathology, in the setting of a sensory neuropathy it is attributed to oxaliplatin-induced hyperexcitability of sensory nerves (Taieb et al., 2002). Oxaliplatin can cause acute onset cold-induced paresthesias in the hands and face.

Diagnostic Evaluation

Nerve conduction studies support a primary sensory axonal neuropathy with reduced or absent sensory nerve responses in the legs with mildly slowed conduction velocities, whereas motor nerve conduction responses are normal.

Management

The neuropathy is dependent upon the accumulated dose, and may subside over time after the drug is stopped, but there can be residual pain. Symptoms frequently continue to worsen for several months (coasting) after stopping the drug (Windebank and Grisold, 2008).

Vinca Alkaloid Drugs

These include vincristine and vindesine.

151

Pathology

Vinca alkaloids interfere with microtubule assembly and axonal transport. Both sensory and motor nerves are affected, and longer nerves are affected to the greatest degree. The cell body is not affected.

Clinical Features

Numbness and paresthesias (which may be painful) develop in the feet, and later the hands, and weakness (which is mild in degree) affects distal extremity muscles in the legs, and later the hands. Tendon reflexes are reduced or absent, first at the ankle but globally over time (DeAngelis et al., 1991). The autonomic nervous system can also be involved.

Diagnostic Evaluation

Sensory and motor responses are reduced, and conduction velocities mildly slowed, supporting a primary axonal sensory greater than motor neuropathy (DeAngelis et al., 1991). Needle EMG shows changes reflecting distal denervation.

Management

Recovery after stopping the drug is good, but the neuropathy may continue after the drug is stopped (Windebank and Grisold, 2008).

Taxanes

These include paclitaxel and docetaxel.

Pathology

Taxanes interfere with normal dynamic microtubule changes and affect axonal transport. Both sensory and motor nerves are affected, but cell bodies are unaffected.

Clinical Features

Sensory symptoms occur in both distal legs and arms with dysesthetic pain, and also distal weakness. Some patients incur an idiosyncratic pattern of proximal weakness of arms and legs (Freilich et al., 1996).

Diagnostic Evaluation

Nerve conduction studies show a distal loss of sensory and motor potentials. Needle EMG of weak proximal muscles may or may not show abnormalities, and abnormalities have been interpreted as both myopathic and neuropathic (Freilich et al., 1996).

Management

Sensory symptoms tend to abate with discontinuation of the drug, as does proximal weakness.

Bortezomib

This drug inhibits proteasome function, and interferes with proteins that promote cell division and proliferation.

Pathology

The mechanism of how bortezomib affects peripheral nerve cells is not clear. Small sensory nerve fibers appear to be preferentially affected.

Clinical Features

There is a distal-predominant sensory neuropathy with neuropathic pain, and the neuropathy can be severe with concomitant use of thalidomide (Cavaletti and Nobile-Orazio, 2007).

Diagnostic Evaluation

Nerve conduction studies support elements of primary demyelination (Thawani et al., 2015).

Management

Symptoms resolve after stopping the drug.

Thalidomide

Aside from thalidomide's original association with teratogenicity when given to pregnant women, it is used to treat myelodyspastic disorders, a number of cancers, and autoimmune disorders.

Pathology

The mechanism of neurotoxicity is not known, but likely involves immunomodulation and antiangiogensis.

Clinical Features

Symptoms are initially a distal-predominant sensory neuropathy, which may include mild weakness. Ankle reflexes are usually absent. A number of patients have a neuropathy prior to treatment with thalidomide due to their underlying disease (multiple myeloma), which worsens with treatment (Cavaletti et al., 2004). The neuropathy occurs more commonly with higher doses, and ranges from 12–44% of patients.

Diagnostic Evaluation

Most are characterized by length-dependent abnormalities, with reduced or absent distal sensory responses and reduced motor responses but preserved conduction velocities. A small portion of patients has evidence for primary demyelination with reduced conduction velocities and partial motor conduction block (Chaudhry et al., 2002).

Management

A partial reverse of symptoms occurs soon after stopping thalidomide, but those with severe neuropathy can take longer (years) (Morawska et al., 2015).

Other Neurotoxic Drugs

Amiodarone

Amiodarone is an antiarrhythmic medication that can cause a peripheral neuropathy, more often when high-maintenance doses were used (>200 mg), but infrequently with current low doses (Orr and Ahlskog, 2009).

Pathology

Amiodarone may be concentrated in nerve tissue and can cause a combination of demyelination or axonal loss (Manji, 2013).

Clinical Features

The neuropathy is characterized by distal sensory loss and motor weakness with reduced distal reflexes, and occasionally by an acute presentation (Fraser et al., 1985).

Diagnostic Evaluation

Nerve conduction studies include reduced sensory and motor response amplitudes and slow conduction velocities consistent with a chronic demyelinating polyradiculopathy (CIDP) (Fraser et al., 1985).

Management

The half-life of amiodarone is long (~30 days) and the concentration of amiodarone may be 80 times higher in nerve than serum, and the neuropathy may not improve with discontinuance of the drug (Fraser et al., 1985).

Colchicine

Colchicine produces a neuromyopathy at customary doses and in the setting of mild renal failure (Kuncl et al., 1987). The myopathic clinical and electrodiagnostic features may be mistaken for an inflammatory muscle disease (polymyositis).

Pathology

The pathology of the neuropathy is most consistent with an axonal process. The pathology of muscle is less clear, and includes vacuolar changes and may reflect a storage abnormality (Kuncl et al., 1987).

Clinical Features

Myopathic features of proximal weakness are more prominent than neuropathy features, which are a mild sensory and motor neuropathy (Kuncl et al., 1987).

Diagnostic Evaluation

Laboratory Features

Serum CK levels are elevated, up to ten times the upper limit of normal (Kuncl et al., 1987).

Electrodiagnostic Features

Nerve conduction findings are reduced or absent distal sensory responses and markedly reduced distal motor responses with relatively preserved conduction velocities. Needle EMG of distal muscles supports neurogenic changes, while in proximal muscles there is evidence for myopathic changes.

Management

There is recovery of the myopathic symptoms and reduction of CK levels within weeks of stopping the drug.

Nitrofurantoin

Nitrofurantoin is used as a long-term prophylactic antibiotic for urinary tract infections and can cause a peripheral neuropathy. The onset is usually within several months of starting the drug (Kammire and Donofrio, 2007).

Pathology

The pathology is not known, but nitrofurantoin interferes with pyruvate oxidation; however, it is unclear if this contributes.

Clinical Features

Symptoms are a distal-predominant loss of sensory perception with paresthesias and dysesthesias, and distal weakness in severe cases (Kammire and Donofrio, 2007). It can also cause a patchy small-fiber neuropathy (Tan et al., 2012).

Diagnostic Evaluation

There are relatively few electrodiagnostic studies available, but the neuropathy is primary axonal. Nerve conduction studies may be normal, and a skin biopsy may show normal fiber density but clustered nerve fiber terminals (Tan et al., 2012).

Management

Recovery varies, dependent upon the severity of axonal loss, from partial to complete, weeks to months after stopping the drug.

Pyridoxine

Both deficiencies and excesses of pyridoxine (vitamin B6) are associated with peripheral neuropathies. Deficiencies occur in the context of drugs to treat specific diseases, such as isoniazid, which may deplete vitamin B6. In the setting of possible drug interactions, pyridoxine supplementation of <6 mg a day may be sufficient. A neuropathy in the setting of primary pyridoxine deficiency due to dietary deficiency is not well described (Ghavanini and Kimpinski, 2014).

Pyridoxine excess occurs in the setting of vitamin supplementation, at times from the patient's feeling that high doses may be more beneficial or when multiple combinations of vitamin tablets are taken (each with B6) (Schaumburg et al., 1983).

Pathology

Biopsies of distal sensory nerve indicate a primary axonal loss. Pathology in experimental animals indicates loss of dorsal root ganglia cells (Schaumburg et al., 1983).

Clinical Features

Elevated pyridoxine causes a dose-dependent sensory neuropathy that can include a sensory dystaxia (Berger et al., 1992). It can occur with doses as low as 200 mg per day (Parry and Bredesen, 1985). With extreme doses (132–183 g over three days), the neuropathy can be profound and prevent ambulation in

the setting of normal strength due to proprioceptive loss (Albin et al., 1987).

Diagnostic Evaluation

Sensory nerve conduction studies show reduced or absent sensory responses (Schaumburg et al., 1983). Motor responses can be mildly reduced. Needle EMG can show scattered changes consistent with mild axonal loss or changes related to disuse from sensory dystaxia (Albin et al., 1987).

Management

Stopping the drug results in slow improvement when the dose is low, but in the extreme a sensory dystaxia can be permanent (Albin et al., 1987).

Human Immunodeficiency Virus Drugs

Human immunodeficiency virus (HIV) and the medications used to treat the condition can separately cause a distal-predominant primary axonal sensory peripheral neuropathy. This section focuses on neuropathies associated with HIV drug treatment, and the neuropathy associated with untreated HIV infection is considered in Chapter 34. It can be difficult to distinguish between the underlying causes in treated patients.

The most neurotoxic antiretroviral drugs are "d drugs" such as didanosine, zalcitabine, and stavudine (causing a neuropathy in ~10%), but these are not commonly used with the availability of newer first-line drugs (Nath, 2015). Amongst newer drugs, the nucleoside reverse transcriptase inhibitors class may cause a peripheral neuropathy due to inhibition of DNA polymerase resulting in interference with mitochondrial DNA synthesis (Kranick and Nath, 2012) Other newer drugs, including non-nucleoside reverse transcriptase inhibitors, protease inhibitors, entry inhibitors, and integrase inhibitors have low nerve toxicity (Margolis et al., 2014).

References

Albin RL, Albers JW, Greenberg HS, Townsend JB, Lynn RB, Burke JM, Jr., et al. Acute sensory neuropathy-neuronopathy from pyridoxine overdose. *Neurology*. 1987;37:1729–32.

Berger AR, Schaumburg HH, Schroeder C, Apfel S, Reynolds R. Dose response, coasting, and differential fiber vulnerability in human toxic neuropathy: a prospective study of pyridoxine neurotoxicity. *Neurology*. 1992;42:1367–70.

Cavaletti G, Beronio A, Reni L, Ghiglione E, Schenone A, Briani C, et al. Thalidomide sensory neurotoxicity: a clinical and neurophysiologic study. *Neurology.* 2004;62:2291–3.

Cavaletti G, Nobile-Orazio E. Bortezomib-induced peripheral neurotoxicity: still far from a painless gain. *Haematologica.* 2007;92:1308–10.

Chaudhry V, Chaudhry M, Crawford TO, Simmons-O'Brien E, Griffin JW. Toxic neuropathy in patients with pre-existing neuropathy. *Neurology.* 2003;60:337–40.

Chaudhry V, Cornblath DR, Corse A, Freimer M, Simmons-O'Brien E, Vogelsang G. Thalidomide-induced neuropathy. *Neurology.* 2002;59:1872–5.

DeAngelis LM, Gnecco C, Taylor L, Warrell RP, Jr. Evolution of neuropathy and myopathy during intensive vincristine/corticosteroid chemotherapy for non-Hodgkin's lymphoma. *Cancer.* 1991;67:2241–6.

Fraser AG, McQueen IN, Watt AH, Stephens MR. Peripheral neuropathy during longterm high-dose amiodarone therapy. *J Neurol Neurosurg Psychiatry.* 1985;48:576–8.

Freilich RJ, Balmaceda C, Seidman AD, Rubin M, DeAngelis LM. Motor neuropathy due to docetaxel and paclitaxel. *Neurology.* 1996;47:115–18.

Ghavanini AA, Kimpinski K. Revisiting the evidence for neuropathy caused by pyridoxine deficiency and excess. *J Clin Neuromuscul Dis.* 2014;16:25–31.

Kammire LD, Donofrio PD. Nitrofurantoin neuropathy: a forgotten adverse effect. *Obstet Gynecol.* 2007;110:510–12.

Kranick SM, Nath A. Neurologic complications of HIV-1 infection and its treatment in the ear of antiretroviral therapy . *Continuum (Minnea; Minn).* 2012;13:319–37.

Kuncl RW, Duncan G, Watson D, Alderson K, Rogawski MA, Peper M. Colchicine myopathy and neuropathy. *N Engl J Med.* 1987;316:1562–8.

Manji H. Drug-induced neuropathies. *Handb Clin Neurol.* 2013;115:729–42.

Margolis AM, Heverling H, Pham PA, Stolbach A. A review of toxicity of HIV medications. *J Med Toxicol.* 2014; 10:26-39.

Morawska M, Grzasko N, Kostyra M, Wojciechowicz J, Hus M. Therapy-related peripheral neuropathy in multiple myeloma patients. *Hematol Oncol.* 2015;33:113–19.

Nath A. Neurologic comlications of human immunodeficiency virus infection. *Continuum (Minnea; Minn).* 2015; 21:1557–76.

Orr CF, Ahlskog JE. Frequency, characteristics, and risk factors for amiodarone neurotoxicity. *Arch Neurol.* 2009;66:865–9.

Parry GJ, Bredesen DE. Sensory neuropathy with low-dose pyridoxine. *Neurology.* 1985;35:1466–8.

Schaumburg H, Kaplan J, Windebank A, Vick N, Rasmus S, Pleasure D, et al. Sensory neuropathy from pyridoxine abuse. A new megavitamin syndrome. *N Engl J Med.* 1983;309:445–8.

Taieb S, Trillet-Lenoir V, Rambaud L, Descos L, Freyer G. Lhermitte sign and urinary retention: atypical presentation of oxaliplatin neurotoxicity in four patients. *Cancer.* 2002;94:2434–40.

Tan IL, Polydefkis MJ, Ebenezer GJ, Hauer P, McArthur JC. Peripheral nerve toxic effects of nitrofurantoin. *Arch Neurol.* 2012;69:265–8.

Thawani SP, Tanji K, De Sousa EA, Weimer LH, Brannagan TH, III. Bortezomib-associated demyelinating neuropathy – clinical and pathologic features. *J Clin Neuromuscul Dis.* 2015;16:202–209.

Windebank AJ, Grisold W. Chemotherapy-induced neuropathy. *J Peripher Nerv Syst.* 2008;13:27–46.

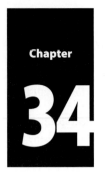

Chapter

34

Neuropathy Associated with Human Immunodeficiency Virus

Introduction

Human immunodeficiency virus (HIV) and the medications used to treat the condition can cause a distal-predominant primary axonal sensory polyneuropathy and other less common forms of neuropathy. This chapter focuses on neuropathies associated with HIV infection, and neuropathies associated with drug treatment are considered in Chapter 33. When antiretroviral drugs are used that have neurotoxic properties, separation between the two underlying causes for a neuropathy becomes clouded.

Both symptomatic and asymptomatic neuropathies can occur before or progress with treatment of HIV, and >30% of patients have a neuropathy (Lee et al., 2015; Robinson-Papp et al., 2015). Risk factors include advanced patient age, concurrent diabetes, and alcohol abuse (Schutz and Robinson-Papp, 2013). Co-infection with hepatitis C is common amongst HIV patients, but seropositivity for hepatitis C is not a risk factor.

Pathology

The underlying pathology of the length-dependent axonal neuropathy is not known. It does not appear to be due to viral infection, but there is evidence for an immune process (Cashman and Hoke, 2015).

Clinical Features

The most common neuropathy is a distal-predominant painful sensory neuropathy that starts in the feet and can progress to the level of the knees. Symptoms include burning in the feet, stabbing pains, and numbness. Signs include reduced perception of pinprick, vibratory and cold, and reduced or absent ankle tendon reflexes (Lee et al., 2015). It should be noted that about one-third of patients with signs of a neuropathy describe no symptoms.

Less common forms include an acute (at the time of infection) or chronic inflammatory demyelinating polyneuropathy, progressive polyradiculopathy (associated with cytomegalovirus), mononeuropathies, and autonomic neuropathies (Wulff et al., 2000; Schutz and Robinson-Papp, 2013).

Diagnostic Evaluation

Laboratory Evaluation

There are correlations, before antiviral drug treatment, with low CD4+ cell counts or high viral loads (Lee et al., 2015). The neuropathy can develop or persist in the setting of drug treatment that lowers these factors

Electrodiagnostic Evaluation

Nerve conduction studies for the common distal-predominant painful sensory neuropathy are remarkable for reduced distal sensory nerve (sural nerve) responses (Amruth et al., 2014). Most patients are diagnosed on clinical features, and nerve conduction studies may not be helpful as they may be normal in patients with sensory symptoms or abnormal in patients without symptoms. Electrodiagnostic studies will be more helpful in the setting of the less common forms of neuropathy (demyelinating neuropathies).

Management

Management focuses on avoiding antiretroviral drugs known to be neurotoxic, such as nucleoside analogues (which are now less commonly used), and to treat symptoms of distal pain. Drugs used to treat neuropathic pain from other causes (Chapter 48) appear to be less effective with HIV-associated distal sensory neuropathy (Phillips et al., 2010).

References

Amruth G, Praveen-kumar S, Nataraju B, Nagaraja BS. HIV Associated Sensory Neuropathy. *J Clin Diagn Res.* 2014;8:MC04–7.

Cashman CR, Hoke A. Mechanisms of distal axonal degeneration in peripheral neuropathies. *Neurosci Lett.* 2015;596:33–50.

Lee AJ, Bosch RJ, Evans SR, Wu K, Harrison T, Grant P, et al. Patterns of peripheral neuropathy in ART-naive patients initiating modern ART regimen. *J Neurovirol.* 2015;21:210–18.

Phillips TJ, Cherry CL, Cox S, Marshall SJ, Rice AS. Pharmacological treatment of painful HIV-associated sensory neuropathy: a systematic review and meta-analysis of randomised controlled trials. *PLoS One.* 2010;5:e14433.

Robinson-Papp J, Sharma S, Dhadwal N, Simpson DM, Morgello S. Optimizing measures of HIV-associated neuropathy. *Muscle Nerve.* 2015;51:56–64.

Schutz SG, Robinson-Papp J. HIV-related neuropathy: current perspectives. *HIV AIDS (Auckl).* 2013;5:243–51.

Wulff EA, Wang AK, Simpson DM. HIV-associated peripheral neuropathy: epidemiology, pathophysiology and treatment. *Drugs.* 2000;59:1251–60.

Leprous Neuropathy

Introduction

Neuropathy from *Mycobacterium lepare* is common in selected regions of the world (India, Brazil, Indonesia, Nigeria), but with ease of travel, patients with leprous neuropathy can be encountered anywhere. The neuropathy results from a bacterial infection and thus is treatable, but without identification and treatment it is progressive.

Unique features of *M. lepare* influence the effect on nerves and the distribution of neuropathic symptoms and signs (Nations et al., 1998; de Freitas and Said, 2013). *M. lepare* is acquired through nasal mucosa and skin contact. There are gradations in the distribution of the bacterium and its effects on nerves, based on an infected individual's innate response to the bacterium, leading to several overlapping classification schemes (Ridley-Jopling is the most common scheme): the range is from the tuberculoid type (with limited involvement) to the lepromatous type (with the greatest distribution of involvement), and intermediate gradations (de Freitas and Said, 2013). The bacterium affects the skin, and has tropism for macrophages and Schwann cells, primarily Schwann cells of unmyelinated fibers. The bacterium does not grow at temperatures higher than 30°C, leading to frequent involvement of nerves in cooler body regions: the face (nose, ear lobes), distal limbs, and buttocks. Within nerves, there is slow multiplication of the bacterium, and the incubation period can be over years or decades. A chronic response occurs within nerves leading to progressive damage to myelinated and unmyelinated fibers.

Pathologic Features

Changes on nerve biopsy vary based on severity, and range from thickening of the perineurium, to inflammation, to fibrosis, with varying degrees of primary axonal loss and secondary demyelination. There may

be bacilli within inflammatory regions (de Freitas and Said, 2013). Nerve enlargement is common.

Clinical Features

There are three classic features and tests: hypopigmented skin lesions with loss of sensory perception within the lesion, palpable thickening of peripheral nerves, and skin-smear positive for acid-fast bacilli. However, the range of pathologic involvement is broad and may be missed. Nerve damage is commonly heralded by skin changes in the form of a rash, affecting cooler regions (the face-nose, ear lobes), and fibrosis can affect facial appearance (leonine facies) or testicular function. Dermal nerves are damaged leading to loss of temperature and touch, and neuropathic pain is common. More proximal nerves are frequently damaged in the following frequency: ulnar nerve at the medial epicondyle, median nerve proximal to the wrist, fibular/peroneal nerve at the fibular head, posterior tibial nerve at the ankle, superficial radial nerve at the wrist, sural nerve, and the greater auricular nerve. There is palpable thickening of nerves. With progression is spread in a stocking-glove distribution. Tendon reflexes tend to be preserved because deep-lying nerves are involved in the reflex arc. A rare neuritic form occurs without skin lesions.

Diagnostic Evaluation

Laboratory Evaluation

Laboratory diagnosis is made by skin and nasal smears showing acid-fast bacilli. Nerve biopsies are generally not necessary as less invasived tissue is usually diagnostic.

Electrodiagnostic Evaluation

Nerve conduction findings relate to the distribution and degree of nerve involvement: there may be slowing of conduction across focal sites (the ulnar nerve at the elbow, the median nerve proximal to the wrist, the peroneal/fibular nerve at the fibular head). Needle EMG shows varying degrees of axonal damage (Nations et al., 1998).

Imaging Evaluation

Leprous neuropathy can present without skin lesions in ~10% of cases (neuritic form), and imaging can help with the differential diagnosis. Ultrasound of nerves can be used to assess nerve enlargement and changes in echogenicity encountered with leprous neuropathy (Jain et al., 2016). The ulnar, median, and peroneal/fibular nerves are the most commonly involved, and showing changes in the appropriate clinical setting is helpful diagnostically. MRI can also be used to demonstrate focal thickening of nerves (Payne et al., 2015).

Management

Patients can experience "reactions," due to increases in their cell-mediated immune response, that alter the stable or chronic course of the disease, and can occur before, during, or after antibiotic treatment (Nations et al., 1998). Antibiotic treatment varies based on the severity of the disease within an individual. The goals are to arrest progressive nerve involvement. Surgical nerve decompression may be helpful (de Freitas and Said, 2013).

References

de Freitas MR, Said G. Leprous neuropathy. *Handb Clin Neurol*. 2013;115:499–514.

Jain S, Visser LH, Suneetha S. Imaging techniques in leprosy clinics. *Clin Dermatol*. 2016;34:70–8.

Nations SP, Katz JS, Lyde CB, Barohn RJ. Leprous neuropathy: an American perspective. *Semin Neurol*. 1998;18:113–24.

Payne R, Baccon J, Dossett J, Scollard D, Byler D, Patel A, et al. Pure neuritic leprosy presenting as ulnar nerve neuropathy: a case report of electrodiagnostic, radiographic, and histopathological findings. *J Neurosurg*. 2015;123:1238–43.

Neuropathy Associated with Nutritional Deficiencies

Introduction

Neuropathies due to nutritional deficiencies are rare in Western countries, but can be encountered in patients from countries where diets may be extreme.

Colbalmin (B12) Deficiency

Colbalmin deficiency has many causes, including atrophic gastritis and hypochlorhydria due to lack of intrinsic factor (pernicious anemia), and perhaps more commonly in the setting of gastric surgery (Kumar, 2014). The classic neurologic condition due to B12 deficiency is subacute combined degeneration with myelopathic features of spasticity and sensory disturbance. Since a myelopathy can include sensory symptoms and signs, it can be difficult to separate sensory loss from central or peripheral pathology, and the question of an isolated peripheral neuropathy remains open (Saperstein and Barohn, 2002; Kumar, 2014). A number of patients with a peripheral neuropathy have B12 levels in the lower range, especially amongst the elderly, and association does not imply causation. Supplementation is not usually effective in reducing symptoms or improving nerve conduction findings (Saperstein and Barohn, 2002), although exceptions are noted (Dalla Torre et al., 2012), and thus it is not clear if B12 deficiency causes a reversible polyneuropathy. This section focuses on features attributed to a polyneuropathy.

Pathology

The pathology is felt to be a primary axonal sensory neuropathy, and may include evidence for motor nerve involvement (Saperstein and Barohn, 2002).

Clinical Features

The neuropathy, when isolated from myelopathic features (that is, absent ankle tendon reflexes), is characterized by distal sensory loss, which can be painful. Clinical clues may be rapid onset and involvement of legs and arms at onset (Kumar, 2014).

Diagnostic Evaluation

Laboratory Evaluation

Further, the role of supportive laboratory tests for associated markers, homocysteine and methyl malonic acid, is not clear (Kumar, 2014). Methylmalonic acid may be a more sensitive marker than homocysteine for B12 deficiency, but neither may be elevated, and blood cell markers may be normal.

Electrodiagnostic Evaluation

There are few electrodiagnostic studies, but a sensory>motor neuropathy is reported (Saperstein and Barohn, 2002), although nerve conduction studies may be normal.

Management

Replacement of B12 when levels are in the lower range of normal (<300–500 ng/L) is reasonable in any patient with an unexplained neuropathy. A slow recovery of symptoms and improvement in sensory nerve response amplitudes has been reported, but patients may not have reduced symptoms (Saperstein and Barohn, 2002; Dalla Torre et al., 2012).

Folic Acid Deficiency

Peripheral neuropathy attributed to a deficiency of folate without concomitant deficiencies in vitamin B12 and thiamine is rare (Botez et al., 1978; Koike et al., 2015). Many countries fortify cereal-grain products with folic acid, but this is not a universal practice.

Pathology

Sural nerve biopsy shows loss of large and small fibers with axonal degeneration but no primary demyelination (Koike et al., 2015).

Clinical Features

Initial symptoms are sensory disturbance starting distally in the legs and progressing proximally over months to years, associated with gait unsteadiness (Koike et al., 2015). Sensory disturbances are loss of vibratory and joint position sense, and tendon reflexes are absent at the ankles and frequently at the knees. A portion of patients exhibits distal weakness.

Diagnostic Evaluation

Nerve conduction studies may show evidence for a primary axonal sensorimotor neuropathy with loss of sensory and motor response amplitudes, but normal conduction velocities (Koike et al., 2015).

Management

Folic acid supplementation can result in improvements in gait stability over months (Koike et al., 2015). Folic acid deficiency frequently coexists with deficiencies of B12 and thiamine, and treatment with all three is reasonable.

References

Botez MI, Peyronnard JM, Bachevalier J, Charron L. Polyneuropathy and folate deficiency. *Arch Neurol.* 1978;35:581–4.

Dalla Torre C, Lucchetta M, Cacciavillani M, Campagnolo M, Manara R, Briani C. Reversible isolated sensory axonal neuropathy due to cobalamin deficiency. *Muscle Nerve.* 2012;45:428–30.

Koike H, Takahashi M, Ohyama K, Hashimoto R, Kawagashira Y, Iijima M, et al. Clinicopathologic features of folate-deficiency neuropathy. *Neurology.* 2015;84:1026–33.

Kumar N. Neurologic aspects of cobalamin (B12) deficiency. *Handb Clin Neurol.* 2014;120:915–26.

Saperstein DS, Barohn RJ. Peripheral Neuropathy Due to Cobalamin Deficiency. *Curr Treat Options Neurol.* 2002;4:197–201.

Chapter 37

Paraneoplastic Sensory Neuropathy

Introduction

Paraneoplastic neurologic syndromes are defined as neurologic dysfunction pathologically linked to a cancer, but remote from the malignancy and sites of metastasis, and after exclusion of other causes of the syndrome. The challenges are in defining the cancer linkage, and the discovery of antibodies (onconeural antibodies) against intracellular neural antigens expressed by the tumor (Table 37.1) has helped with well-established cancer-antibody linkages. Diagnostic criteria are available to support definite and possible paraneoplastic syndromes (Graus et al., 2004). Criteria for definite paraneoplastic syndrome include one of the following: presence of a classic syndrome (Table 37.1) and cancer that develops within five years, without requirement for antibodies; a non-classic syndrome with improvement with cancer treatment; a non-classic syndrome but a classic type of cancer that develops within five years, with antibodies; or a classic or non-classic syndrome with no cancer, but with classic antibodies. Criteria for possible paraneoplastic syndrome require less rigorous connections between the syndrome, a cancer, and antibodies. Peripheral nerves are the primary neurologic structure involved in approximately one-third of paraneoplastic syndromes, and sensory neuronopathies are the focus of this chapter (Giometto et al., 2010). Chronic inflammatory demyelinating polyradiculoneuropathies (CIDP) associated with plasma cell dyscrasias are discussed in Chapter 25).

Clinical points to bear in mind when considering a paraneoplastic neuropathy are: the neuropathy commonly occurs before the detection of the cancer; symptoms follow a subacute time course and may involve upper extremity and facial nerves early on, and may also include involvement of the central nervous system; paraneoplastic neuropathies are very rare (0.01% of cancers); and clinical features suggestive of paraneoplastic neuropathy occur more commonly

Table 37.1 Paraneoplastic Syndromes Involving Peripheral Nerves

Classic paraneoplastic peripheral nerve syndromes
Sensory neuropathy: small cell lung cancer, lymphoma, adenocarcinoma; anti-H (antineuronal nuclear antibody type 1 – ANNA-1), anti-CV2 (collapsin response-mediator protein-5 – CRMP-5)
Autonomic neuropathies: small-cell lung cancer, adenocarcinoma, thymoma; anti-Hu, anti-ganglionic nicotinic acetylcholine receptor
Neuropathies with vasculitis: solid organ cancers, lymphoma; seronegative
Less well-established paraneoplastic peripheral nerve syndromes
Motor neuropathy
Sensorimotor neuropathy
Plexopathies
Primary demyelinating neuropathies (acute and chronic)

Top: Classic syndromes and associated cancers and paraneoplastic antibodies. Bottom: Less well established paraneoplastic syndromes.

as idiopathic neuropathies or associated with autoimmune disorders, or due to drug neurotoxicity. The relationship between antibodies, antibody titers, and an associated cancer varies amongst patients, and antibody data must be interpreted in context to reduce false-positive results and unnecessary testing (Muppidi and Vernino, 2014).

Pathology

Sensory neuronopathies are due to antibody-mediated destruction of dorsal root cell bodies (Koike and Sobue, 2013). At postmortem examination, the degree of sensory neuronal loss varies and frequently is asymmetric. Either large sensory fibers or small fibers can be preferentially involved, correlating with ataxic and painful clinical features, respectfully. Antibodies can be directed concurrently at central nervous system structures such as the cerebellum, cerebral cortex, and brainstem.

Clinical Features

Paraneoplastic sensory neuronopathies commonly follow a subacute time course (weeks to months) and most have asymmetric patterns. A clinical clue is that the location of symptoms is based on the involved dorsal root ganglia and does not follow a length-dependent polyneuropathy pattern: sites include face, scalp, trunk, hands, arms, or proximal legs before feet. Loss of large-diameter sensory neurons is felt to account for loss of touch perception and proprioception resulting in dystaxia of involved limbs, and loss of small-fiber neurons for pain, and elements of both symptoms can be present. Tendon reflexes in the involved nerve are reduced or absent. Motor nerves are involved in a percentage, as are autonomic nerves causing urinary retention, constipation, or orthostatic hypotension, and the presence of these features does not exclude the diagnosis.

Diagnostic Evaluation

Laboratory Evaluation

Paraneoplastic antibody testing helps confirm the diagnosis, and sensory neuronopathies are most commonly associated with small-cell lung cancer, and with anti-Hu (antineuronal nuclear antibody type 1 – ANNA-1) or anti-CV2 (collapsin response-mediator protein-5 – CRMP-5) antibodies, although ~15% have no antibodies. However, patients with paraneoplastic neuropathies may not have a detectable antibody. Identification of a classic underlying cancer is important, and testing should include assessment of risk factors, a thorough general medical examination (in women, breast and pelvic examination), imaging studies of chest, abdomen, and pelvis, and colonoscopy. A positron emission tomography (PET) scan may be helpful when no malignancy is found with routine testing (Gwathmey, 2016). If no malignancy

is found, PET scans should be repeated twice yearly for four years.

Electrodiagnostic Evaluation

Paraneoplastic sensory neuronopathies involve the dorsal root ganglia and SNAP responses will be reduced or absent in involved nerves, while generally motor components of the same nerve will be normal. However, motor involvement in paraneoplastic sensory neuronopathies occurs, and is detected by reduced CMAP amplitude and denervation on needle EMG.

Management

Early detection of a cancer is the first goal, and with treatment of the cancer progression of the paraneoplastic neuropathy may be arrested. There are little data to guide direct treatment of the paraneoplastic neuropathy (Giometto et al., 2012) due to no randomized and controlled trials. Medications used include immunomodulatory therapies (intravenous immune globulin, corticosteroids, plasma exchange, cyclophosphamide, and rituximab).

References

Giometto B, Grisold W, Vitaliani R, Graus F, Honnorat J, Bertolini G. Paraneoplastic neurologic syndrome in the PNS Euronetwork database: a European study from 20 centers. *Arch Neurol.* 2010;67:330–5.

Giometto B, Vitaliani R, Lindeck-Pozza E, Grisold W, Vedeler C. Treatment for paraneoplastic neuropathies. *Cochrane Database Syst Rev.* 2012;12:CD007625.

Graus F, Delattre JY, Antoine JC, Dalmau J, Giometto B, Grisold W, et al. Recommended diagnostic criteria for paraneoplastic neurological syndromes. *J Neurol Neurosurg Psychiatry.* 2004;75:1135–40.

Gwathmey KG. Sensory neuronopathies. *Muscle Nerve.* 2016;53:8–19.

Koike H, Sobue G. Paraneoplastic neuropathy. *Handb Clin Neurol.* 2013;115:713–26.

Muppidi S, Vernino S. Paraneoplastic neuropathies. *Continuum (Minneap Minn).* 2014;20:1359–72.

Small Fiber Neuropathy

Introduction

Small-fiber neuropathies are defined as symptoms, clinical findings, and laboratory test abnormalities attributed to thinly myelinated A-delta and unmyelinated C-fibers. This definition excludes concurrent involvement of large-diameter sensory or motor fibers. Of note, the frequency of associated diseases results in a disproportionate number of small-fiber neuropathies in the elderly.

Pathology

There are many causes of small-fiber neuropathies, and they can be divided into those associated with concurrent diseases and those that have a hereditary basis. Concurrent diseases include diabetes mellitus type 2, infections (human immunodeficiency virus, hepatitis), autoimmune diseases (Sjögren syndrome, systemic lupus, celiac disease), and systemic amyloidosis. Hereditary neuropathies include Fabry disease, sodium channelopathies, and amyloidosis (see Chapters 44 and 45). Skin hypersensitivity may be part of the fibromyalgia syndrome. Despite efforts to find an underlying cause, none will be found in a percentage of patients (25–90%) (Chan and Wilder-Smith, 2016).

Underlying pathology is largely unknown, except for those associated with autoimmune diseases and channelopathies. For autoimmune diseases, there is likely an inflammatory element, but given the high frequency of these diseases and the low frequency of small-fiber neuropathies amongst patients, triggering factors are unknown. For channelopathies, mutations in voltage-gated sodium channels (Nav1.7, Nav1.8, Nav1.9) are associated with increased excitability of dorsal root ganglion cells (Chan and Wilder-Smith, 2016). Hyperexcitability leads to increased nerve discharges, but the subsequent cause of nerve damage is not known. Mutations have been found in a small number of patients with idiopathic small-fiber neuropathies (Hoeijmakers et al., 2015).

Clinical Features

Symptoms are pain, frequently burning in nature, and allodynia or hyperalgesia. Disagreeable sensations to contact by bed sheets and clothes may occur. The distribution is more commonly a length-dependent pattern, but can be a patchy distribution involving face, arms, or the trunk. Clinical testing discloses hypersensitivity to light touch, impaired or heightened perception to noxious stimuli (pin prick), altered perception of high- or low-temperature probes, and greater uncomfortable sensations to repeated stimuli (wind-up phenomena). In contract, sensory perception of light touch, vibration, and joint position, conveyed by large nerve fibers, is intact, as is strength and tendon reflexes (Chan and Wilder-Smith, 2016).

Diagnostic Evaluation

Nerve conduction studies are normal, as the diagnosis requires an intact sural nerve response. Supportive laboratory tests are abnormalities on quantitative sensory testing or reduced intraepidermal nerve fiber density on skin biopsies.

There is a set of formal diagnostic criteria and levels of certainty (Chan and Wilder-Smith, 2016). Definite small-fiber neuropathy requires length-dependent pattern with normal sural response and reduced density of intraepidermal nerve fibers at the ankle or abnormal quantitative sensory testing results at the foot. Probable small-fiber neuropathy requires clinical features and normal sural response. Possible small-fiber neuropathy requires only the clinical features.

Management

Treating the underlying condition may result in reduced symptoms. Since neuropathic pain is the primary symptom, treatment focuses on drugs that treat nerve-based pain (see Chapter 48). A very small percentage of patients may have an immune-based cause and will respond to intravenous immune globulin or corticosteroids, but reliance on a subjective treatment endpoint may be challenging, especially when using immunoglobulin. The long-term prognosis has not been studied, and such a study will be challenging given the spectrum of causes.

References

Chan AC, Wilder-Smith EP. Small fiber neuropathy: Getting bigger! *Muscle Nerve*. 2016;53:671–82.

Hoeijmakers JG, Faber CG, Merkies IS, Waxman SG. Painful peripheral neuropathy and sodium channel mutations. *Neurosci Lett*. 2015;596:51–9.

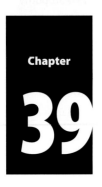

Uremic Neuropathy

Introduction

The relationship between chronic renal failure and the development of a polyneuropathy has been recognized and studied from the 1960s, when hemodialysis was available to prolong survival. The prevalence of peripheral neuropathy in end-stage renal disease is 60–100%, dependent upon diagnostic criteria for subclinical and clinical neuropathy (Krishnan and Kiernan, 2007). Given that end-stage renal failure is commonly due to diabetes, the concurrence of both etiologic factors for a neuropathy likely explains the infrequent request for neurologic and electrodiagnostic consultation. However, acute onset neuropathy in the setting of uremia may not be widely appreciated (see below).

Pathology

Sural nerve biopsies reveal a spectrum of changes, including axonal loss with regenerating axonal sprouts and both primary and secondary demyelination (Said et al., 1983). The underlying cause is not clear as the presence of regenerating axonal sprouts supports the possibility of improvement, and improvements are observed in the setting of renal transplant.

Clinical Features

The neuropathy in chronic renal failure follows a length-dependent pattern with sensory symptoms exceeding motor symptoms, but in some patients, distal leg and arm weakness can be marked (Krishnan and Kiernan, 2007). There is loss of large-fiber modalities with reduced light touch perception, reduced or absent tendon reflexes, and atrophic weakness of distal muscles. Distal leg cramps are common. There can also be symptoms of autonomic dysfunction, supporting small-fiber involvement (Said, 2013). In the setting of diabetes, it is not possible to separate the effects of diabetes from uremia as clinical and pathologic features overlap.

Progression is slow, and there may be improvements in symptoms with dialysis (Said, 2013). With renal transplantation, there is a two-phase improvement, the first soon after surgery and the second over months, and overall, symptoms and signs (including some nerve conduction metrics) can improve (Bolton, 1976).

Acute Neuropathy

A severe and accelerated uremic neuropathy occurs, leading to a non-ambulatory state that can mimic the time course of acute inflammatory demyelinating polyradiculoneuropathy (AIDP) (Ropper, 1993). Nerve conduction studies reflect both axonal loss and slow conduction velocities, mimicking that observed with AIDP. Nerve biopsy supports both axonal and myelin loss. The etiology is uncertain, and given the small number of patients reported, there are varied clinical circumstances.

Diagnostic Evaluation

The diagnosis is usually straightforward in the setting of end-stage renal failure with or without diabetes, except in acute forms.

Laboratory Evaluation

Polyneuropathy symptoms rarely begin with creatinine levels <4.0–6.0 mg/dl (glomerular filtration rates ~18–29 ml/min), and the neuropathy becomes symptomatic with creatinine levels >8 mg/dl (filtration rate ~6 ml/min) (severe to end stage chronic renal disease).

Electrodiagnostic Evaluation

Nerve conduction studies show a reduction or loss of SNAP amplitude, and to lesser extent CMAP amplitudes, and mild degrees of conduction velocity slowing (Krishnan and Kiernan, 2007). The absence of distal sensory and motor responses parallels the clinical degree of neuropathy symptoms and signs. The effects on nerve conduction values of long-term (five years) hemodialysis and peritoneal dialysis are stabilization, but no predictable improvement (Ogura et al., 2001). However, with renal transplantation there is an improvement in conduction velocity and response amplitude based on the severity of the neuropathy before transplantation (Bolton, 1976).

Management

The severity of the neuropathy depends also upon comorbid factors such as presence of diabetes and management of renal function. Management of renal failure is by dialysis, and clinical and nerve conduction abnormalities that follow are dependent upon long-term dialysis, with greatest benefit from transplantation.

References

Bolton CF. Electrophysiologic changes in uremic neuropathy after successful renal transplantation. *Neurology.* 1976;26:152–61.

Krishnan AV, Kiernan MC. Uremic neuropathy: clinical features and new pathophysiological insights. *Muscle Nerve.* 2007;35:273–90.

Ogura T, Makinodan A, Kubo T, Hayashida T, Hirasawa Y. Electrophysiological course of uraemic neuropathy in haemodialysis patients. *Postgrad Med J.* 2001;77:451–4.

Ropper AH. Accelerated neuropathy of renal failure. *Arch Neurol.* 1993;50:536–9.

Said G. Uremic neuropathy. *Handb Clin Neurol.* 2013;115:607–12.

Said G, Boudier L, Selva J, Zingraff J, Drueke T. Different patterns of uremic polyneuropathy: clinicopathologic study. *Neurology.* 1983;33:567–74.

Neuropathy Associated with Gluten Sensitivity

Introduction

Celiac disease in its classic form is an autoimmune disorder affecting the small intestine, triggered in genetically susceptible individuals by ingestion of gluten. Gluten is a mixture of proteins in wheat, barley, rye, and oats, and causes an inflammatory response in the gut with villous atrophy, crypt hyperplasia, and intraepithelial lymphocytes. The pathologic changes in the intestines cause symptoms of abdominal bloating, diarrhea, and changes to skin. There is also a spectrum of other symptoms, including neurologic disorders of cerebellar ataxia and peripheral neuropathies (length-dependent, sensorimotor primary axonal neuropathies, and dorsal root ganglionopathies) (Hadjivassiliou et al., 2016). The prevalence of celiac disease is ~1%. Antibodies are produced that serve as markers.

A related condition, gluten-related diseases or non-celiac gluten sensitivity, with no villus changes or antibodies, has been associated with gastrointestinal symptoms and affected individuals may have neurologic involvement (Aziz et al., 2015). When antibody testing is negative, the diagnosis of a gluten-related condition as a cause of a neuropathy is difficult, and further challenging as a gluten-free diet may or may not result in an improvement in the neuropathy. It is also difficult to envision improvement in the setting of a primary axonal neuropathy or ganglionopathy.

The incidence of neuropathy associated with celiac or non-celiac gluten sensitivity varies: a 2.5-fold risk of developing a peripheral neuropathy among people with celiac disease was found from a population study (Thawani et al., 2015); extensive evaluation of patients with an idiopathic neuropathy revealed a diagnosis of celiac disease in <2% (Farhad et al., 2016), while another study revealed an incidence of 34%, with three-quarters having a diagnosis of non-celiac gluten sensitivity (Aziz et al., 2015).

Pathology

Peripheral nerve biopsies show sparse lymphocytic infiltrates with perivascular cuffing, and similar changes to dorsal root ganglia from autopsies. These changes are felt to represent antibody-mediated pathology (Hadjivassiliou et al., 2014).

Clinical Features

A spectrum of peripheral nerve disorders attributed to gluten sensitivity ranges from sensorimotor axonal neuropathy, mononeuropathy multiplex, motor neuropathy, and small-fiber neuropathy (Hadjivassiliou et al., 2014). Onset is in adulthood and progresses over years, yet gluten enteropathy is frequently diagnosed in childhood.

Diagnostic Evaluation

Celiac disease is diagnosed by a duodenal biopsy showing villous atrophy as the most specific test, and video capsule endoscopy is an alternative (Rashid and Lee, 2016). The diagnosis can be supported by serum antibody tests for anti-tissue tranglutaminase antibody and anti-deamindated gliadin antibody. An IgA deficiency is more common in patients with celiac disease, and low IgA levels can cause false-negative antibody tests as the test are for IgA-based antibodies; thus, with low IgA levels (<0.2 gm/l), IgG anti-deamindated gliadin antibody should be assessed. There are associate HLA types, and the presence of HLA-DQ2 is found in 95% and HLA-DQ8 in 5%, and thus not finding these findings is against celiac disease.

Management

Treatment is by eliminating gluten from the diet, which leads to resolution of pathologic changes in the gut. Symptoms associated with peripheral neuropathies frequently resolve with such a diet, and an increase in sural SNAP amplitude has been reported (the improvement was 0.76 μV, a value within the noise level of sensory responses) (Hadjivassiliou et al., 2006). Gluten-free diets are less difficult to manage with the increased availability of gluten-free food products and restaurants featuring gluten-free dishes, and a trial diet is reasonable.

References

Aziz I, Hadjivassiliou M, Sanders DS. The spectrum of noncoeliac gluten sensitivity. *Nat Rev Gastroenterol Hepatol.* 2015; 12(9):516–26.

Farhad K, Traub R, Ruzhansky KM, Brannagan TH, III. Causes of neuropathy in patients referred as "idiopathic neuropathy." *Muscle Nerve.* 2016; 53(6):856–61.

Hadjivassiliou M, Duker AP, Sanders DS. Gluten-related neurologic dysfunction. *Handb Clin Neurol.* 2014; 120:607–19.

Hadjivassiliou M, Kandler RH, Chattopadhyay AK, Davies-Jones AG, Jarratt JA, Sanders DS, et al. Dietary treatment of gluten neuropathy. *Muscle Nerve.* 2006; 34(6):762–6.

Hadjivassiliou M, Rao DG, Grinewald RA, Aeschlimann DP, Sarrigiannis PG, Hoggard N, et al. Neurological Dysfunction in Coeliac Disease and Non-Coeliac Gluten Sensitivity. *Am J Gastroenterol.* 2016; 111(4):561–7.

Rashid M, Lee J. Serologic testing in celiac disease: Practical guide for clinicians. *Can Fam Physician.* 2016; 62(1):38–43.

Thawani SP, Brannagan TH, III, Lebwohl B, Green PH, Ludvigsson JF. Risk of Neuropathy Among 28,232 Patients With Biopsy-Verified Celiac Disease. *JAMA Neurol.* 2015; 72(7):806–11.

Neuropathy Associated with Lyme Neuroborreliosis

Introduction

Lyme neuroborreliosis is caused by the tick-born spirochete *Borrelia burgdorferi*, which occurs as different genospecies in North America and Europe, which may explain differences in clinical features of neuroborreliosis (Hansen et al., 2013). Tick vectors are primarily deer and mice. Infection is common in the northern hemisphere of both continents, but with geographic variances: within the USA, rates are much higher in the North East and much lower in more western regions, and in Europe rates are higher in Scandinavia and central regions. There is a seasonal component, with ticks active only in warm weather.

There are issues recognizing human infection, as a history of a tick bite is frequently not recalled, and serologic testing does not establish the time of infection. Accordingly, it has been difficult to determine the epidemiology of Lyme peripheral nerve involvement.

Pathology

Infection with *B. burgdorferi* follows three stages: early localization with the characteristic erythema migrans rash (in most but not all patients) and systemic clinical features; followed by an early disseminated stage (2–4 weeks after the bite) with possible spreading to the central and peripheral nervous system; and if untreated a late dissemination stage, which is uncommon in North America (Hansen et al., 2013). There are three genospecies in Europe and only one in North America (*B. burgdorferi* sensu stricto). In Europe, there may be an association between site of bite and site of neurological involvement. The spirochete is tissue-based and localizes to meninges, and in peripheral nerve to the endoneurium. Animal models and rare human postmortem studies show inflammation of nerve roots and dorsal root ganglia. Sensory nerve biopsies show perivascular cellular infiltrates in vessels with thrombotic occlusions leading to axonal loss.

Clinical Features

More clinical data are available from patients in Europe than in North America, and differences in clinical presentation are worth reviewing in the setting of international travel (Pachner and Steiner, 2007; Hansen et al., 2013). The first stage is the classic erythema migrans rash, but not all patients recognize a rash. Overall, a low percentage of patients experience neurologic involvement in Europe, and an even lower percentage in North America. The most common neurologic involvement in Europe is acute painful meningoradiculitis. Approximately half develop a palsy of the seventh cranial nerve (mostly unilateral), and other cranial neuropathies are rare. A small percentage of patients experience limb weakness in a nerve root or plexus pattern. The frequency of an isolated length-dependent neuropathy is very low in Europe. In North America, subacute meningitis occurs within a few weeks of erythema migrans, but it is not clear how often a length-dependent polyneuropathy occurs. Descriptions of peripheral nerve involvement in North America suggest a variety of patterns, including distal paresthesias and radicular pain (Logigian and Steere, 1992). However, generalizations cannot be made from these data as the interval from proposed infection to development of peripheral nerves varied from 0 to 165 months and 60% had been treated with appropriate antibiotics, which clouds the certainty of the relation to Lyme infection.

Diagnostic Evaluation

Laboratory Evaluation

In North America, serum antibody testing alone is more commonly performed than in Europe, where comparisons between cerebral spinal fluid and serum antibody titers are performed due to high background seroprevalence and multiple genospecies. A two-step antibody is recommended in North America with an initial ELISA test, which if positive is followed by a western blot test (Moore et al., 2016). There are complexities in interpreting tests results, leading to possible false positive tests. Positive tests cannot readily distinguish between active (recent) infection and previous exposure, but a negative test in the setting of neurologic symptoms excludes infection, as neurologic symptoms follow infection by weeks.

Electrodiagnostic Evaluation

Pooled data from patients suggest mild slowing of motor and sensory nerves, but as presented, specifics of nerve conduction abnormalities are not available (Logigian and Steere, 1992). Findings expected for a length-dependent polyneuropathy appear to be rare.

Painful radiculopathy or distal radiculopathy in the setting of recent erythema migrans and a positive two-step antibody test performed ~4 weeks after the rash is supportive of Lyme neuroborreliosis, and treatment is appropriate.

Management

Data on treatment is mostly from patients with meningitis and rarely from patients with peripheral nerve involvement. An evidence-based review supports treatment with antibiotics, cephalosporins, or penicillin in North America and doxycycline in Europe, with recent studies supporting efficacy of oral doxycycline for all genospecies of the spirochete (Halperin et al., 2007).

The issue of chronic Lyme disease requiring long-term treatment is controversial, and there is no compelling evidence that prolonged symptoms attributed to *B burgdorferi* are due to treatment-resistant spirochetes.

References

Halperin JJ, Shapiro ED, Logigian E, Belman AL, Dotevall L, Wormser GP, et al. Practice parameter: treatment of nervous system Lyme disease (an evidence-based review): report of the Quality Standards Subcommittee of the American Academy of Neurology. *Neurology*. 2007;69:91–102.

Hansen K, Crone C, Kristoferitsch W. Lyme neuroborreliosis. *Handb Clin Neurol*. 2013;115:559–75.

Logigian EL, Steere AC. Clinical and electrophysiologic findings in chronic neuropathy of Lyme disease. *Neurology*. 1992;42:303–11.

Moore A, Nelson C, Molins C, Mead P, Schriefer M. Current guidelines, common clinical pitfalls, and future directions for laboratory diagnosis of Lyme disease, United States. *Emerging Infectious Diseases*. 2016;10:1169–77.

Pachner AR, Steiner I. Lyme neuroborreliosis: infection, immunity, and inflammation. *Lancet Neurol*. 2007;6:544–52.

Hereditary Neuropathies

Hereditary neuropathies are caused by alterations or absences of structural or functional proteins in peripheral nerves due to gene mutations. Mutations can be passed to offspring, most commonly by an autosomal dominant inheritance pattern, less commonly an x-linked pattern, and least commonly an autosomal recessive pattern. Spontaneous mutations occur, and, for certain genes, point mutations account for ~30% of hereditary neuropathies. Over 1,000 mutations in 80 genes have been identified, some common but many rare. Mutations in the same gene can follow different inheritance patterns and can be associated with different pathologic features. The expression of neuropathic symptoms and signs can vary within a family, reflecting poorly understood modifying or epigenetic factors. The incidence of hereditary neuropathies is difficult to determine because few patients are tested for gene mutations, and there are ethnic differences in some mutation frequencies that affect epidemiologic studies. For families with onset of symptoms late in life, a hereditary pattern may not be considered. Prevalence estimates are ~1:2,500–3,300 (Bird, 1993; Gutmann and Shy, 2015). It has been estimated that 20% of patients presenting to a neuromuscular clinic with an unclassified chronic neuropathy have CMT (Charcot Marie Tooth) type 1A.

Families with polyneuropathies were recognized in the late 1800s, and clearly described in 1886 by J-M Charcot and P Marie in an article (Charcot and Marie, 1886) and by H Tooth (Tooth, 1886) in a medical dissertation. The nomenclature has evolved over time, and the most common forms are referred to as Charcot Marie Tooth or CMT, but there are less common hereditary forms referred to by older terms (hereditary sensory and autonomic neuropathies) or by singular names (hereditary amyloidosis, porphyric neuropathies, and Fabry neuropathy).

References

Bird TD. *Charcot-Marie-Tooth Hereditary Neuropathy Overview.* In: Pagon RA, Adam MP, Ardinger HH, Wallace SE, Amemiya A, Bean LJH, et al., eds. Seattle, WA: GeneReviews(R), 1993.

Charcot J-M, Marie P. Sur une forme particulière d'atrophie musculaire progressive souvent familial debutant par les pieds et les jambs et atteignant plus tard les mains. *Rev. Méd (Paris)* 1886;6:97.

Gutmann L, Shy M. Update on Charcot-Marie-Tooth disease. *Curr Opin Neurol.* 2015;28:462–7.

Tooth HH. The peroneal type of progressive muscular atrophy. *London, HK Lewis & Co,* 1886.

Hereditary Neuropathies (Charcot Marie Tooth Neuropathies)

Introduction

Hereditary neuropathies are considered when there is a family history of a polyneuropathy or when the neuropathy started relatively early in life (first two decades). However, a hereditary neuropathy may also begin during adult life, and should be considered in a patient who has a slowly progressive polyneuropathy and life-long high arches and hammer toes (Brewerton et al., 1963) (see Chapter 3). Electrophysiological investigations in the mid-1900s recognized families with two ranges of motor nerve conduction velocities: type 1 with slow velocities (<38 m/s in arm nerves), and type 2 with low-normal or mildly slowed conduction velocities (>38 m/s). Nerve conduction features of type 1 suggest uniform slowing and are considered to be a demyelinative form, and features of type 2 are considered to be an axonal form. In addition, families have been described with intermediate range (25–50 m/s) conduction velocities.

The nomenclature of hereditary neuropathies has shifted over time. The most consistent is division into types 1 and 2 based on nerve conduction studies, although intermediate range conduction velocities have been described and genotype/phenotype correlations have blurred the dichotomy. At one point, naming was based on which types of peripheral nerves are involved: hereditary neuropathies with both motor and sensory nerves affected were called HMSN types 1 and 2, and forms with sensory or autonomic fibers or motor fibers were called HSN or HSAN or HMN. With the identification of specific mutations, the nomenclature has largely (but not completely) changed to CMT followed by numbers based on nerve conduction velocities (type 1 or 2) and by letters based on the order of gene mutation discovery (Table 42.1) (Rossor et al., 2015). HSN, HMN or HSAN nomenclature remains for neuropathies involving these specific types of nerves. Inspection of Table 42.1 reveals

that mutations in the same gene can lead to autosomal dominant or recessive patterns, and that there are a large number of rare mutations.

There are also rare families who have, in addition to a polyneuropathy, ataxia, spasticity, and other central nervous system features. This chapter focuses on the more common hereditary polyneuropathies and does not consider syndromes, which includes the above additional features.

Pathologic Features

The initial division of hereditary neuropathies into demyelinating and axonal forms was based in part on observed abnormalities of myelin in type 1 with shorter myelin segments and onion bulb formations with varying degrees of loss of large-diameter fibers, while in type 2 there were few changes in myelin but a prominent loss of axons in distal nerve segments. Slow conduction alone does not account for progressive weakness and sensory loss in type 1, as patients can function well with conduction velocities in the mid-teen range, and secondary axonal loss explains symptoms and signs of weakness and sensory loss and progression over time (Lawson et al., 2003). The underlying genetic-based pathologic mechanism is not known for any mutation, but likely involves defects in maintenance of the structure of myelin (Schwann cells) or the axon (Gutmann and Shy, 2015).

Clinical Features

The clinical pattern is slow progression of motor and sensory fiber loss leading to a stocking-glove distribution of weakness and sensory loss. Motor nerve loss and weakness usually predominate over sensory loss. Early motor nerve loss leads to changes in the shape of the foot with high arches and hammer toes, although flat feet can occur (Wicart, 2012). It is to be noted that not all individuals who have high arches and hammer

Table 42.1 Table of Known Mutations Associated with CMT Neuropathies

Name	Proportion of CMT Type	Protein Product (Gene)
CMT1: Autosomal dominant		
CMT1A	~75%	Peripheral myelin protein (PMP-22)
CMT1B	~10%	Myelin P 0 protein (MPZ)
CMT1C		Lipopolysaccharide-induced tumor necrosis factor-alpha factor (LITAF)
CMT1F		Neurofilament light polypeptide (NEFL)
CMT2: Autosomal Dominant		
CMT2A	~20%	Mitofusin-2 (MFN2)
CMT2B		Ras-related protein Rab-7 (RAB7)
CMT2C		Transient receptor potential cation channel subfamily V member 4 (TRPV4)
CMT2D	~3%	Glycyl-tRNA synthetase (GARS)
CMT2E	~4%	Neurofilament light polpeptide (NEFL)
CMT2F		Heat-shock protein beta-1 (HSPB1)
CMT2I/2J		Myelin P 0 protein (MPZ)
CMT2L		Heat-shock protein beta-8 (HSPB8)
CMT Intermediate: Autosomal Dominant		
DI-CMTA		
DI-CMTB		Dynamin 2 (DNM2)
DI-CMTC		Tyrosyl-tRNA synthetase (YARS)
DI-CMTD		Myelin P 0 protein (MPZ)
Di-CMTF		Intermediate CMT focal segmental glomerulosclerosis (IFN2)
DI-CMTF		Guanine mucleotide-binding protein subunit beta-4 (GNB4)
CMT4: Autosomal Recessive CMT1		
CMT4A		Ganglioside-induced differentiation-associated protein 1 (GDAP1)
CMT4B1		Myotubularin-related protein 2 (MTMR2)
CMT4B2		Myotubularin-related protein 13 (SBF2)
CMT4B3		Myotubularin-related protein 1 (SBF1)
CMT4C		SH3 domian & tetratricopeptice repeats-containing progein 2 (SHCTC2)
CMT4D		Protein NDGR1 (NDGR1)
CMT4E		Early growth response protein 2 (ERG2)
CMT4F		Periaxin (PRX)
CMT4H		FYVE, RhoGEF & PH domain-containing progein 4 (FGD4)
CMT4J		Phosphatidylinositol 3, 5 biphosphate (FIG4)
CMTX: X-linded		
CMTX1	~90%	Gap junction beta-1 protein (GJB1)
CMTX4		Apoptosis-inducing factor 1 (AIFM1)
CMTX5		Ribose-phosphate pyrophosphokinase 1 (PRPS1)
CMTX6		Pyruvate dehydrogenase kinase isoform 3 (PDK3)
HNPP: Autosomal Dominant		
		Peripheral myelin protein (PMP-22)

Table 42.1 (*continued*)

Name	Proportion of CMT Type	Protein Product (Gene)
HSN/HSAN: Autosomal Dominant		
HAS/HSAN1A	Most common	Serine palmitoyltransferase 1 (SPTLC1)
HSN/HSAN1B		*Ras-related protein 7 (FAB7)*
HSN/HSAN1C or type 3		*Serine palmitoyltransferase 2 (SPTLC2)*
HSN/HSAN1D or type 4		*Atlastin-1 (ATL1)*
HSN/HSAN1E		*DNA (cytosine-5)-methytrasferase 1 (DNMT1)*
HSN/HSAN1F		*Atlastin-3 (ATL3)*

Note: Rare mutations in italics.

Table 42.2 Clinical Features Supportive of Hereditary Neuropathy

Early onset (first, second, or third decade) of neuropathy or foot problems:

    Inability to run easily

    Need to wear special shoes

Presence of high arches and hammer toes from young age

Distal leg muscle atrophy; hand muscle atrophy if neuropathy severe

Distal-predominant pattern sensory and motor loss

Chronic and progressive course

Absent ankle reflexes

Electrodiagnostic studies supporting very chronic denervation

Diagnosis of an acquired neuropathy resistant to treatment

toes have a hereditary neuropathy, but such foot changes in the setting of a neuropathy raise the possibility of a hereditary neuropathy (Brewerton et al., 1963). There is frequent progression of structural foot changes with calluses along the lateral aspect of the foot leading to discomfort when walking. Atrophy of distal leg muscles can be marked, leading to prominence of the leading edge of the tibia bone, and the description of "saber shins." With further progression in some individuals there is atrophy of intrinsic hand muscles and flexion contractures of the fingers. Most aspects of the neuropathy are symmetric, but ~10% have asymmetries (Piscosquito et al., 2014), and asymmetry was noted in a drawing in H Tooth's dissertation.

Examination reveals weakness of toe extension and flexion, ankle dorsiflexion and eversion of the feet, and, in some individuals, weakness of finger abduction and extension. The peroneal distribution leads to walking on the lateral sides of the foot and frequent complaints of ankle instability. Foot drop varies in degree, and may be profound. Distal sensory loss is evident with deficiencies of light touch perception, but loss is usually mild and less prominent than distal weakness. Tendon reflexes are usually absent at the ankles.

The clinical diagnosis of CMT is straightforward when a hereditary pattern is clear from the family history and patient examination, and genetic conformation can be considered. When a familial pattern is not obvious, but a patient's clinical features are suggestive of a longstanding course (Table 42.2), needle EMG findings described below can support a longer time course than a patient appreciates. Family data may not be recognized by the patient, but may be teased out by querying features described in Chapter 3 for each grandparent, parent and sibling. A hereditary pattern can be obscured by mild symptoms in a parent or early death, and small sibships of parents and the patient. Recessive patterns are difficult to detect with small sibships, but are rare and more likely in societies in which consanguineous relationships occur.

Diagnostic Evaluation
Laboratory Evaluation
There are no distinct general laboratory features, and alternative metabolic disorders are to be excluded. In older individuals, comorbid neuropathies can coexist (diabetic neuropathy) with a hereditary neuropathy, and it can be difficult to separate the clinical effects of the two.

Gene testing can be diagnostic, but point mutations can be missed with certain test techniques, and new mutations continue to be discovered; thus, a negative genetic test does not exclude an inherited neuropathy. Methods of testing for gene mutations are evolving, and whole exome sequencing is becoming financially reasonable. However, such testing may disclose a mutation of unknown significance, which can complicate interpretation. The diagnostic yield is higher amongst type 1 forms. It is appropriate to follow a focused algorithm of testing, with the first step to determine arm motor nerve conduction velocities and the second step to test for genes associated with the most common mutations for known type 1 or type 2 mutations (Table 38.1) (Rossor et al., 2015). The frequency of gene mutations varies amongst studies due to referral patterns, but mutations for peripheral myelin protein 22 (PMP-22), GJB1, myelin P zero (MPZ), and MFN2 genes are most common, and should be tested for initially, with other less-common gene mutations tested second (DiVincenzo et al., 2014). Overall, the diagnostic yield for patients with a suspected hereditary neuropathy referred for genetic testing varies from 44% to 87% (Rudnik-Schoneborn et al., 2016).

Electrodiagnostic Evaluation

The first step is to determine motor nerve conduction velocities in the arm (as responses may be low or absent in the legs): <38 m/s without abnormal temporal dispersion is associated with CMT type 1; 25–50 m/s are intermediate velocities associated with CMTX; 45–55 m/s is associated with type 2, but are not specific and overlap with non-hereditary neuropathies. It is to be appreciated that with greater numbers of identified genes, classic phenotypic distinctions between types 1 and 2 neuropathies may become blurred. When conduction velocities are in the slow range there may be concern that they represent chronic demyelinating polyradiculoneuropathy (CIDP), and a feature unique to CMT 1 is the lack of abnormal temporal dispersion that is prominent in CIDP (Figure 42.1). Needle EMG shows axonal loss for both forms. Chronicity is associated with all forms of hereditary neuropathy, and is supported on needle EMG by observation of very reduced recruitment of motor unit that have high amplitudes but simple waveforms (Figure 42.2).

Management

Hereditary neuropathies cause disabilities to varying degrees but do not involve other organs and do not shorten life (note, some genetic disorders can involve other portions of the nervous system in addition to peripheral nerves, but are not considered here). At this time, there is no disease modifying treatment, and exercise has not been found to be helpful in slowing the course of progression (Gutmann and Shy, 2015). Pain is described and is considered to be neuropathic and treated as such, but pain from orthopedic causes also occurs. Orthopedic issues affecting the feet and ankle are common and patients may benefit from

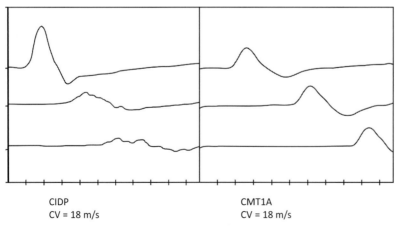

CIDP
CV = 18 m/s

CMT1A
CV = 18 m/s

Figure 42.1 Ulnar motor nerve conduction contrasting CMAP waveforms in chronic inflammatory demyelinating polyradiculoneuropathy (CIDP) with Charcot Marie Tooth neuropathy Type 1A (CMT1A). Left panel: CIDP; right panel: CMT1A; conduction velocity ~18 m/s for both. There is marked abnormal temporal dispersion with CIDP and normal dispersion with CMT1A.

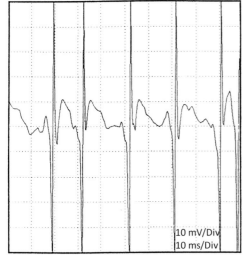

Figure 42.2 EMG recording of single motor unit from anterior tibialis muscle in a patient with a chronic neuropathy. Clues to a possible hereditary neuropathy are high discharge rate (approximate 50 Hz), high amplitude (approximately 10 KmV), and simple configuration.

surgical corrective procedures (Wicart, 2012). Many people have functionally significant foot drop and can benefit from braces across the ankles (ankle-foot arthosis – AFO) (Ramdharry et al., 2012). It is rare for a patient to become nonambulatory. The question of greater weakness due to overwork or over-exercise is commonly asked, but for CMT1A, there is no supportive evidence that either is a concern (Piscosquito et al., 2014), and is likely generalizable to other mutations.

CMT1 (Autosomal Dominant)

This is the most common category of hereditary neuropathy, and accounts for 40–50% among Europeans and their descendants. Within the category, CMT1A is singly the most common (70–80%), and is caused by a duplication of the peripheral myelin protein 22 (PMP-22) gene, and less commonly by a point mutation. CMT1B is the next most common (10–12%), and is due to mutations of the myelin P zero (MPZ) gene. The remaining CMT1 autosomal dominant forms are rare (Bird, 1993a).

CMT1 can be suspected when there are slow conduction velocities with uniform slowing. An affected individual's conduction velocities do not change over time (years) (Gutmann et al., 1983). Thus, suspected family members with subclinical or mild neuropathies can be identified by slow conduction velocities.

CMT2 (Autosomal Dominant)

Clinical features of CMT2 overlap with those of CMT1, but are usually less severe. The distinguishing feature is normal or near-normal motor nerve conduction velocities. CMT2A is the most common form within this category (20%), and is due to mutations in the mitofusin-2 (MFN2) gene. Other mutations are rare (Bird, 1993a).

Dominant Intermediate CMT

This form is rare, and characterized by motor nerve conduction velocities 25–50 m/s, which are between type 1 (<38 m/s) and type 2 (~50 m/s) (Liu and Zhang, 2014).

CMT4 (Autosomal Recessive)

This type is primarily distinguished by a recessive inheritance pattern, and the clinical features are similar to other forms of CMT. Nerve conduction studies include axonal and demyelination features. A clinical subtype, Dejerine–Sottas syndrome, with early onset in infancy and childhood has been linked to a number of mutations, and is no longer considered a separate entity (Bird, 1993a).

CMTX (X-linked)

CMTX is characterized by a moderate to marked neuropathy in affected males and no or mild findings in female carriers. Symptoms occur in childhood to adolescence. Nerve conduction studies reveal an intermediate range of velocities. Carriers may have nerve conduction slowing. CMTX1 is the most common x-linked form (90%), and others are rare. Overall, CMTX is the second-most common form of CMT (Yiu et al., 2011).

Hereditary Neuropathy with Predisposition to Pressure Palsies (Autosomal Dominant)

Hereditary neuropathy with predisposition to pressure palsies (HNPP) is an autosomal dominant neuropathy characterized most commonly by transient and occasionally permanent nerve damage following relative mild trauma to the nerve. It is due to a duplication of the PNP22 gene or a point mutation, and 20% represent *de novo* mutations.

Clinical features are transient paresthesias or weakness following mild trauma over a nerve, and repeated trauma can accumulate over time, leading to permanent deficits. Episodes generally occur in the first and second decades of life and nerve damage may be subclinical. Ankle reflexes are frequently absent in the setting of a mild diffuse neuropathy.

Nerve biopsy studies are characterized by focal swelling of myelin, tomacula, on individual nerve fibers (Bird, 1993b). Nerve conduction studies show a mild generalized length-dependent neuropathy characterized by mild slowing of sensory nerve more than motor nerves, with focal slowing across common nerve entrapment sites (Andersson et al., 2000).

HSN/HSAN

HSN/HSAN type 1 is an autosomal dominant type of neuropathies involving predominantly sensory nerves, but also autonomic nerves to varying degrees, accounting for the variable nomenclatures (HSAN when there is a marked degree of autonomic fiber involvement). HSN/HSAN type 2 neuropathies are autosomal recessive forms, which include two congenital syndromes, Riley-Day syndrome and congenital insensitivity to pain and anhidrosis. Another category is mutations in voltage-gated sodium channels.

Nerve pathology shows fiber loss with graded severity: unmyelinated > small myelinated > myelinated fibers. Clinical features for both types are progressive, distal-predominant sensory loss, painless distal soft tissue injuries that may become infected, and skin changes. Poor healing can lead to distal amputations. There can be considerable associated pain. There may be marked muscle atrophy, especially with type 1. Proximal pathologic studies show loss of dorsal root ganglion cells and motor neurons. Nerve conduction studies are remarkable for absent sensory responses, and motor responses may be low but conduction velocities are normal. Management focuses on foot care; special shoes, detection, and attention to skin breakdown (see Chapter 47). Pain may be marked and is felt to be neuropathic, and can be treated with appropriate medications (see Chapter 48).

References

Andersson PB, Yuen E, Parko K, So YT. Electrodiagnostic features of hereditary neuropathy with liability to pressure palsies. *Neurology*. 2000;54:40–4.

Bird TD. *Charcot-Marie-Tooth Hereditary Neuropathy Overview*. In: Pagon RA, Adam MP, Ardinger HH, Wallace SE, Amemiya A, Bean LJH, et al., eds. Seattle, WA: GeneReviews(R), 1993a.

Bird TD. *Hereditary Neuropathy with Liability to Pressure Palsies*. In: Pagon RA, Adam MP, Ardinger HH, Wallace SE, Amemiya A, Bean LJH, et al., eds. Seattle, WA: GeneReviews(R), 1993b.

Brewerton DA, Sandifer PH, Sweetnam DR. "Idiopathic" Pes Cavus: An Investigation into Its Aetiology. *Br Med J*. 1963;2:659–61.

DiVincenzo C, Elzinga CD, Medeiros AC, Karbassi I, Jones JR, Evans MC, et al. The allelic spectrum of Charcot-Marie-Tooth disease in over 17,000 individuals with neuropathy. *Mol Genet Genomic Med*. 2014;2:522–9.

Gutmann L, Fakadej A, Riggs JE. Evolution of nerve conduction abnormalities in children with dominant hypertrophic neuropathy of the Charcot-Marie-Tooth type. *Muscle Nerve*. 1983;6:515–19.

Gutmann L, Shy M. Update on Charcot-Marie-Tooth disease. *Curr Opin Neurol*. 2015;28:462–7.

Lawson VH, Gordon Smith A, Bromberg MB. Assessment of axonal loss in Charcot-Marie-Tooth neuropathies. *Exp Neurol*. 2003;184:753–7.

Liu L, Zhang R. Intermediate Charcot-Marie-Tooth disease. *Neurosci Bull*. 2014;30:999–1009.

Piscosquito G, Reilly MM, Schenone A, Fabrizi GM, Cavallaro T, Santoro L, et al. Is overwork weakness relevant in Charcot-Marie-Tooth disease? *J Neurol Neurosurg Psychiatry*. 2014;85:1354–8.

Ramdharry GM, Day BL, Reilly MM, Marsden JF. Foot drop splints improve proximal as well as distal leg control during gait in Charcot-Marie-Tooth disease. *Muscle Nerve*. 2012;46:512–19.

Rossor AM, Evans MR, Reilly MM. A practical approach to the genetic neuropathies. *Pract Neurol*. 2015;15:187–98.

Rudnik-Schoneborn S, Tolle D, Senderek J, Eggermann K, Elbracht M, Kornak U, et al. Diagnostic algorithms in Charcot-Marie-Tooth neuropathies: experiences from a German genetic laboratory on the basis of 1206 index patients. *Clin Genet*. 2016;89:34–43.

Wicart P. Cavus foot, from neonates to adolescents. *Orthop Traumatol Surg Res*. 2012;98:813–28.

Yiu EM, Geevasinga N, Nicholson GA, Fagan ER, Ryan MM, Ouvrier RA. A retrospective review of X-linked Charcot-Marie-Tooth disease in childhood. *Neurology*. 2011;76:461–6.

Chapter 43

Neuropathies Associated with Porphyria

Introduction

Porphyric neuropathies result from inherited enzyme defects in the synthesis of heme, resulting in accumulation of one or more intermediary molecules. There are eight enzymes in the biosynthetic pathway, and the porphyrias can be divided biochemically into hepatic and erythropoietic organ sites in which intermediary molecules accumulate, or clinically into acute or cutaneous by sites where symptoms occur. Four forms of acute porphyria cause neurologic symptoms: acute intermittent porphyria (AIP) (autosomal dominant), hereditary coproporphyria (autosomal dominant), variegate porphyria (autosomal dominant), and ALAD (δ-aminolevulinate dehydratase) deficiency (autosomal recessive). This chapter focuses on adult forms, and although ALAD occurs in infancy it will not be considered.

While most enzymatic disorders are inherited in an autosomal recessive pattern, which accounts for very low levels of enzymatic activity (~5%), three of the above porphyric neuropathies are autosomal dominant, and ~50% of enzymatic activity is insufficient to prevent disease (Albers and Fink, 2004). The genetic-clinical spectrum of porphyric disorders is complex, as a large number of mutations are associated with some forms of porphyric neuropathy (acute intermittent porphyria). Overall prevalence rates vary, from case reports to rates from 0.5–2/100,000, and some mutations have a local (country) founder effect. Further, penetrance can be as low as 10% (Lin et al., 2013). Lastly, there are a large number of precipitating factors that influence clinical expression of a neuropathy, such as drugs, hormones, and diet.

Acute Porphyrias

The three enzymatic deficiencies responsible for neuropathies (acute intermittent porphyria [AIP], hereditary coproporphyria, and variegate porphyria) have similar clinical neurologic presentations, and the primary difference is the presence of skin lesions with hereditary coproporphyria and variegates porphyria.

AIP is the most common form causing neurologic symptoms, and is linked to over 300 mutations. Prevalence rates are 1–2/100,000, higher in Scandinavia and the British Isles. Hereditary coproporphyria has mutations unique to individual families. Variegate porphyria, while rare, has a high prevalence in South African White populations.

Pathology

The pathologic process of how accumulation of heme products affect nerves is not known (Albers and Fink, 2004). The pathologic findings are primary proximal motor neuron loss, with lesser loss of dorsal root ganglion cells. Any changes to myelin are thought to be secondary to axonal loss.

Clinical Features

There is a classic clinical triad during an attack that generally follows a pattern of initial abdominal pain, followed by behavioral/psychiatric symptoms, and somewhat later by peripheral neuropathy (Albers and Fink, 2004). Abdominal symptoms are abrupt and severe with visceral pain that is not readily localizable. Constipation is common and not infrequently the abdomen is explored surgically. The behavioral/psychiatric symptoms are not well described as they may not be the clinical focus, but include anxiety, restlessness, insomnia, depression, and psychosis. Other symptoms are aggressive or impulsive behavior, delusions, emotional lability (Crimlisk, 1997). With the somatic peripheral neuropathy is an autonomic neuropathy, which may account for the abdominal pain and constipation and rare bladder and bowel incontinence (Albers and Fink, 2004). There is also labile hypertension that may complicate the behavioral/psychiatric symptoms.

The neuropathy generally occurs later, within a month (3–75 days) of the onset of abdominal pain

Table 43.1 Acute Porphyrias and Metabolic Abnormalities

Type	Enzyeme Deficiency	Urine Metabolites	Stool Metabolites
ALA (δ-aminolevulinate dehydratase) deficiency	δ-aminolevulinate dehydratase	⇑ δ-aminolevulinate dehydratase Coproporphyrinogen	Normal
Acute intermittent	Porphobilinogen	⇑ δ-aminolevulinate dehydratase Porphobilinogen Uroporphyrinogen	Normal

(Ridley, 1969). The neuropathy predominantly involves motor nerves, and the pattern is unique, with prominent weakness of arm muscles and onset in the arms in 50%, and weakness may be asymmetric in distribution. The neuropathy can be severe, resulting in quadriparesis, and occasionally respiratory failure. Sensory disturbances are not common, and may have a proximal distribution.

Diagnostic Evaluation

Laboratory Evaluation

Elevated amounts of heme metabolites are excreted in urine and stool during an attack, and quantitative measures can be made from 24-hour collections (Table 43.1). However, there may not be specificity of excreted metabolites to distinguish among the forms of porphyria during an attack, but the diagnosis of a porphyric neuropathy is unlikely if heme metabolites are normal during an attack. Conversely, other conditions are associated with elevated heme metabolites, and include diabetes, liver disease, and iron-deficiency anemia (Albers and Fink, 2004).

Electrodiagnostic Evaluation

Nerve conduction studies document reduced motor responses with conduction velocities reflecting axonal loss and not primary demyelination. Sensory nerve responses occasionally are reduced or absent, but most patients with profound motor nerve pathology (quadriparesis) have normal sensory responses. Needle EMG supports acute denervation at the time of an attack, and later reinnervation (Albers et al., 1978).

Management

Management of an acute attack includes efforts to abort the attack and manage symptoms (Albers and Fink, 2004). Maintaining adequate carbohydrates is the first step as glucose inhibits ALA synthesis. Intravenous administration of heme is also an inhibitor of ALA synthesis and can be administered if carbohydrate load is not effective. Management of symptoms includes treatment of abdominal pain, which may require opiod analgesics, and management of autonomic instability. In the extreme, there can be respiratory failure. After an attack and recognition of the disorder, prevention focuses on not taking medications that induce cytochrome P450 enzymes. Lists are available from the American Porphyria Foundation, and common items to be avoided are alcohol, barbiturates, calcium channel blockers, and a number of anticonvulsant medications.

References

Albers JW, Fink JK. Porphyric neuropathy. *Muscle Nerve*. 2004;30:410–22.

Albers JW, Robertson WC, Jr., Daube JR. Electrodiagnostic findings in acute porphyric neuropathy. *Muscle Nerve*. 1978;1:292–6.

Crimlisk HL. The little imitator – porphyria: a neuropsychiatric disorder. *J Neurol Neurosurg Psychiatry*. 1997;62:319–28.

Lin CS, Park SB, Krishnan AV. Porphyric neuropathy. *Handb Clin Neurol*. 2013;115:613–27.

Ridley A. The neuropathy of acute intermittent porphyria. *Q J Med*. 1969;38:307–33.

Hereditary Amyloid Neuropathy

Introduction

Neuropathies due to deposition of amyloid can be divided into hereditary forms (familial amyloid polyneuropathy – FAP, which is the most common) and rare acquired forms, which are discussed in Chapter 29 (Shin and Robinson-Papp, 2012). FAP is most commonly associated with mutations in the transthyretin gene (TTR-FAP), but other rare genetic forms occur with mutations in the gene coding for apolipoprotein A-1 (Iowa form, based on a family in Iowa) and mutations in the gelsolin gene. TTR-FAP neuropathy may occur without systemic clues to an amyloid pathology (no involvement or subclinical involvement of other organs that make the genetic condition life-threatening). The age of onset of nerve involvement ranges from the second to ninth decades. All hereditary forms follow an autosomal dominant inheritance pattern.

Pathologic Features

Transthyretin is a plasma transport protein (for retinol and thyroxine) and misfolding leads to aggregation and accumulation in a variety of organs. TTR-FAP was originally discovered in Portugal, associated with a Val30Met mutation in the transthyretin gene, but subsequently has been found to occur worldwide and can be caused by 120 different mutations (single or double mutations or deletions) (Ando et al., 2013). Penetrance is variable, and a hereditary pattern may be missed, and the polyneuropathy can also occur without a family history. Some mutations are associated with cardiomyopathy and others with polyneuropathy.

Apolipoprotein A1 mutations can cause amyloid deposition, but involvement of peripheral nerves is not common, or is not the predominant clinical feature (Shin and Robinson-Papp, 2012). A number of mutations are described, but not all lead to amyloid deposition.

Gelsolin is an actin-modulating protein. Gelsolin-related amyloid polyneuropathy is due to one of two mutations in the gelosolin gene that results in increased amyoidogenesis (Kiuru-Enari and Haltia, 2013).

Amyloid accumulation in peripheral nerves is patchy within fascicles and causes nerve damage by mechanical compression, and also within microvessels resulting in focal ischemia, or possibly by toxic effects of amyloid (Shin and Robinson-Papp, 2012; Koike et al., 2016). Amyloidosis is confirmed by demonstrating amyloid deposits by Congo red stain.

Clinical Features

TTR-FAP polyneuropathy begins with involvement of small myelinated and unmyelinated fibers causing a painful polyneuropathy in a stocking-glove distribution that steadily progresses over four to five years to include the hands. Large myelinated sensory and motor fibers then become involved, leading to sensory loss and ambulatory issues (Dohrn et al., 2013). Median mononeuropathy at the wrist (carpal tunnel syndrome) is felt to be common.

Initial clinical and electrodiagnostic features can lead to a diagnosis of chronic inflammatory demyelinating polyradiculoneuropathy (CIDP) (Rajabally et al., 2016). However, the neuropathy in these patients progresses despite adequate treatment, and thus in the setting of treatment-unresponsiveness CIDP, additional features of autonomic neuropathy, previous carpal tunnel syndrome, and weight loss should prompt consideration for TTR-FAP. Other clues to the correct diagnosis include a review of family members for involvement of other organs, including autonomic neuropathy (orthostatic hypotension, impotence, change in sweating), gastrointestinal dysfunction (severe constipation, alternating diarrhea, and constipation), cardiac issues (cardiomyopathy), and renal failure.

Apolipoprotein A1 neuropathy is a length-dependent sensory > motor neuropathy associated with painful sensations (Van Allen et al., 1969).

Gelsolin-related amyloid polyneuropathy predominantly involves sensory nerves, and motor involvement is mild and follows a length-dependent course (Kiuru-Enari and Haltia, 2013). There are other more predominant features, including slowly progressive facial weakness (cranial nerve VII) resulting in distinctive facial skin folds and laxity of skin out of proportion to aging.

Diagnostic Evaluation

The initial diagnosis for all types of amyloid neuropathy is by showing deposition of amyloid in tissue by Congo red staining. However, nerve biopsies do not always stain positive for amyloid, and an aspirate of subcutaneous abdominal fat has a higher diagnostic yield. The amount of amyloid found (semiquantitative scoring) has been associated with extent of involvement of other organs (van Gameren et al., 2006). Of note, amyloid may not be found in familial cases with late onset of neuropathy (Dohrn et al., 2013). In the eye, deposition of amyloid leads to corneal lattice dystrophy.

Genetic confirmation is by gene testing, after considering diagnostic features to refine the type of group of mutations to test for.

Electrodiagnostic Evaluation

The primary findings are an axonal neuropathy, although there may be elements of demyelination or mixed changes to myelin and axons (Mariani et al., 2015). Median mononeuropathy at the wrist is reported to be common in TTR-FAP, but a prospective study supports a length-dependent slowing of both distal median and ulnar sensory segments compared to slowing of the former in classic carpal tunnel syndrome (Koike et al., 2009).

Management

Transthyretin variants are produced in the liver, and liver transplantation is the most effective therapy, but may not halt cardiac involvement. Pharmacologic treatment of misfolded amyloid is by tafamidis and diflunisal, and gene-modifying drugs (FNA interference and antisense nucleotides) (Ando et al., 2013). Clinical management falls into two categories: one is management of involvement of other organs (heart, kidneys, gastrointestinal organs) and the other is management of symptoms from peripheral nerve involvement. These include medications for neuropathic pain (see Chapter 48), and carpal tunnel surgery for median nerve entrapment,

References

Ando Y, Coelho T, Berk JL, Cruz MW, Ericzon BG, Ikeda S, et al. Guideline of transthyretin-related hereditary amyloidosis for clinicians. *Orphanet J Rare Dis.* 2013;8:31.

Dohrn MF, Rocken C, De Bleecker JL, Martin JJ, Vorgerd M, Van den Bergh PY, et al. Diagnostic hallmarks and pitfalls in late-onset progressive transthyretin-related amyloid-neuropathy. *J Neurol.* 2013;260:3093–108.

Kiuru-Enari S, Haltia M. Hereditary gelsolin amyloidosis. *Handb Clin Neurol.* 2013;115:659–81.

Koike H, Morozumi S, Kawagashira Y, Iijima M, Yamamoto M, Hattori N, et al. The significance of carpal tunnel syndrome in transthyretin Val30Met familial amyloid polyneuropathy. *Amyloid.* 2009;16:142–8.

Koike H, Ikeda S, Takahashi Y, Iijima M, Misumi Y, Ando Y, et al. Schwann cell and endothelial cell damage in transthyretin familial amyloid polyneuropathy. *Neurology.* 2016;87:2220–9.

Mariani LL, Lozeron P, Theaudin M, Mincheva Z, Signate A, Ducot B, et al. Genotype-phenotype correlation and course of transthyretin familial amyloid polyneuropathies in France. *Ann Neurol.* 2015;78:901–16.

Rajabally YA, Adams D, Latour P, Attarian S. Hereditary and inflammatory neuropathies: a review of reported associations, mimics and misdiagnoses. *J Neurol Neurosurg Psychiatry.* 2016;87:1051–60.

Shin SC, Robinson-Papp J. Amyloid neuropathies. *Mt Sinai J Med.* 2012;79:733–48.

Van Allen MW, Frohlich JA, Davis JR. Inherited predisposition to generalized amyloidosis. Clinical and pathological study of a family with neuropathy, nephropathy, and peptic ulcer. *Neurology.* 1969;19:10–25.

van Gameren II, Hazenberg BP, Bijzet J, van Rijswijk MH. Diagnostic accuracy of subcutaneous abdominal fat tissue aspiration for detecting systemic amyloidosis and its utility in clinical practice. *Arthritis Rheum.* 2006;54:2015–21.

Chapter

45

Neuropathy Associated with Fabry Disease

Introduction

Fabry disease is an x-linked lysosomal disorder due to a mutation in the GLA gene resulting in a reduction or absence of the enzyme α-galactosidase A, which leads to an accumulation of globotriaosylceramide (ceramidetrihexoside) within lysosomes (El-Abassi et al., 2014). Accumulation occurs in multiple organs, including endothelial cells, kidneys, heart, and dorsal root ganglia. Females can be affected due to x-chromosome inactivation.

Pathology

The cause of nerve damage is not clear, and may result from ceramide accumulation in dorsal root ganglia, causing a ganglinopathy. There may also be nerve ischemia due to accumulation in microvessels perfusing nerves.

Clinical Features

Features depend upon the level of α-galactosidase A activity and are divided into classic with no enzyme activity, and non-classic with low amounts of activity. In the classic form, symptoms of burning pain and hypo- or hyperhydrosis occur in addition to transient and permanent cerebrovascular changes, cardiomyopathy, renal failure, and angiokeratomas. Symptoms begin in the first decade of life. In the non-classic group, symptoms occur with the fourth to sixth decade and are milder, and usually affect one organ system.

Pain attributed to loss of small myelinated and unmyelinated fibers is common, and follows a symmetric length-dependent pattern affecting the soles and palms first. Pain may be episodic in the form of a crisis, progressing from distal to proximal in the body, and precipitated by fever, exercise, and rapid changes in temperature. Crises are superimposed on chronic pain in a length-dependent pattern.

Diagnostic Evaluation

Nerve conduction studies are usually normal, as large fibers are not affected. Quantitative sensory testing will be abnormal. Skin biopsy commonly shows reduced intraepidermal nerve fiber density in 50% of patients. Gene testing is available, and, in the appropriate clinical setting, a dried blood spot can be used to screen for α-galactosidase A activity, and if activity is absent or reduced the findings can be confirmed by GLA gene mutation analysis. Gene dysfunction can occur by a large number of mutations (El-Abassi et al., 2014). Routine screening for Fabry disease in patients with isolated small-fiber painful neuropathies and no features suggestive of Fabry has an extremely low yield (de Greef et al., 2016).

Management

Fabray disease can be treated with enzyme replacement therapy, which is focused on treating the multiple organs involved. With respect to the peripheral nervous system, treatment has reduced neuropathic pain, but the degree may be influenced by the concomitant effect on peripheral nerves of involvement of other organs, such as renal function (Uceyler et al., 2011). Since enzyme replacement therapy does not markedly reduce pain, concurrent treatment of neuropathic pain is required (see Chapter 48). Factors that precipitate a painful crisis should be avoided. Fabray disease remains a challenging disease even with enzyme replacement therapy that was introduced in 2001–2003, and long-term follow up is dependent upon the degree of cardiac and renal involvement pending, and death occurs from failure of these organs.

References

de Greef BT, Hoeijmakers JG, Wolters EE, Smeets HJ, van den Wijngaard A, Merkies IS, et al. No Fabry Disease in Patients Presenting with Isolated Small Fiber Neuropathy. *PLoS One.* 2016;11:e0148316.

El-Abassi R, Singhal D, England JD. Fabry's disease. *J Neurol Sci.* 2014;344:5–19.

Uceyler N, He L, Schonfeld D, Kahn AK, Reiners K, Hilz MJ, et al. Small fibers in Fabry disease: baseline and follow-up data under enzyme replacement therapy. *J Peripher Nerv Syst.* 2011;16:304–14.

Neuropathies Associated with Rare Conditions and Uncertain Associations

Introduction

Determining the cause of a neuropathy is the goal, but efforts should be based on sound principles. There should be a clear association between the peripheral neuropathy and the underlying condition, with documentation of a consistent type of neuropathy associated with the condition, a degree of understanding of underlying pathology as it relates to the condition, and a documented response to treatment or, if not treatable, a biomarker that links neuropathy severity to the underlying condition. For a number of medical conditions commonly raised in the differential diagnosis of peripheral neuropathies, the above associations are not clear or the medical conditions are rarely associated with peripheral neuropathy. Several rare and uncertain associations are discussed here, and medical conditions with specific laboratory tests are considered in Chapter 5 on Diagnostic Testing.

Neuropathies Associated with Rare Conditions and Uncertain Associations

Inflammatory Bowel Disease

The association between inflammatory bowel disease (Crohn disease and ulcerative colitis) and peripheral neuropathy is difficult to define, and incidence rates in the literature vary markedly (0–39%) (Garcia-Cabo and Moris, 2015). A clear association is frequently confounded by factors such as comorbities strongly associated with peripheral neuropathies (diabetes mellitus type 2), a long time duration between diagnosis of bowel disease and neuropathy (which blurs cause-and-effect relationships), possible associated nutritional deficiencies, and use of neurotoxic drugs to treat inflammatory bowel disease. Overall, the incidence is likely very low (Figueroa et al., 2013).

Neurosarcoidosis

Literature reviews indicate that the nervous system is affected in ~5% of patients with sarcoidosis (neurosarcoidosis), and, within neurosarcoidosis, peripheral nerves are involved in ~15% (Fritz et al., 2016). The diagnosis of sarcoidosis is difficult to make, with no pathognomonic clinical or laboratory features, resulting in frequent over-diagnosis (Govender and Berman, 2015). In this setting, the spectrum of peripheral nerve disease ascribed to sarcoidosis includes mononeuropathies, polyradiculopathies, polyneuropathies, Guillain-Barré syndrome, chronic inflammatory demyelinating polyradiculoneuropathy, and non-length-dependent sensory neuropathy. Many are from case reports or retrospective series, and the diagnosis of sarcoid is only secure (definite versus probable neurosarcoidosis) in about 25% of reported patients (Fritz et al., 2016).

Pathology

Pathologic demonstration of peripheral nerve neurosarcoidosis is based on finding granulomas in involved tissue, but their location is rarely such as to directly affect peripheral nerves in the above neuropathy patterns (Burns et al., 2006). Convincing pathology are granulomas with direct pressure on a nerve or a vasculitic process affecting small vessels in nerve or muscle (Said et al., 2002). Muscle frequently includes inflammation and granulomas.

Clinical Features

Peripheral nerve involvement includes cranial nerves (most frequently cranial nerve VII), but other kinds of neuropathies are less clearly documented. In the setting of positive biopsies for sarcoidosis, mononeuropathy (median, ulnar, fibular/peroneal nerves), polyradiculoneuropathy, and polyneuropathy are described (Burns et al., 2006). Symptom onset is usually rapid, and may precede or follow symptoms of sarcoidosis in other organs after varying intervals (months to a decade or more) (Said et al., 2002). Painful, non-length-dependent small-fiber neuropathies are described in the setting of cutaneous sarcoidosis, but appear to be rare (Khan and Zhou, 2012).

Diagnostic Evaluation

Laboratory Evaluation

Serum angiotensin converting enzyme (ACE) levels are elevated in only 25% of patients. The most common non-neural tissues with granulomas are lung, skin, and mediastinal lymph nodes; and the sural nerve is most informative for peripheral nerve involvement (Burns et al., 2006). Skin biopsies have reduced intraepidermal nerve fiber densities (Khan and Zhou, 2012), and can show perineural granulomas (Munday et al., 2015).

Electrodiagnostic Evaluation

Nerve conduction studies usually show axonal loss in the above patterns, and rare elements of demyelination.

EMG findings of denervation in paraspinal muscles can be used to support a polyradiculopathy (Burns et al., 2006).

Management

There are few controlled trials. The response to treatment (most commonly high-dose corticosteroids) is variable, with some patients showing improvement, others no change, or some progression (Burns et al., 2006).

Thyroid Disease

Autoimmune thyroid disease includes both hyperthyroid (Graves disease) and hypothyroid function (thyroiditis), and also subclinical thyroid dysfunction. Laboratory testing in a large sample of the general population reveals an incidence of hypothyroidism (elevated TSH) at 4.6% (4.3% clinical and 0.3% subclinical) and hyperthyroidism (elevated T4) at 1.3% (0.5% clinical and 0.7% subclinical) (Hollowell et al., 2002). Primary care providers commonly order thyroid function tests, and the majority of patients with thyroid disease are likely being treated. Amongst patients evaluated for causes of a neuropathy, a small percentage have abnormal thyroid tests; but when full consideration is given, alternative causes (non-thyroid disease) are not found but the contribution of thyroid disease is not clear (Gallagher et al., 2013).

Pathology

The underlying pathology has not been defined.

Clinical Features

Patient series find large numbers of patients with distal sensory symptoms (29% who were hypothyroid; 14% who were hyperthyroid) as well as weakness (Duyff et al., 2000a).

Diagnostic Evaluation

Laboratory Evaluation

Abnormal thyroid tests are defining for thyroid dysfunction, as above.

Electrodiagnostic Evaluation

Small differences in nerve conduction velocity values have been found, but the values are within the laboratory limit of normal (Duyff et al., 2000b).

Management

Treatment resulted in reduced symptoms in patients with electrodiagnostic evidence for a primary axonal neuropathy, an unexpected finding with this pathology. Thus, the correlation between thyroid dysfunction and polyneuropathy is not strong.

Rheumatologic Diseases

Rheumatologic diseases represent inflammatory disorders of joints and soft tissues, and frequently include involvement of multiple organs. Constitutional symptoms of pain in joints and muscles are common, making distinctions of peripheral nerve disease difficult (Nouh et al., 2014). There are a number of non-specific laboratory tests available, and a review indicates that the most common abnormal tests are antineutrophil cytoplasmic antibody (ANCA) and anti-nuclear antibody (ANA); both of these are non-specific, and are elevated in a substantial percentage of the general elderly population (Gallagher et al., 2013).

References

Burns TM, Dyck PJ, Aksamit AJ, Dyck PJ. The natural history and long-term outcome of 57 limb sarcoidosis neuropathy cases. *J Neurol Sci*. 2006;244:77–87.

Duyff RF, Van den Bosch J, Laman DM, van Loon BJ, Linssen WH. Neuromuscular findings in thyroid dysfunction: a prospective clinical and electrodiagnostic study. *J Neurol Neurosurg Psychiatry*. 2000a;68:750–5.

Duyff RF, Van den Bosch J, Laman DM, van Loon BJ, Linssen WH. Neuromuscular findings in thyroid dysfunction: a prospective clinical and electrodiagnostic study. *J Neurol Neurosurg Psychiatry*. 2000b;68:750–5.

Figueroa JJ, Loftus EV, Jr., Harmsen WS, Dyck PJ, Klein CJ. Peripheral neuropathy incidence in inflammatory bowel disease: a population-based study. *Neurology*. 2013;80:1693–7.

Fritz D, van de Beek D, Brouwer MC. Clinical features, treatment and outcome in neurosarcoidosis: systematic review and meta-analysis. *BMC Neurol*. 2016;16:220.

Gallagher G, Rabquer A, Kerber K, Calabek B, Callaghan B. Value of thyroid and rheumatologic studies in the evaluation of peripheral neuropathy. *Neurol Clin Pract*. 2013;3:90–8.

Garcia-Cabo C, Moris G. Peripheral neuropathy: an underreported neurologic manifestation of inflammatory bowel disease. *Eur J Intern Med*. 2015;26:468–75.

Govender P, Berman JS. The Diagnosis of Sarcoidosis. *Clin Chest Med*. 2015;36:585–602.

Hollowell JG, Staehling NW, Flanders WD, Hannon WH, Gunter EW, Spencer CA, et al. Serum TSH, T(4), and thyroid antibodies in the United States population (1988 to 1994): National Health and Nutrition Examination Survey (NHANES III). *J Clin Endocrinol Metab*. 2002;87:489–99.

Khan S, Zhou L. Characterization of non-length-dependent small-fiber sensory neuropathy. *Muscle Nerve*. 2012;45:86–91.

Munday WR, McNiff J, Watsky K, DiCapua D, Galan A. Perineural granulomas in cutaneous sarcoidosis may be associated with sarcoidosis small-fiber neuropathy. *J Cutan Pathol*. 2015;42:465–70.

Nouh A, Carbunar O, Ruland S. Neurology of rheumatologic disorders. *Curr Neurol Neurosci Rep*. 2014;14:456.

Said G, Lacroix C, Plante-Bordeneuve V, Le Page L, Pico F, Presles O, et al. Nerve granulomas and vasculitis in sarcoid peripheral neuropathy: a clinicopathological study of 11 patients. *Brain*. 2002;125:264–75.

Management of Peripheral Neuropathies

After a structured approach to evaluating and diagnosing peripheral neuropathies comes management. A cause is determined in approximately 50–60% of neuropathies, but a disease-modifying treatment is available for only a fraction of neuropathies. Thus, patient education, management of concurrent diseases, management and prevention of complications, and treatment of neuropathic pain remain important elements.

Chapter 47

Management of Peripheral Neuropathies

Patient Education

The vocabulary, concepts, and terms associated with peripheral neuropathies are broad and may be confusing for patients. Providing clear written information or Internet sources is helpful. However, the Internet includes miracle treatment offers that are unproven, and it is not unexpected that with no disease-modifying treatment for most neuropathies many patients seek alternative treatment. It is important to be open and non-judgmental in answering queries by patients for these treatments.

Physical Care

Some forms of polyneuropathy, diabetic neuropathy in particular, are associated with foot complications due to loss of sensory perception leading to unsuspected trauma, skin breakdown, formation of ulcers, and complications of poor wound healing (Schaper et al., 2016). Prevention is key and includes the following factors: identification of patients with risk factors, determining severity of a sensory neuropathy (testing with 10-gm monofilament), proper foot care (daily washing and foot inspection), use of appropriate shoes (not too tight, with deep toe box), proper cutting of toe nails (preferably by a podiatrist), and aggressive treatment of pre-ulcerative signs.

Devices to Assist Function

Ankle-foot-orthoses (AFOs) are braces to compensate for weak ankle dorsiflexion (foot drop). Clinically significant foot drop occurs with longstanding and severe polyneuropathies, most notably hereditary (Charcot Marie Tooth) neuropathies. The simplest approach is use of lightweight high-top shoes that provide ankle joint support (Carter, 2005). The next is use of elastic or lace-up fabric braces that support the ankle and are worn under or over socks and not outwardly visible. When foot drop is marked, AFOs have the potential to improve gait, reduce stumbling and falls, reduce stress on the ankle joint, and aid overworked muscles. A variety of AFO designs (ready-made to custom-molded) and construction materials (plastic to carbon fiber) are available, and proper and comfortable fitment is best accomplished by an orthotist. A practical approach is for a patient to bring to the orthotic shop loose-fitting athletic shoes (AFOs take up space in the shoe) and "test walk" ready-made AFOs by walking around the shop; if the AFO helps gait, the patient is more likely to use it. However, despite potential benefits, many patients with CMT do not wear their AFOs, largely due to altered self-image, which can be a challenge to overcome (Vinci and Gargiulo, 2008).

The question arises as to whether use of an AFO accelerates effect the rate of progression of distal leg weakness? This cannot be tested in slowly progressive primary axonal polyneuropathies, but has been assessed in fibular/peroneal mononeuropathies with secondary axonal damage, and there is no evidence for slower recovery of strength attributed to AFO use (Geboers et al., 2001). By extrapolation to polyneuropathies, there are only positive functional benefits from using an AFO.

Four-wheeled walkers can assist poor balance, but are not commonly needed. It is very rare for a patient with peripheral neuropathy to require a wheelchair, but occasional use can reduce fatigue of walking exceptionally long distances (airports, vacations). A handicapped parking permit also reduces walking distances.

Exercise

Mild exercise is generally beneficial, but focused exercise will not increase strength or improve altered gait to a functional degree (Carter, 2005). There is a small risk of damaging weak muscles if exercise is overly intense (to muscle exhaustion).

Exercise may be beneficial for patients with diabetic neuropathy for several reasons. The onset and severity of diabetic neuropathies are influenced by elements of the metabolic syndrome, and reduction of one or more syndrome elements by exercise is beneficial (Singleton et al., 2015). Body mass index (BMI) and waist circumference are the most modifiable elements with exercise, but lowering triglyceride and hemoglobin A1c levels can also occur. Exercise can lead to an increase in intraepidermal nerve endings and less pain in patients with painful diabetic neuropathy. However, exercise must be maintained for continued benefit.

References

Carter GT. Rehabilitation management of peripheral neuropathy. *Semin Neurol.* 2005;25:229–37.

Geboers JF, Janssen-Potten YJ, Seelen HA, Spaans F, Drost MR. Evaluation of effect of ankle-foot orthosis use on strength restoration of paretic dorsiflexors. *Arch Phys Med Rehabil.* 2001;82:856–60.

Schaper NC, Van Netten JJ, Apelqvist J, Lipsky BA, Bakker K. Prevention and management of foot problems in diabetes: a Summary Guidance for Daily Practice 2015, based on the IWGDF Guidance Documents. *Diabetes Metab Res Rev.* 2016;32 Suppl 1:7–15.

Singleton JR, Smith AG, Marcus RL. Exercise as Therapy for Diabetic and Prediabetic Neuropathy. *Curr Diab Rep.* 2015;15:120.

Vinci P, Gargiulo P. Poor compliance with ankle-foot-orthoses in Charcot-Marie-Tooth disease. *Eur J Phys Rehabil Med.* 2008;44:27–31.

Chapter 48

Pharmacologic Management of Peripheral Neuropathies

Introduction

The ability to slow, halt, or reverse the progression of polyneuropathies in the form of disease-modifying treatments is limited to immune-mediated neuropathies. Toxic neuropathies will generally stop progressing (but some agents are associated with progression for a limited period of time – called coasting) and may improve when the neuropathic agent is stopped, but the degree of recovery is variable. For entrapment neuropathies, there are limited surgical interventions, but some that are attributed to focal nerve entrapment (anterior and posterior interosseous syndromes) may be due to other causes and may not respond to surgery (see Chapters 8, 9, and 10). At this time, the majority of length-dependent axonal polyneuropathies have no reliably effective disease-modifying treatments. Many neuropathies cause pain, and there are effective medications that reduce neuropathic pain.

Neuropathy Assessment

It is useful to assess the status of a peripheral neuropathy in individual patients. Approximations of severity can be obtained from a patient's symptoms and verified by clinical sign, but standardized assessment instruments are useful. They are essential for studies that determine the prevalence of neuropathies in a population. They allow for more accurate determination of severity when making treatment management decisions (Hanewinckel et al., 2016).

Assessment Scales

Most assessment scales focus on sensory > motor length-dependent polyneuropathies. The most common uses of screening scales are to estimate the frequency of neuropathy in the general population or in the elderly, and to estimate the prevalence of diabetic neuropathies because these neuropathies are frequently mild in degree and may not be appreciated by the patient. Scales vary in scope and detail and can include the following elements singly or in combination: patient questionnaires about symptoms; clinical signs; data from routine laboratory tests; data from special test procedures, and assessment of patient function (Table 48.1) (Hanewinckel et al., 2016). Consequently, scales can be brief (four screening questions) or involved (45 minutes with the need for specialized testing equipment). Given the large number of available scales and variety of uses it is difficult to make specific recommendations for particular tests for screening for length-dependent neuropathies.

Scales have also been developed for motor > sensory neuropathies, such as immune-mediated polyneuropathies, and can be used to make treatment decisions based on assessing change in neuropathy severity over time or after treatment. They differ from screening scales used for length-dependent polyneuropathies because immune-mediated neuropathies may include upper limb involvement or an asymmetric pattern of involvement (van Nes et al., 2008). When scales are used to judge improvements in function, the question arises of what values of change in the scale represent meaningful changes for the patient and whether the changes have an impact on quality of life. These scales generally assess a patient's ability to perform daily functions. The INCAT (Inflammatory Cause and Treatment) and RODS (Rasch-Build Overall Disability Scale) are useful for chronic inflammatory demyelinating polyradiculoneuropathy (CIDP) (Hughes et al., 2001; van Nes et al., 2011), and the MMN-RODS is specific for multifocal motor neuropathy (Table 48.2) (Vanhoutte et al., 2015).

Assessment of Strength

Assessment of strength (qualitative manual muscle testing or quantitative handheld dynamometry) can be used to judge efficacy of treatment, and applied

Table 48.1 Screening Scales Used to Identify the Presence of a Neuropathy or to Scale the Severity

Scale: Sensory > Motor	Utility	Practicality
Based on Symptoms		
Neuropathy Symptom Score (NSS)	Detection, severity	Time consuming
Neuropathy Symptom Profile (NSP)	Characterization, severity	Time consuming
Neuropathy Symptoms & Change (NSC)	Change	Time consuming
Diabetic Neuropathy Symptom (DNS)	Characterization	Rapid
Based on Signs		
Neuropathy Disability Score (NDS)/Neuropathy Impairment Score (NIS)	Detection, severity	Weighted to motor dysfunction
Utah Early Neuropathy Scale (UENS)	Detection	Rapid
Early Neuropathy Scale (ENS)	Detection	Rapid
Based on Symptoms & Signs		
Michigan Neuropathy Screening Instrument (MNSI)	Detection, severity	Rapid
Michigan Diabetic Neuropathy Score (MDNS)	Detection, severity	Time consuming
Toronto Clinical Neuropathy Score (TCNS)	Detection, severity	Rapid
Total Neuropathy Score (TNS)	Detection, severity	Time consuming
Scale: Motor > Sensory or Motor Only		
Based on Function		
Modified Rankin Scale	Severity	Originally for stroke, weighted to leg funcction
Inflammatory Cause and Treatment (INCAT)	Severity	Assesses arm & leg function
Rasch-build Overall Disability Scale (RODS)	Severity	Assesses arm & leg function
Rasch-Build Overall Disability Scale for Multifocal Motor Neuropathy (MMN-RODS)	Severity	Assesses arm & leg function

to functionally affected muscle groups or as summed strength of the legs or arms. There are issues comparing normal or near-normal strength assessed by the ordinal numbers in the MRC ratings of "4" or "5" strength, with cardinal numbers obtained by quantitative testing, and the latter is more sensitive (Aitkens et al., 1989). Although not a global assessment, quantitative measurement of grip strength using a grip dynamometer is an alternative measure that correlates with global patient function (RODS scale) (Draak et al., 2016).

Nerve Conduction Studies

Nerve conduction studies are valuable in determining underlying pathology in immune-mediated neuropathies, and it may seem reasonable to use follow-up studies to guide therapy. The practical issues are that nerve conduction data may not reveal the full extent of pathology along the whole length of nerves (in particular, proximal segments) or identify functionally significant abnormalities. Data from serial nerve conduction studies in an IVIG treatment trial comparing patients who did or did not respond to treatment is instructive. Significantly more subjects who became weaker on placebo developed new nerve conduction abnormalities compared to subjects who did respond to IVIG and had improved nerve conduction measures; however, most who did respond also developed new abnormalities in some nerves (Chin et al., 2015). Thus, for the individual patient, repeat nerve conduction studies do not provide clinically useful data compared to clinical assessment or functional scales. There is an exception for acute immune-mediated neuropathies, and repeat studies may change or clarify the diagnosis of acute inflammatory demyelinating polyradiculoneuropathy (AIDP) versus acute motor axonal neuropathy (AMAN) (Chapters 19 and 21) (Uncini and Kuwabara, 2012)

Disease-modifying Treatments

Treatments that alter immune function can halt or reverse progression of immune-mediated

Table 48.2 Functional Scales to Aid in Managing Patients with Chronic Immune-mediated Neuropathies

Rasch-build Overall Disability Scale (R-ODS)			
	Impossible to Perform	**Performed with Difficulty**	**Ealisly Performed**
Read newspaper/book			
Eat			
Brush teeth			
Wash upper body			
Sit on toilet			
Make sandwich			
Dress upper body			
Wash lower body			
Move a chair			
Turn key in loci			
Go to physician			
Take shower			
Do dishes			
Do shopping			
Catch object (ball)			
Bend, pick up object			
Walk one flight of stairs			
Travel by public transportation			
Walk, avoid obstacales			
Walk outside <1 km			
Carry, put down heavy object			
Dance			
Stand for hours			
Run			

Inflammatory Neuropathy Cause and Treatment Group (INCAT) Scale	
Arm Disability: Score	**Leg Disability: Score**
No upper limb problems: 0	Walking not affected: 0
Symptoms in one or two arms but able to perform all daily functions: 1	Walking affected but walks independently outdoors: 1
Symptoms in one or two arms affecting but not preventing functions: 2	Usually uses unilateral support walking outdoors: 2
Symptoms in one or two arms preventing some daily functions: 3	Usually uses bilateral support walking outdoors: 3
Symptoms in one or two arms preventing performing functions but some purposeful movement: 4	Usually uses wheelchair outdoors, but able to stand/walk few steps: 4
No purposeful arm movement: 5	Restricted to wheelchair, unable to stand/walk few steps: 5

Source: Modified from van Nes et al. (2011) and Hughes et al. (2001).

polyneuropathies. Acute immune-mediated neuropathies such as Guillain-Barré syndrome are relatively common and accurately diagnosed, with good data on treatment options and outcomes (see Chapter 19). This chapter focuses on treatment of chronic immune-mediated neuropathies such as CIDP, which are less common and frequently misdiagnosed, while multifocal motor neuropathy with conduction block is very rare and likely over-diagnosed (Allen and Lewis, 2015). Consequently, there are few randomized controlled Class I or II trials for first line therapies and most assess efficacy over short time periods. Reports on long-term treatment effects are usually derived from retrospective chart reviews, and factors complicating interpretations are patients who may have received multiple medications over the reviewed time period. Other factors that affect treatment outcomes are differences in underlying pathologies amongst immune-mediated neuropathies within a diagnostic category, and also the degree of secondary axonal damage. Data for second-line therapies for refractory patients are based on very small trials and less predictable results.

Therapy programs for immune-mediated neuropathies are generally handed down during physician training, and modified by personal experience. It is valuable to review principles and certain historic features of first-line treatment modalities as they relate to management strategies. An important principle is to have clear endpoint measures to assess response to therapy and guide changes. Assessments, as discussed above, can be by clinical evaluation, scales, or measurement of strength.

Chronic Immune-Mediated Polyneuropathies

Corticosteroids

Adrenal corticotrophic hormone (ACTH) was used in the 1950s as the first medication shown to be effective in CIDP, and was followed in the 1980s by prednisone (Bromberg and Carter, 2004). A single short randomized controlled trial yielded results of questionable significance, but overall there is empiric evidence for a reliable effect in most patients (Hughes and Mehndiratta, 2015). Initial doses vary and range from 40–100 mg daily or 80–200 mg every other day, maintained for 3–4 weeks, and then tapered.

Prednisone taper schedules vary markedly, are based on arbitrary formulae, and modified by clinical factors (Bromberg and Carter, 2004). The biologic half-life of corticosteroids is longer than the pharmacokinetic half-life, and low doses may be immunologically effective. There are no biomarkers of efficacy, and the lowest effective dose may not become apparent until the next lower dose is associated with a relapse. There are a number of side effects from corticosteroid use, and most are manageable. Support is weak for alternative-day dosing causing fewer side effects than daily dosing.

Immune Globulin

Intravenous Immune Globulin

IVIG was reported in 1985 to be effective in patients with CIDP. Comparisons between IVIG and corticosteroids (prednisone, prednisolone, methylprednisolone) show equal efficacy but fewer side effects with IVIG. Response to IVIG tends to be more rapid while the duration of remission is longer with corticosteroids (Adrichem et al., 2016).

IVIG is given as an initial high-induction dose followed by a lower-maintenance dose for a period of time and then attempts are made at tapering. The induction dose of 2 g/kg is almost universal, but its origins are based on empiric treatment of a few patients with both immune deficiency and concomitant thrombocytopenia where the monthly immune deficiency maintenance dose of 0.4 g/kg was extended (because platelet counts continued rise) during the five-day workweek for a total of 2 g/kg (Berger and Allen, 2015). As a consequence, the initial dose is usually infused 0.4 g/kg daily for five days; however, experience from a large trial shows that it can be comfortably and safely infused over two or three days (Hughes et al., 2008). The initial dose can be based on ideal body weight in patients weighing over 80 kg (Anderson and Olson, 2015). There are no robust trials assessing lower initial doses (Adrichem et al., 2016). The maintenance dose is customarily 1 g/kg, and maintenance dosing schedule of every 3–4 weeks is based on IVIG half-life. Factors that influence the metabolism (pharmacokinetics) of IVIG include tissue receptor interactions with the Fc portion of the IgG antibody. Fc-receptors in endothelial cells link to the antibody and become saturated by the infused IVIG, thereby reducing exogenous IgG catabolism. Considerable variability exists among patients receiving the same amount of IVIG (Rajabally et al.,

2013). This may be attributed to variability in the capacity of Fc-receptors in individual patients due to polymorphisms in the Fc-receptor gene.

A large placebo-controlled IVIG trial for CIDP conducted over a long duration (24 weeks with cross-over to a second 24 weeks) and based on 2 g/kg initial dosing followed by 1 g/kg every three weeks revealed several factors of clinical utility (Hughes et al., 2008). Most patients who responded to IVIG showed clinical improvement within six weeks (Latov et al., 2010). Clinical improvement continued while on every three-week IVIG therapy, and reached a plateau at about six months despite continued therapy. However, ~50% of subjects who responded to IVIG during the first 24 weeks did not relapse when re-randomized to placebo during the second 24 weeks, and thus did not need IVIG. Other studies support a similar high percentage of patients who initially respond to IVIG but did not relapse when IVIG is withdrawn (Adrichem et al., 2016). Thus, it is important to determine the continued need for IVIG therapy on an individual patient basis.

Tapering IVIG can be based on IgG half-life (by holding the interval at three to four weeks and lowering the dose from 1 g/kg) or based on patient convenience (by stretching out the interval holding the dose at 1 g/kg) (Adrichem et al., 2016). There is no consensus for which plan is more appropriate, and patient preference (fewer venipunctures) may favor the latter. A recent taper algorithm has been proposed (Lunn et al., 2016).

Subcutaneous Immune Globulin

The half-life of IgG is the same whether administered subcutaneously or intravenously, and the same total dose administered in lower subcutaneous doses more frequently leads to more stable levels of IgG levels and reduced infusion side effects (Rajabally, 2014). Patients can manage their infusions for CIDP and multifocal motor neuropathy (MMN) on their own schedule. There are no differences in efficacy for CIDP and MMN when administered by either route (Racosta et al., 2017).

Short-term Treatment: Plasma Exchange

Plasma exchange has been shown to be effective for treating CIDP and is usually performed as a series of exchanges (4–6), but the response may be short-lived as the procedure removes plasma-based proteins of the immune system that may be active in the underlying pathology, but the immune system remains active and the pathologic proteins are replaced (Mehndiratta et al., 2015). The procedure requires access to two veins, and can be performed through peripheral access, but more commonly through use of a central venous catheter, and placement may cause complications and thus hospital admission for several days to complete the series.

Refractory CIDP

Some patients do not respond to corticosteroids or IVIG, and a large percentage may have an alternative diagnosis (Kaplan et al., 2017). Among those with a clinically confirmed diagnosis of CIDP a variety of treatment regimens and medication were successful in most, but not all, patients, and included more frequent IVIG infusions, or addition of mycophenolate mofitil, or pulse cyclophosphamide therapy.

Treatment of Painful Neuropathies

Damage to sensory nerves can result in painful symptoms. A variety of causes and factors are likely involved that depend on the nature of nerve damage and subsequent changes in the central nervous system. Pain from peripheral nerve damage is called neuropathic pain, in contrast to nociceptive pain that arises from damage to tissue (Baron et al., 2010). Neuropathic pain can be very disabling and affect quality of life, and can constitute a patient's chief complaint. Few peripheral neuropathies can be halted or reversed, and pain management is an important intervention.

Pathologic Features

Major challenges exist to investigating the origins and factors in treating nociceptive pain (Baron et al., 2010; Gilron et al., 2015). Several mechanisms may be present in a given patient. Brief paroxysmal pain in the absence of external stimuli likely reflects ectopic spontaneous nerve activity, which has been recorded by microneurography. Ectopic activity occurs in thinly myelinated and unmyelinated nerve fibers, and both damaged and undamaged neighboring fibers may be activated. Nerve damage can lead to increases in voltage-gated sodium channels (and possibly other ion channels), which may account for spontaneous ectopic nerve action potentials. Hyperalgesia and allodynia may be due to increases in receptor proteins as a consequence of nerve damage.

Ectopic paroxysmal or otherwise-inappropriate sensory nerve action potentials reach the dorsal horn of the spinal cord. Synaptic connections there are complex, and different fiber types (thinly myelinated and unmyelinated nerve fibers) make specific connections to second-order projection neurons. Central sensitization is due to changes in second-order (or later order) neurons to the damaged peripheral neurons and contributes to the abnormal nerve activity reaching higher cortical levels. Mechanisms include increased release of excitatory amino acids neurotransmitters and neuropeptides in the dorsal horn, which could bring about changes in receptors.

Descriptions of painful sensations can differ among patients who have the same clinical peripheral neuropathy diagnosis; for example, among those with painful diabetic neuropathy some describe squeezing feelings, others burning and others stabbing. This has led to attempts at classifying neuropathic pain on type of pain (sensory profile) rather than on the clinical type of neuropathy, based on the theory that different mechanisms elicit specific types of pain and treatment should be based on proposed mechanisms underlying types of pain. Classification is based on patient surveys and testing paradigms (Baron et al., 2010). How this can be used to selective treatment options is not yet clear.

Principles of Treatment

Treatment of neuropathic pain frequently requires a broad approach, especially when severe. Pain is a complex clinical entity and patient perceptions and responses to treatment vary. Education on the underlying features of the painful neuropathy is important. Setting goals for an appropriate response to treatment is essential, and a pain reduction of 50% is a reasonable goal (Finnerup et al., 2015). Various scales for assessing and managing treatment are available, and the traditional pain level scale (0 = no pain to 10 = worst imaginable) and similar response relief scale (0 = no relief to 10 = complete relief), are useful (Gilron et al., 2015). When pain treatment is challenging, especially when first-line medications (see below) are not effective and when strong opioid medications are being considered, referral to a multidisciplinary pain clinic is appropriate as they include a variety of providers (physical therapist, counselor/psychologist).

Non-pharmacologic Treatment

The effects of exercise on perceived pain are not fully understood, but are felt to be positive. Many changes occur within the spinal cord with exercise due to increased muscle afferent nerve activity (Baron et al., 2010). There are many patient factors affecting participation, including motivation, risk of injury to feet in the setting of reduced tactile sensations, pain from exercise, and interest or enthusiasm for the type of the exercise. For diabetic neuropathy, aerobic exercise has been shown to increase intraepidermal fiber densities (Singleton et al., 2015). For diabetic neuropathy associated with the metabolic syndrome, exercise can reduce syndrome risk factors (lower blood pressure, glucose levels, lipid levels, weight loss) (see Chapter 28). Finally, exercise in any form has positive effects on mental health that are difficult to quantify, such as taking charge, having time to think, and achieving a sense of well-being. As for all exercise, dedication is key for long-term effects.

Pharmacologic Treatment

Pharmacologic options are the next step when non-pharmacologic efforts alone are not successful. While a number of different polyneuropathies have painful features, most trial data are from painful diabetic neuropathies. Class I–II studies focus on treatment outcomes that achieved a >30–50% change in baseline over placebo or in comparison to another treatment (Bril et al., 2011; Finnerup et al., 2015; Gilron et al., 2015). Other aspects considered are the number of patients needed to treat (NNT) to achieve the optimum outcome. A limited number of first line drugs are listed in Table 48.3.

Guidelines for reaching therapeutic doses include starting with low doses and increasing very slowly. Patients are concerned with side effects and slow dose increases reduce the incidence of side effects and allow for reaching therapeutic doses. It is appropriate to try to achieve a suitable dose before abandoning a drug and moving to another. Combination therapy with drugs from two different classes may be more successful than either alone (for example, gabapentin and amitriptyline). Issues with elderly patients include increased incidence of polyneuropathy with age, the presence of comorbidities resulting in frequent polypharmacotherapy, and age-related changes in metabolism and clearance of drugs. These factors may lead to patient confusion and falls when pain-relieving drugs are given (Brouwer et al., 2015).

Table 48.3 Drugs to Treat Neuropathic Pain

Anticonvulsant Drugs		
Drug	Dose	Schedule
Pregablin	300–600 mg	2 divided doses
Gabapentin	900–3600 mg	3 divided doses
Antidepressant Drugs		
Venlafaxine	75–225 mg	2 divided doses
Duloxitine	60–120 mg	1–2 divided doses
Amitriptyline	25–100 mg	1–2 divided doses
Narcotic Drugs		
Tramadol	50–200 mg	1–4 divided doses
Topical Drugs		
Capsaicin	0.075%	3–4 doses
Lidoderm	0.50%	1 dose

Anticonvulsant Drugs

Pregabalin is modestly effective relative to placebo (~10% reduction) and the NNT for a 50% reduction in pain is ~4. There is improvement in quality of life. Gabapentin has a similar degree of effectiveness and a positive change in patient quality of life compared to placebo.

Antidepressant Drugs

Venlafaxine is effective relative to placebo (~20% reduction) with an NTT of ~5. Duloxetine is less effective (8% reduction). Both venlafaxine and duloxetine improve quality of life. Amitriptyline has a large effect (~40% reduction) compared to placebo.

Opioid Drugs

Tramadol is effective relative to placebo (~15% reduction). Opioid drugs are associated with side effects of sedation, nausea, and constipation. Importantly, there is the potential for tolerance and the need for dose escalation, and possible addiction.

Other Pharmacologic Drugs

Capsaicin is effective (~40% reduction) compared to placebo, but challenging to apply. Lidoderm patch is effective with ~25% reduction in pain.

References

Adrichem ME, Eftimov F, van Schaik IN. Intravenous immunoglobulin treatment in chronic inflammatory demyelinating polyradiculoneuropathy, a time to start and a time to stop. *J Peripher Nerv Syst.* 2016;21:121–7.

Aitkens S, Lord J, Bernauer E, Fowler WM, Jr., Lieberman JS, Berck P. Relationship of manual muscle testing to objective strength measurements. *Muscle Nerve.* 1989;12:173–7.

Allen JA, Lewis RA. CIDP diagnostic pitfalls and perception of treatment benefit. *Neurology.* 2015;85:498–504.

Anderson CR, Olson JA. Correlation of weight-based i.v. immune globulin doses with changes in serum immunoglobulin G levels. *Am J Health Syst Pharm.* 2015;72:285–9.

Baron R, Binder A, Wasner G. Neuropathic pain: diagnosis, pathophysiological mechanisms, and treatment. *Lancet Neurol.* 2010;9:807–19.

Berger M, Allen JA. Optimizing IgG therapy in chronic autoimmune neuropathies: a hypothesis driven approach. *Muscle Nerve.* 2015;51:315–26.

Bril V, England J, Franklin GM, Backonja M, Cohen J, Del Toro D, et al. Evidence-based guideline: Treatment of painful diabetic neuropathy: report of the American Academy of Neurology, the American Association of Neuromuscular and Electrodiagnostic Medicine, and the American Academy of Physical Medicine and Rehabilitation. *Neurology.* 2011;76:1758–65.

Bromberg MB, Carter O. Corticosteroid use in the treatment of neuromuscular disorders: empirical and evidence-based data. *Muscle Nerve.* 2004;30:20–37.

Brouwer BA, de Greef BT, Hoeijmakers JG, Geerts M, van Kleef M, Merkies IS, et al. Neuropathic Pain due to Small Fiber Neuropathy in Aging: Current Management and Future Prospects. *Drugs Aging.* 2015;32:611–21.

Chin RL, Deng C, Bril V, Hartung HP, Merkies IS, Donofrio PD, et al. Follow-up nerve conduction studies in CIDP after treatment with IGIV-C: Comparison of patients with and without subsequent relapse. *Muscle Nerve.* 2015.

Draak TH, Gorson KC, Vanhoutte EK, van Nes SI, van Doorn PA, Cornblath DR, et al. Correlation of the patient's reported outcome Inflammatory-RODS with an objective metric in immune-mediated neuropathies. *European journal of neurology.* 2016;23:1248–53.

Finnerup NB, Attal N, Haroutounian S, McNicol E, Baron R, Dworkin RH, et al. Pharmacotherapy for neuropathic pain in adults: a systematic review and meta-analysis. *Lancet Neurol.* 2015;14:162–73.

Gilron I, Baron R, Jensen T. Neuropathic pain: principles of diagnosis and treatment. *Mayo Clin Proc.* 2015;90:532–45.

Hanewinckel R, Ikram MA, van Doorn PA. Assessment scales for the diagnosis of polyneuropathy. *J Peripher Nerv Syst.* 2016;21:61–73.

Hughes R, Bensa S, Willison H, Van den Bergh P, Comi G, Illa I, et al. Randomized controlled trial of intravenous immunoglobulin versus oral prednisolone in chronic inflammatory demyelinating polyradiculoneuropathy. *Ann Neurol.* 2001;50:195–201.

Hughes RA, Donofrio P, Bril V, Dalakas MC, Deng C, Hanna K, et al. Intravenous immune globulin (10% caprylate-chromatography purified) for the treatment of chronic inflammatory demyelinating polyradiculoneuropathy (ICE study): a randomised placebo-controlled trial. *Lancet Neurol.* 2008;7:136–44.

Hughes RA, Mehndiratta MM. Corticosteroids for chronic inflammatory demyelinating polyradiculoneuropathy. *Cochrane Database Syst Rev.* 2015;1:CD002062.

Kaplan A, Brannagan TH. Evaluation of patients with refractory chronic inflammatory demyelinating polyneuropathy. *Muscle Nerve.* 2017; 55:476–82.

Latov N, Deng C, Dalakas MC, Bril V, Donofrio P, Hanna K, et al. Timing and course of clinical response to intravenous immunoglobulin in chronic inflammatory demyelinating polyradiculoneuropathy. *Arch Neurol.* 2010;67:802–7.

Lunn MP, Ellis L, Hadden RD, Rajabally YA, Winer JB, Reilly MM. A proposed dosing algorithm for the individualized dosing of human immunoglobulin in chronic inflammatory neuropathies. *J Peripher Nerv Syst.* 2016;21:33–7.

Mehndiratta MM, Huges RA, Prichard J. Plasma exchange for chronic inflammatory demyelinating polyradiculoneuropathy. *Cochrand Database System Rev.* 2015;CD003906.

Racosta JM, Sposato LA, Kimpinski K. Subcutaneous vs. Intravenous Immunoglobulin for Chronic Autoimmune Neuropathies: A Meta-analysis. *Muscle Nerve.* 2017;55:802–9.

Rajabally YA. Subcutaneous immunoglobulin therapy for inflammatory neuropathy: current evidence base and future prospects. *J Neurol Neurosurg Psychiatry.* 2014;85:631–7.

Rajabally YA, Wong SL, Kearney DA. Immunoglobulin G level variations in treated chronic inflammatory demyelinating polyneuropathy: clues for future treatment regimens? *J Neurol.* 2013;260:2052–6.

Singleton JR, Smith AG, Marcus RL. Exercise as Therapy for Diabetic and Prediabetic Neuropathy. *Curr Diab Rep.* 2015;15:120.

Uncini A, Kuwabara S. Electrodiagnostic criteria for Guillain-Barre syndrome: a critical revision and the need for an update. *Clin Neurophysiol.* 2012;123:1487–95.

van Nes SI, Faber CG, Merkies IS. Outcome measures in immune-mediated neuropathies: the need to standardize their use and to understand the clinimetric essentials. *J Peripher Nerv Syst.* 2008;13:136–47.

van Nes SI, Vanhoutte EK, van Doorn PA, Hermans M, Bakkers M, Kuitwaard K, et al. Rasch-built Overall Disability Scale (R-ODS) for immune-mediated peripheral neuropathies. *Neurology.* 2011;76:337–45.

Vanhoutte EK, Faber CG, van Nes SI, Cats EA, Van der Pol WL, Gorson KC, et al. Rasch-built Overall Disability Scale for Multifocal motor neuropathy (MMN-RODS((c))). *J Peripher Nerv Syst.* 2015;20:296–305.

Index